MW01050429

Differential Diagnoses in Surgical Pathology:
Cytopathology

DIFFERENTIAL DIAGNOSES IN SURGICAL PATHOLOGY SERIES

Series Editor: Jonathan I. Epstein

Differential Diagnoses in Surgical Pathology: Genitourinary System
Jonathan I. Epstein and George J. Netto, 2014

Differential Diagnoses in Surgical Pathology: Gastrointestinal System
Elizabeth A. Montgomery and Whitney M. Green, 2015

Differential Diagnoses in Surgical Pathology: Pulmonary Pathology
Rosane Duarte Achcar, Steve D. Groshong and Carlyne D. Cool, 2016

Differential Diagnoses in Surgical Pathology: Head and Neck
William H. Westra and Justin A. Bishop, 2016

Differential Diagnoses in Surgical Pathology: Breast
Jean F. Simpson and Melinda E. Sanders, 2016

Differential Diagnoses in Surgical Pathology:
Cytopathology

Christopher J. VandenBussche, MD, PhD

Associate Director, Division of Cytopathology
Associate Professor of Pathology and Oncology
The Johns Hopkins University School of Medicine
Baltimore, Maryland

Syed Z. Ali, MBBS, MD

Director, Division of Cytopathology
Professor of Pathology and Radiology
The Johns Hopkins University School of Medicine
Baltimore, Maryland

SERIES EDITOR

Jonathan I. Epstein, MD

Professor of Pathology, Urology and Oncology
The Reinhard Professor of Urological Pathology
Director of Surgical Pathology
The Johns Hopkins Medical Institutions
Baltimore, Maryland

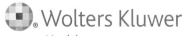
. Wolters Kluwer
Health

Philadelphia • Baltimore • New York • London
Buenos Aires • Hong Kong • Sydney • Tokyo

Acquisitions Editor: Keith Donnellan
Development Editor: Ariel S. Winter
Editorial Coordinator: Julie Kostelnik
Marketing Manager: Julie Sikora
Production Project Manager: Kim Cox
Design Coordinator: Joan Wendt
Manufacturing Coordinator: Beth Welsh
Prepress Vendor: TNQ Technologies

9 8 7 6 5 4 3 2 1

Printed in China

Library of Congress Cataloging-in-Publication Data

ISBN-13: 978-1-975113-14-8

Cataloging in Publication data available on request from publisher.

shop.lww.com

PREFACE

The practice of cytopathology revolves around the creation of a differential diagnosis. Often, without the benefit of the level of architecture seen in histologic sections, the cytopathologist must use the smallest cytomorphologic clues—and even look beyond cells and into the surrounding background—to narrow the differential diagnosis or even arrive at a singular diagnosis.

This book compares similar entities that are often in the differential diagnosis together and focuses on those small details that can help favor one entity over another. In addition to high yield, bulleted cytomorphologic descriptions and representative images, the book also includes important clinical differences between lesions, as well as the latest molecular alterations associated with each entity, when known.

Some of the presented entities are common, while others are rare. This book may be used to learn about a given entity in more detail, to broaden a differential diagnosis, or eliminate less likely diagnoses from a differential. Whether used in a pinch or read from cover-to-cover, we hope this book will become a trusted reference for the reader when cytopathology specimens are encountered.

**Christopher J. VandenBussche and
Syed Z. Ali**

CONTENTS

Gynecologic Cytopathology

	Low-Grade Squamous Intraepithelial Lesion (LSIL)	High-Grade Squamous Intraepithelial Lesion (HSIL)
Age	Any age but more likely to be transient infection in younger women	Any age
Location	Cervix (also vagina, anus, and vulva)	Cervix (also vagina, anus, and vulva)
Signs and symptoms	None; detected on routine screening or on colposcopy	None; detected on routine screening or on colposcopy
Etiology	Premalignant lesion associated with both low- and high-risk HPV	Premalignant lesion more commonly associated with high-risk HPV types
Cytomorphology	• Squamous cells with enlarged nuclei *(Figures 1.1.1 and 1.1.2)* • Irregular nuclear borders and/or "raisinoid" nucleus *(Figures 1.1.3 and 1.1.4)* • Occasional binucleation *(Figure 1.1.5)* • Koilocytes have, in addition to the above features, a well-defined polygonal perinuclear halo with sharp edges and central clearing *(Figures 1.1.3 and 1.1.4)*	• Cellular fragments and dispersed single cells *(Figures 1.1.6 and 1.1.7)* • High N/C ratio due to increased nuclear size and decreased amounts of cytoplasm *(Figure 1.1.8)* • Hyperchromatic nuclei without prominent nucleoli *(Figure 1.1.8)* • Markedly irregular nuclear borders *(Figure 1.1.9)* • Anisonucleosis may be present *(Figure 1.1.2)* • Dense, opaque cytoplasm in individual cells *(Figure 1.1.9)*
Special studies	HPV studies	HPV studies
Molecular alterations	Under investigation; mostly driven by HPV oncogenes	Under investigation; mostly driven by HPV oncogenes
Treatment	Colposcopy to exclude the presence of HSIL	Complete excision
Clinical implications	Often regresses, especially in young women	May progress to squamous cell carcinoma if incompletely excised

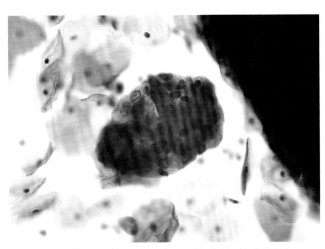

Figure 1.1.1　Low-grade squamous intraepithelial lesion (LSIL). A fragment of atypical squamous cells. The amount of cytoplasm is maintained, but the nuclei are significantly larger than those seen in adjacent intermediate cells.

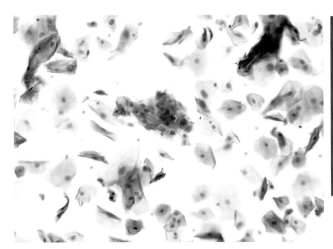

Figure 1.1.2　Low-grade squamous intraepithelial lesion (LSIL). The cells in this central fragment have polygonal cytoplasm and their nuclei are enlarged compared with adjacent intermediate cells. Examination at higher magnification is required to determine whether perinuclear halos are present, but greatly increased nuclear size alone is sufficient for a diagnosis of LSIL.

Figure 1.1.3　Low-grade squamous intraepithelial lesion (LSIL). These cells are koilocytes because they have nuclear atypia (hyperchromasia, enlargement, and binucleation) and perinuclear clearing (halo) with sharp edges.

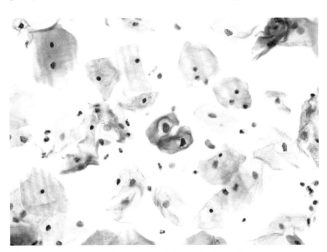

Figure 1.1.4　Low-grade squamous intraepithelial lesion (LSIL). These koilocytes have enlarged nuclei with irregular borders ("raisinoid nuclei"), hyperchromasia, and polygonal shaped, well-defined perinuclear halos.

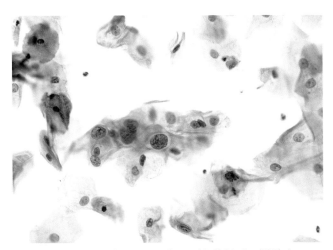

Figure 1.1.5　Low-grade squamous intraepithelial lesion (LSIL). A group of LSIL cells that demonstrate nuclear enlargement, binucleation, hyperchromasia, anisonucleosis, and irregular nuclear borders. Well-defined perinuclear halos are absent but are not needed to diagnose LSIL in this case, given the presence of other atypical features.

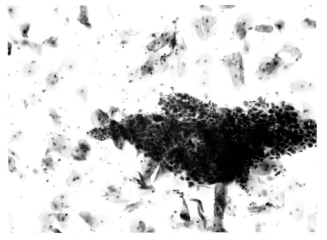

Figure 1.1.6　High-grade squamous intraepithelial lesion (HSIL). A fragment of small, hyperchromatic cells. The cells have very little cytoplasm and appear to have irregular shapes, causing concern for HSIL. Examination at higher magnification is required to confirm these cells as HSIL versus other entities that can cause hyperchromatic crowded groups.

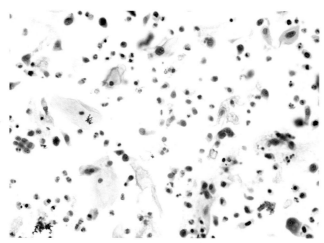

Figure 1.1.7   High-grade squamous intraepithelial lesion (HSIL). The cells in this field are predominantly dispersed. Several cells have high N/C ratios and enlarged dark nuclei with irregular nuclear borders. If such cells are seen in sufficient numbers, a diagnosis of HSIL can be made.

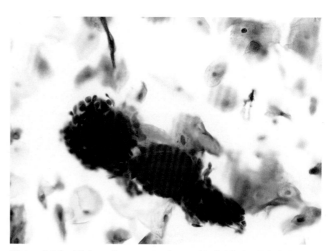

Figure 1.1.8   High-grade squamous intraepithelial lesion (HSIL). This fragment contains cells with hyperchromasia and very little cytoplasm. HSIL cells are often much smaller than LSIL cells, since LSIL cells usually maintain their cytoplasm.

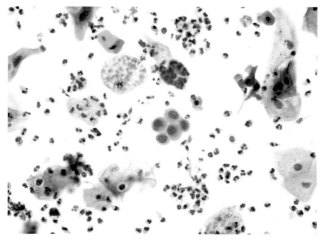

Figure 1.1.9   High-grade squamous intraepithelial lesion (HSIL). The five cells seen centrally are concerning for HSIL, as they have enlarged dark nuclei with irregular nuclear borders. The cytoplasm has a dense opaque look, suggesting these cells have arisen from an area of squamous metaplasia and at very least represent atypical immature squamous metaplasia.

	High-Grade Squamous Intraepithelial Lesion (HSIL)	Squamous Cell Carcinoma
Age	Any age	Any age
Location	Cervix (also vagina, anus, and vulva)	Cervix (also vagina, anus, and vulva)
Signs and symptoms	None; detected on routine screening or on colposcopy	Dyspareunia; bleeding; vaginal discharge; mass on colposcopy; may be asymptomatic
Etiology	Premalignant lesion more commonly associated with high-risk HPV types	Progression of HSIL secondary to HPV infection (usually high-risk subtype)
Cytomorphology	• Cellular fragments and/or dispersed single cells *(Figures 1.2.1* and *1.2.2)* • High N/C ratio due to increased nuclear size and decreased amounts of cytoplasm *(Figures 1.2.3* and *1.2.4)* • Hyperchromatic nuclei without prominent nucleoli *(Figures 1.2.3* and *1.2.4)* • Markedly irregular nuclear borders may be present • Anisonucleosis may be present *(Figure 1.2.5)* • Dense, opaque cytoplasm in individual cells	• Malignant cells in fragments and/or present singly *(Figures 1.2.6* and *1.2.7)* • Enlarged cells with large nuclei and high N/C ratios *(Figure 1.2.8)* • Nuclear contour irregularities *(Figure 1.2.7)* • Anisonucleosis *(Figure 1.2.9)* • Cells may be keratinizing, with pink cytoplasm and irregular cytoplasmic extensions and pyknotic nuclei *(Figure 1.2.10)* • Necrosis may be present *(Figure 1.2.9)*
Special studies	HPV studies	None; a cytomorphologic diagnosis
Molecular alterations	Under investigation; mostly driven by HPV oncogenes	Most commonly mutations in PIK3CA, KRAS, and EGFR
Treatment	Complete excision	Depends on stage; conization, hysterectomy, pelvic lymph node dissection, and/or chemoradiation
Clinical implications	May progress to squamous cell carcinoma if incompletely excised	Depends on stage; best if complete surgical removal

Figure 1.2.1 High-grade squamous intraepithelial lesion (HSIL). These tissue fragments contain numerous crowded, hyperchromatic nuclei. At this magnification, these cells could represent either HSIL or squamous cell carcinoma, but no features of squamous cell carcinoma are seen to allow such a diagnosis. In many instances, it can be difficult to distinguish HSIL from squamous cell carcinoma on a Pap test, but both diagnoses require rapid clinical follow-up.

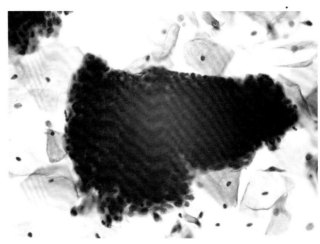

Figure 1.2.2 High-grade squamous intraepithelial lesion (HSIL). This fragment contains numerous crowded, hyperchromatic nuclei and forms a three-dimensional structure. The nuclei have high N/C ratios and appear disorganized within the fragment.

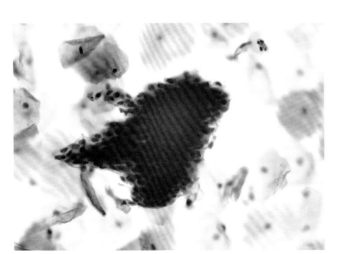

Figure 1.2.3 High-grade squamous intraepithelial lesion (HSIL). These hyperchromatic cells have opaque cytoplasm, irregular nuclear borders, and oval-to-elongated nuclei. No additional features suggestive of squamous cell carcinoma can be seen, such as necrosis, keratinization, greatly enlarged nuclei, prominent pleomorphism, or anisonucleosis.

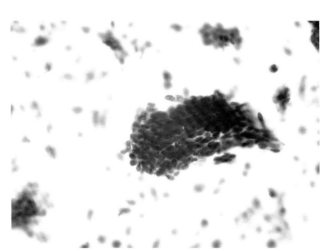

Figure 1.2.4 High-grade squamous intraepithelial lesion (HSIL). The nuclei in this fragment have only mild irregularities in their contours and the nuclei are all around the same size.

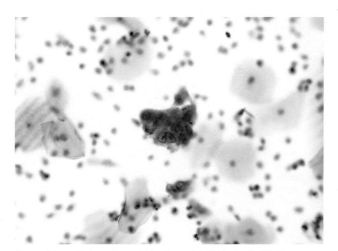

Figure 1.2.5 High-grade squamous intraepithelial lesion (HSIL). These atypical cells have more cytoplasm than in the previous figures, but have enlarged nuclei with hyperchromasia, are pleomorphic, and demonstrate nuclear size variation. The N/C ratios are more compatible with HSIL than LSIL.

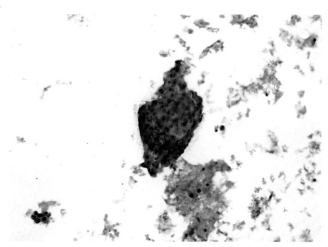

Figure 1.2.6 Squamous cell carcinoma. This tissue fragment contains cells with pink cytoplasm, indicating keratinization. While this could represent atypical parakeratosis, the cells have dark and crowded nuclei, and the background contains abundant necrosis.

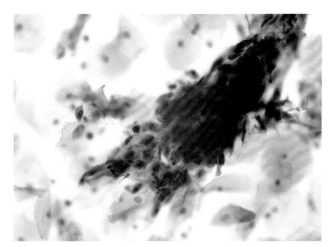

Figure 1.2.7 Squamous cell carcinoma. The cells in this fragment are enlarged and have large nuclei and high N/C ratios. The nuclei are dark and have markedly irregular nuclear borders. There is prominent variation in nuclear size. While HSIL is in the differential, the features are concerning for a possible squamous cell carcinoma.

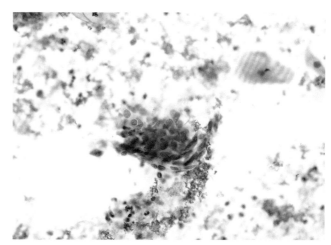

Figure 1.2.8 Squamous cell carcinoma. The cells have high N/C ratios and irregular nuclear shapes. They are crowded and disorganized within the fragment. They could represent HSIL, but the presence of "clinging diathesis" (necrotic granular debris attached to the fragment) raises suspicion for squamous cell carcinoma.

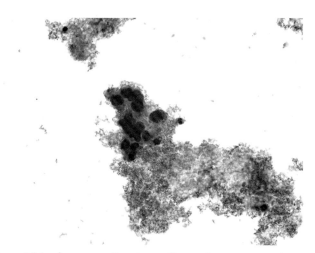

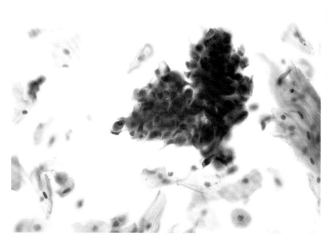

Figure 1.2.9   Squamous cell carcinoma. These cells appear as carcinoma would be seen elsewhere in the body: large cells with enlarged nuclei, high N/C ratios, hyperchromasia, anisonucleosis, and markedly irregular nuclear contours.

Figure 1.2.10   Squamous cell carcinoma. This fragment contains cells with crowded, hyperchromatic nuclei. Some of the cells demonstrate frank keratinization, a feature that favors a squamous cell carcinoma over HSIL.

	High-Grade Squamous Intraepithelial Lesion (HSIL)	Endocervical Adenocarcinoma
Age	Any age	Any age
Location	Cervix (also vagina, anus, and vulva)	Cervix
Signs and symptoms	None; detected on routine screening or on colposcopy	Dyspareunia; bleeding; vaginal discharge; mass on colposcopy; may be asymptomatic
Etiology	Premalignant lesion more commonly associated with high-risk HPV types	HPV infection, most commonly HPV 16 and/or 18; may be associated with adenocarcinoma in situ
Cytomorphology	• Cellular fragments and/or dispersed single cells *(Figures 1.3.1* and *1.3.2)* • High N/C ratio due to increased nuclear size and decreased amounts of cytoplasm *(Figure 1.3.3)* • Hyperchromatic nuclei without nucleoli *(Figure 1.3.4)* • Nuclear border irregularities *(Figure 1.3.5)* • Anisonucleosis may be present *(Figure 1.3.5)* • Dense, opaque cytoplasm in individual cells	• Malignant cells in fragments or present singly *(Figures 1.3.6* and *1.3.7)* • Three-dimensional fragments with columnar cells *(Figures 1.3.8* and *1.3.9)* • Enlarged cells with large nuclei and high N/C ratios *(Figures 1.3.8* and *1.3.9)* • Nuclear contour irregularities may be present • Anisonucleosis *(Figure 1.3.9)* • Prominent nucleoli *(Figure 1.3.10)* • Necrosis may be present
Special studies	HPV studies	None; a cytomorphologic diagnosis
Molecular alterations	Under investigation; mostly driven by HPV oncogenes	Under investigation
Treatment	Complete excision	Depends on stage; conization, hysterectomy, pelvic lymph node dissection, and/or chemoradiation
Clinical implications	May progress to squamous cell carcinoma if incompletely excised	Depends on stage; best if complete surgical removal is possible

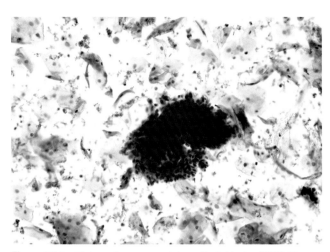

Figure 1.3.1   High-grade squamous intraepithelial lesion (HSIL). The cells in this tissue fragment have enlarged, crowded, and hyperchromatic nuclei. Examination at higher magnification is required to assess the nature of this hyperchromatic crowded group, but the amount of hyperchromasia is concerning for HSIL.

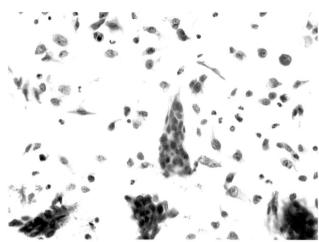

Figure 1.3.2   High-grade squamous intraepithelial lesion (HSIL). This field contains small fragments of HSIL as well as dispersed HSIL cells. The cells have high N/C ratios and dark chromatin. HSIL cells may look elongated in some preparations, emulating the columnar shapes of cells with glandular differentiation.

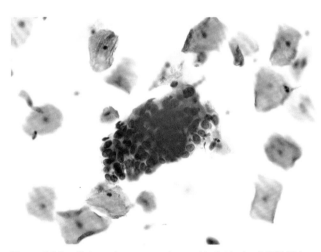

Figure 1.3.3   High-grade squamous intraepithelial lesion (HSIL). This fragment contains numerous crowded, dark nuclei. The nuclei are oval shaped and vary in size.

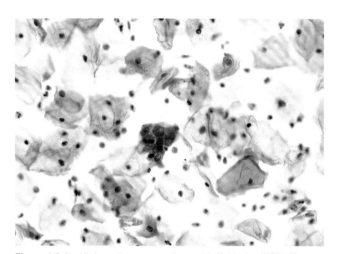

Figure 1.3.4   High-grade squamous intraepithelial lesion (HSIL). The nuclei in this small fragment of HSIL have prominent variation in size and mild nuclear contour irregularities. Nucleoli are absent and should not be seen in HSIL.

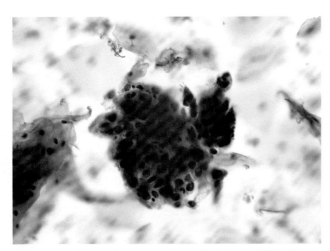

Figure 1.3.5 High-grade squamous intraepithelial lesion (HSIL). This fragment emulated a squamous cell carcinoma, as some nuclei have markedly irregular borders, nuclear size variation is prominent, and some cells adjacent appear to be keratinized. Despite being rare, keratinizing HSIL lesions do exist.

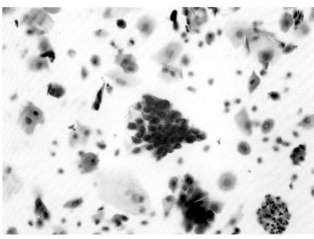

Figure 1.3.6 Endocervical adenocarcinoma. A small fragment of cells emulates HSIL. The cells are small, with high N/C ratios and dark nuclei. There is little size variation between the nuclei.

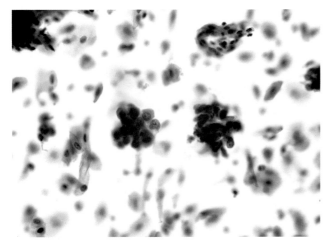

Figure 1.3.7 Endocervical adenocarcinoma. The hyperchromatic cells in this field have little size variation, oval-to-elongated nuclei, and high N/C ratios. While HSIL remains in the differential, the presence of elongated nuclei and nucleoli (though small) should cause consideration of an adenocarcinoma.

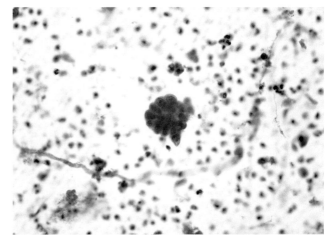

Figure 1.3.8 Endocervical adenocarcinoma. This tissue fragment has a smooth, scalloped border that is not usually seen with squamous differentiation. The cells are three-dimensional and have small nucleoli, additional features that are more suggestive of glandular differentiation.

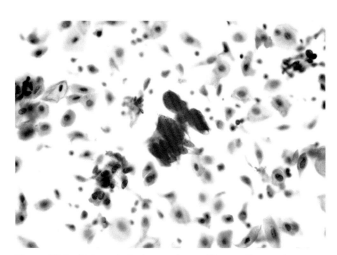

Figure 1.3.9   Endocervical adenocarcinoma. These cells are columnar and have large, hyperchromatic, elongated nuclei. The differential diagnosis includes endocervical adenocarcinoma as well as adenocarcinoma in situ.

Figure 1.3.10   Endocervical adenocarcinoma. This tissue fragment is three-dimensional and contains cells with prominent nucleoli. Some cells have a columnar shape. The differential diagnosis includes endocervical adenocarcinoma as well as cells with marked reactive atypia.

	Squamous Cell Carcinoma	Endocervical Adenocarcinoma
Age	Any age	Any age
Location	Cervix (also vagina, anus, and vulva)	Cervix
Signs and symptoms	Dyspareunia; bleeding; vaginal discharge; mass on colposcopy; may be asymptomatic	Dyspareunia; bleeding; vaginal discharge; mass on colposcopy; may be asymptomatic
Etiology	Progression of HSIL secondary to HPV infection (usually high-risk subtype)	HPV infection, most commonly HPV 16 and/or 18; may be associated with adenocarcinoma in situ
Cytomorphology	• Malignant cells in fragments or present singly *(Figure 1.4.1)* • Enlarged cells with large nuclei and high N/C ratios *(Figure 1.4.2)* • Nuclear contour irregularities *(Figure 1.4.3)* • Anisonucleosis *(Figures 1.4.2 and 1.4.3)* • Cells may be keratinizing, with pink cytoplasm and irregular cytoplasmic extensions and pyknotic nuclei • Necrosis may be present *(Figures 1.4.4 and 1.4.5)*	• Malignant cells in fragments or present singly *(Figures 1.4.6 and 1.4.7)* • Three-dimensional fragments with columnar cells *(Figure 1.4.7)* • Enlarged cells with large nuclei and high N/C ratios *(Figure 1.4.8)* • Nuclear contour irregularities *(Figure 1.4.2)* • Anisonucleosis *(Figure 1.4.9)* • Prominent nucleoli *(Figure 1.3.10)* • Necrosis may be present *(Figure 1.4.10)*
Special studies	None; a cytomorphologic diagnosis	None; a cytomorphologic diagnosis
Molecular alterations	Most commonly mutations in PIK3CA, KRAS, and EGFR	Under investigation
Treatment	Depends on stage; conization, hysterectomy, pelvic lymph node dissection, and/or chemoradiation	Depends on stage; conization, hysterectomy, pelvic lymph node dissection, and/or chemoradiation
Clinical implications	Depends on stage; best if complete surgical removal is possible	Depends on stage; best if complete surgical removal is possible

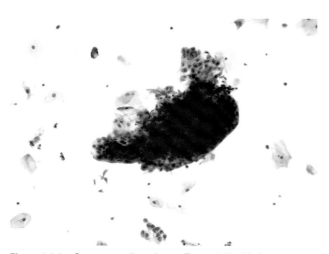

Figure 1.4.1   Squamous cell carcinoma. The nuclei in this fragment are hyperchromatic and crowded. The cells have significant anisonucleosis and carcinoma is suspected. An examination at higher magnification will help determine whether these cells have squamous or glandular features.

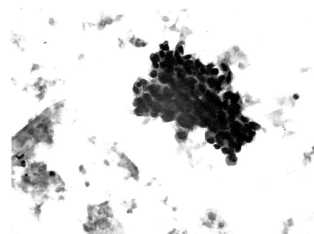

Figure 1.4.2   Squamous cell carcinoma. These carcinoma cells have dark, enlarged nuclei with markedly irregular borders. They have polygonal cytoplasm, which favors a squamous cell carcinoma over an adenocarcinoma. There is abundant necrotic debris in the background.

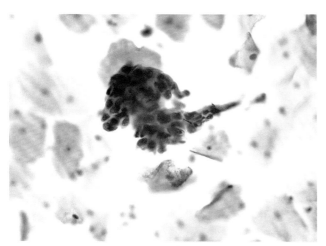

Figure 1.4.3   Squamous cell carcinoma. These cells resemble HSIL but have severe nuclear atypia: nuclear enlargement and anisonucleosis. The cytoplasm appears dense and opaque, favoring a squamous cell carcinoma over an adenocarcinoma.

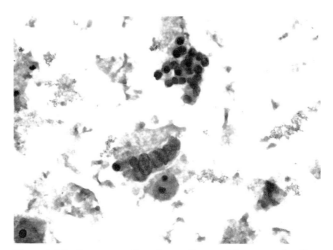

Figure 1.4.4   Squamous cell carcinoma. Two small fragments of malignant cells are seen amid necrotic debris. One fragment contains cells with enlarged, elongated nuclei that suggests a glandular differentiation. However, these cells are from a patient with squamous cell carcinoma. It can be difficult to differentiate a squamous cell carcinoma from an adenocarcinoma in some situations, although squamous cell carcinoma is found more often.

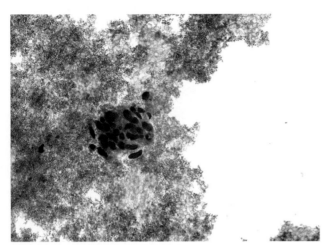

Figure 1.4.5   Squamous cell carcinoma. Cells with dark, elongated nuclei are found in a background of granular debris. The elongated nuclei may cause one to consider a glandular lesion, but elongated nuclei can be found in HSIL and squamous cell carcinoma.

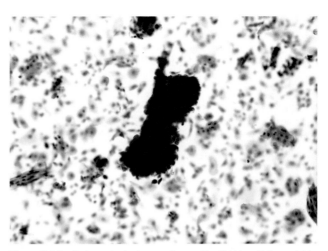

Figure 1.4.6   Endocervical adenocarcinoma. The field is cellular and this fragment of adenocarcinoma contains overlapping, hyperchromatic nuclei. Some edges of the fragment have a feathery appearance because the nuclei are elongated and palisaded along the fragment edges.

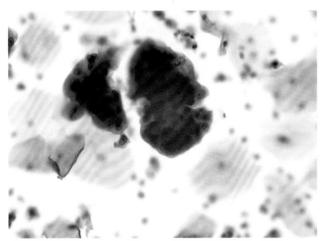

Figure 1.4.7   Endocervical adenocarcinoma. The nuclei seen here have irregular contours and are of different sizes. One clue to the glandular differentiation of these cells is the tissue fragment's smooth edges. Fragments of squamous cell carcinoma are more likely to have jagged edges.

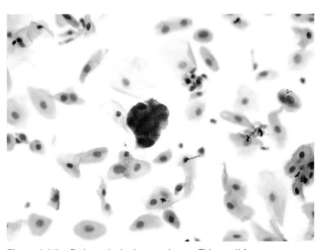

Figure 1.4.8   Endocervical adenocarcinoma. This small fragment contains cells with very dark nuclei and irregular nuclear contours. The tissue fragment contains smooth edges.

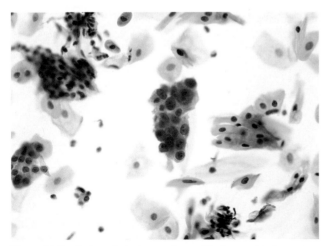

Figure 1.4.9   Endocervical adenocarcinoma. The fragment in the center of the field contains cells with prominent anisonucleosis and nucleoli. The cell cytoplasm is not opaque but instead has a foamy quality, suggesting a glandular differentiation.

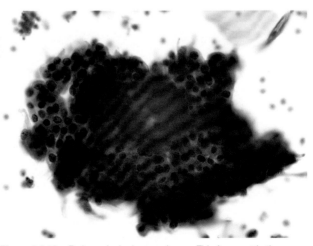

Figure 1.4.10   Endocervical adenocarcinoma. This fragment is three-dimensional and contains cells with enlarged nuclei and prominent nucleoli.

	High-Grade Squamous Intraepithelial Lesion (HSIL)	Adenocarcinoma in Situ
Age	Any age	Younger, reproductive age women
Location	Cervix (also vagina, anus, and vulva)	Cervix
Signs and symptoms	None; detected on routine screening or on colposcopy	Usually asymptomatic
Etiology	Premalignant lesion more commonly associated with high-risk HPV types	HPV infection, most commonly HPV 16 and/or 18
Cytomorphology	• Cellular fragments and dispersed single cells (Figures 1.5.1 and 1.5.2) • High N/C ratio due to increased nuclear size and decreased amounts of cytoplasm (Figures 1.5.2 and 1.5.3) • Hyperchromatic nuclei without nucleoli (Figures 1.5.2 and 1.5.3) • Markedly irregular nuclear borders • Anisonucleosis may be present (Figure 1.5.4) • Dense, opaque cytoplasm in individual cells (Figure 1.5.5)	• Primarily cellular fragments and occasionally single cells (Figures 1.5.6 and 1.5.7) • Monotonous columnar-shaped cells (Figure 1.5.8) • Oval-shaped nuclei with minimal cytoplasm (Figure 1.5.9) • Hyperchromasia, powdery chromatin, and smooth nuclear borders (Figure 1.5.10) • Nuclei may palisade and project from the tissue edge, causing a "feathering" effect (Figures 1.5.1 and 1.5.2)
Special studies	HPV studies	None; a cytomorphologic diagnosis
Molecular alterations	Under investigation; mostly driven by HPV oncogenes	Under investigation
Treatment	Complete excision	Conization or hysterectomy
Clinical implications	May progress to squamous cell carcinoma if incompletely excised	May progress to adenocarcinoma if incompletely excised

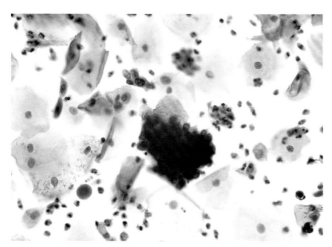

Figure 1.5.1   High-grade squamous intraepithelial lesion (HSIL). Crowded cells with overlapping, hyperchromatic nuclei and high N/C ratios. Some oval-shaped nuclei project from the tissue edges, emulating the "feathering" sometimes seen in AIS.

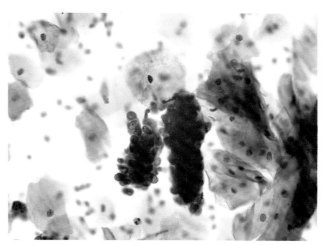

Figure 1.5.2   High-grade squamous intraepithelial lesion (HSIL). The nuclei seen here have some nuclear border irregularities and nuclear size variation. Many are oval-shaped and have scant cytoplasm, causing difficulty in identifying their squamous differentiation.

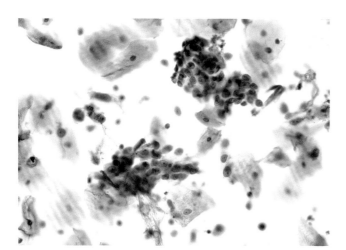

Figure 1.5.3   High-grade squamous intraepithelial lesion (HSIL). Two fragments of HSIL containing enlarged nuclei with hyperchromasia and nuclear border irregularities. Some cells are elongated, giving them a columnar appearance.

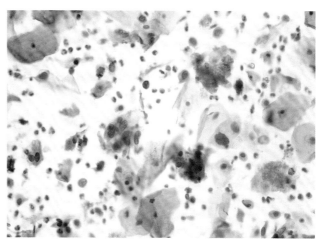

Figure 1.5.4   High-grade squamous intraepithelial lesion (HSIL). The small fragment in the center of the field has elongated, enlarged nuclei that might suggest glandular differentiation. However, there are several atypical squamous cells in the background that are more suggestive of a squamous lesion. One confounding factor is the coexistence of squamous and glandular lesions in the same specimen, as both are caused by HPV.

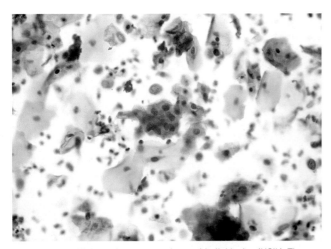

Figure 1.5.5 High-grade squamous intraepithelial lesion (HSIL). These atypical cells are easily identified as squamous given their abundant, polygonal cytoplasm that is keratinized (pink-staining). While a rare occurrence, HSIL can sometimes appear keratinized.

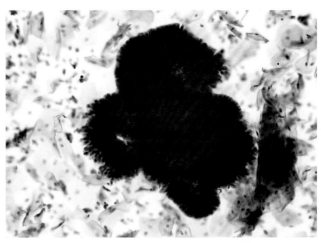

Figure 1.5.6 Adenocarcinoma in situ (AIS). A large fragment of crowded, hyperchromatic cells. The columnar shapes of the cells can be identified around the tissue fragment edges, and some dark nuclei project from the fragment, causing a "feathering" effect.

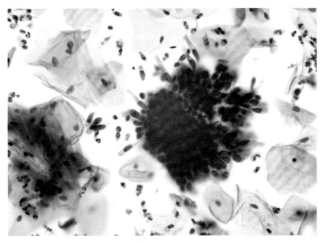

Figure 1.5.7 Adenocarcinoma in situ (AIS). The lesional cells are present in a small tissue fragment as well as singly in the background. The cells are distinctly columnar. While the differential includes reactive endocervical cells, the powdery chromatin appearance should cause concern for AIS.

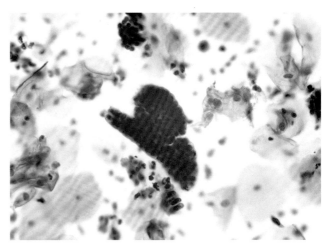

Figure 1.5.8 Adenocarcinoma in situ (AIS). A three-dimensional fragment of hyperchromatic cells. The smooth edges suggest a glandular rather than squamous lesion. The differential diagnosis includes adenocarcinoma as well as AIS.

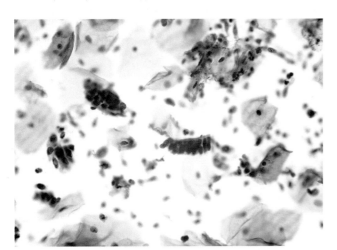

Figure 1.5.9 Adenocarcinoma in situ (AIS). Small strips of cells, with crowded, enlarged, dark nuclei that are poorly aligned within each fragment.

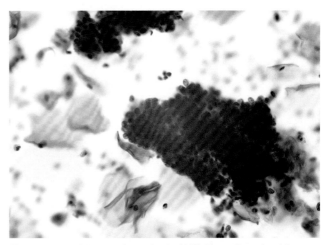

Figure 1.5.10 Adenocarcinoma in situ (AIS). Three-dimensional fragments of cells with high N/C ratios, hyperchromasia, and irregular nuclear borders. Note the projection of nuclei at the tissue fragment edges ("feathering").

1.6 HIGH-GRADE SQUAMOUS INTRAEPITHELIAL LESION (HSIL) VERSUS SQUAMOUS METAPLASIA

	High-Grade Squamous Intraepithelial Lesion (HSIL)	Squamous Metaplasia
Age	Any age	Any age
Location	Cervix (also vagina, anus, and vulva)	Cervix
Signs and symptoms	None; detected on routine screening or on colposcopy	Asymptomatic
Etiology	Premalignant lesion more commonly associated with high-risk HPV types	Common and benign transition of endocervical glandular epithelium to squamous metaplastic epithelium in the transformation zone
Cytomorphology	• Cellular fragments and dispersed single cells *(Figures 1.6.1 and 1.6.2)* • High N/C ratio due to increased nuclear size and decreased amounts of cytoplasm *(Figures 1.6.3 and 1.6.4)* • Hyperchromatic nuclei without nucleoli *(Figure 1.6.4)* • Markedly irregular nuclear borders *(Figures 1.6.4 and 1.6.5)* • Anisonucleosis may be present *(Figures 1.6.1 and 1.6.2)* • Dense, opaque cytoplasm in individual cells *(Figure 1.6.4)*	• Small cellular fragments and single cells *(Figures 1.6.6 and 1.6.7)* • Cells in fragments have "tiling" effect in which small spaces are seen between cells *(Figure 1.6.8)* • Polygonal-shaped cells *(Figure 1.6.9)* • Dense, opaque cytoplasm *(Figure 1.6.10)* • Slightly enlarged nuclei with regular contours *(Figures 1.6.7 and 1.6.8)* • Hyperchromasia should not be prominent *(Figures 1.6.7 and 1.6.8)*
Special studies	HPV studies	None; a cytomorphologic diagnosis
Molecular alterations	Under investigation; mostly driven by HPV oncogenes	N/A
Treatment	Complete excision	N/A
Clinical implications	May progress to squamous cell carcinoma if incompletely excised	N/A

Figure 1.6.1   High-grade squamous intraepithelial lesion (HSIL). Numerous crowded tissue fragments with hyperchromatic cells. The small fragment of cells in the center has opaque cytoplasm but enlarged, dark nuclei with irregular contours and significant size variation.

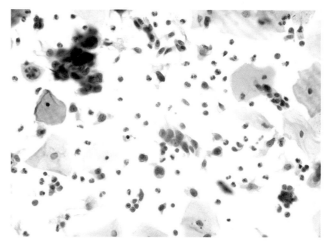

Figure 1.6.2   High-grade squamous intraepithelial lesion (HSIL). The lesional cells have high N/C ratios, hyperchromasia, and irregular nuclear borders.

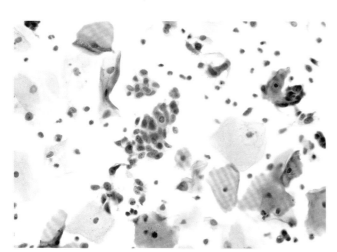

Figure 1.6.3   High-grade squamous intraepithelial lesion (HSIL). The cells have high N/C ratios and dark nuclei. Squamous metaplastic cells usually have a moderate amount of cytoplasm and N/C ratios below 0.5.

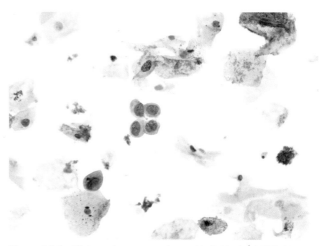

Figure 1.6.4   High-grade squamous intraepithelial lesion (HSIL). These cells have a metaplastic appearance due to their dense cytoplasm, oval shapes, and loosely cohesive nature. The nuclei are too enlarged and dark, and the nuclear contours are too irregular, for these cells to represent simply benign metaplastic cells.

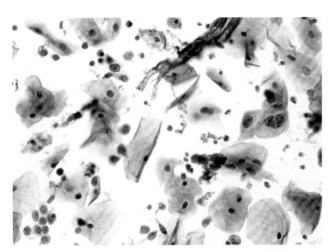

Figure 1.6.5 High-grade squamous intraepithelial lesion (HSIL). Numerous single cells with dense cytoplasm and high N/C ratios. These cells can easily be missed as they are small and dispersed throughout the background.

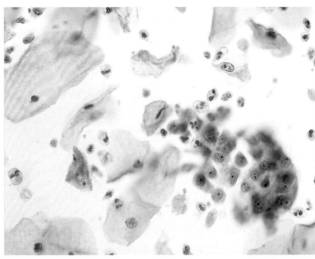

Figure 1.6.6 Squamous metaplasia. A fragment of loosely cohesive cells (lower right-hand side of the field). The cells have a moderate amount of cytoplasm and the nuclei are of similar size and have regular nuclear contours, favoring benign squamous metaplasia.

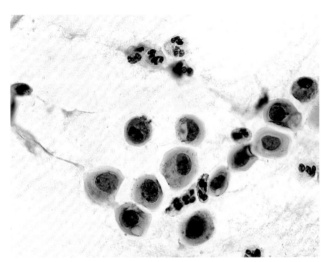

Figure 1.6.7 Squamous metaplasia. Singly dispersed metaplastic cells. Despite having some hyperchromasia and enlarged nuclei, these cells have low N/C ratios and are not diagnostic of HSIL. Their polygonal shapes and dense cytoplasm are features compatible with a squamous metaplastic zone origin.

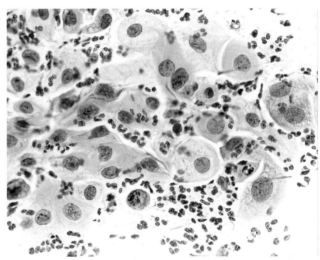

Figure 1.6.8 Squamous metaplasia. A monolayer tissue fragment of squamous metaplastic cells with abundant cytoplasm, polygonal shapes, and small empty spaces between adjacent cells. The latter features reflect an attempt at forming intercellular junctions.

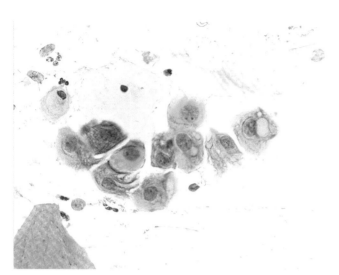

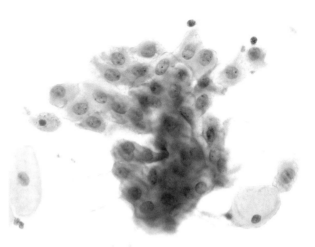

Figure 1.6.9 Squamous metaplasia. Squamous metaplastic cells are seen adjacent to an intermediate cell. Their nuclei are enlarged compared with the intermediate cell nucleus, and their cytoplasm appears more dense and opaque.

Figure 1.6.10 Squamous metaplasia. A fragment of metaplastic squamous cells with dense cytoplasm, polygonal shapes, and similarly sized nuclei with regular nuclear borders.

	Glycogenated Cells	Low-Grade Squamous Intraepithelial Lesion (LSIL)
Age	Premenopausal women	Any age but more likely to be transient infection in younger women
Location	Cervix	Cervix (also vagina, anus, and vulva)
Signs and symptoms	None	None; detected on routine screening or on colposcopy
Etiology	Accumulation of glycogen; associated with postpartum period, late menstrual cycle, and pregnancy	Premalignant lesion associated with both low- and high-risk HPV
Cytomorphology	• Parabasal or intermediate cells with perinuclear clearing ("halo") containing glycogen (Figures 1.7.1 and 1.7.2) • Halos are usually seen in large number of cells within the specimen (Figure 1.7.3) • Halos often have round and/or have regular borders (Figures 1.7.4 and 1.7.5)	• Squamous cells with enlarged nuclei (Figure 1.7.6) • Irregular nuclear borders and/or "raisinoid" nucleus • Occasional binucleation (Figures 1.7.7 and 1.7.8) • Koilocytes have, in addition to the above features, a well-defined polygonal perinuclear halo with sharp edges and central clearing (Figures 1.7.9 and 1.7.10)
Special studies	N/A	HPV studies
Molecular alterations	N/A	Under investigation; mostly driven by HPV oncogenes
Treatment	N/A	Colposcopy to exclude the presence of HSIL
Clinical implications	N/A	Often regresses, especially in young women

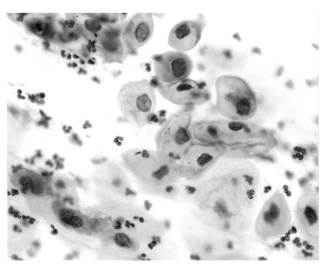

Figure 1.7.1   Glycogenated cells. These parabasal cells are atypical enough to be diagnosed as ASC-US or ASC-H, as they have enlarged nuclei, mild nuclear contour irregularities, and hyperchromasia. Several cells are binucleated. The presence of glycogen, seen as large and ill-defined halos in the cell cytoplasm, may contribute to an overdiagnosis of LSIL.

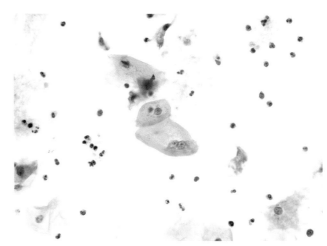

Figure 1.7.2   Glycogenated cells. These intermediate cells are binucleated, a finding that can be seen in both dysplastic and reactive processes. The cells have large areas of ill-defined pale-staining cytoplasm due to glycogenation, creating a false picture of LSIL.

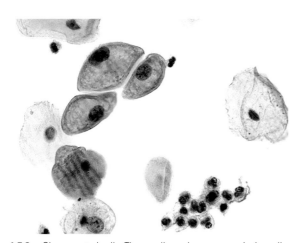

Figure 1.7.3   Glycogenated cells. These cells are known as navicular cells. They are boat-shaped intermediate cells containing well-defined glycogen halos. They are seen during pregnancy and late in the menstrual cycle.

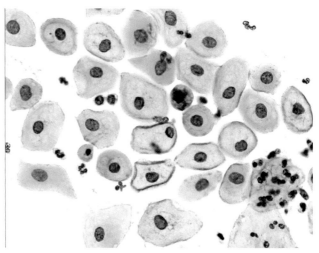

Figure 1.7.4   Glycogenated cells. The field is filled with numerous navicular cells. Several cells contain areas of glycogen surrounded by well-defined, smooth borders and only a thin rim of uninvolved cytoplasm.

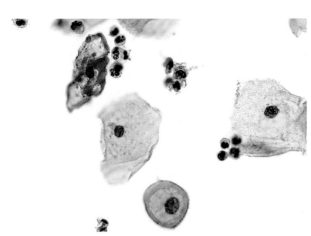

Figure 1.7.5   Glycogenated cells. The cell at the bottom has a round and large perinuclear halo. The nucleus is not much larger than those of the nearby intermediate cells and its contours are regular.

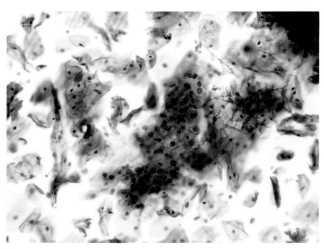

Figure 1.7.6   Low-grade squamous intraepithelial lesion (LSIL). While perinuclear halos are not identified at this magnification, this fragment contains cells with enlarged nuclei and irregular borders. Significantly increased nuclear size is sufficient for a diagnosis of LSIL even in the absence of koilocytes.

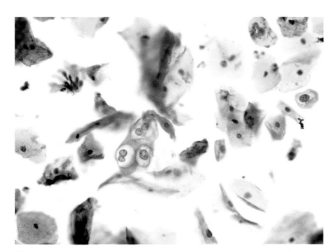

Figure 1.7.7   Low-grade squamous intraepithelial lesion (LSIL). Several cells with both perinuclear halos and nuclear atypia (enlargement and binucleation) are present. The halos are well defined and some have a polygonal shape.

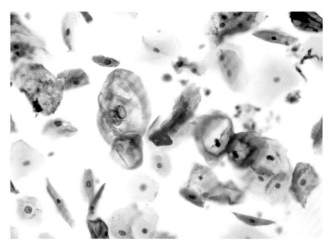

Figure 1.7.8   Low-grade squamous intraepithelial lesion (LSIL). Several koilocytes with perinuclear halos and binucleation can be seen. One cell has significantly enlarged nuclei compared with other koilocytes.

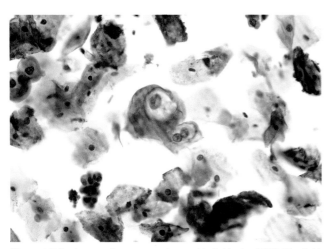

Figure 1.7.9 Low-grade squamous intraepithelial lesion (LSIL). The field contains several dysplastic cells, but the koilocytes (central field) stand out from the rest. Their halos have sharp edges and irregular shapes.

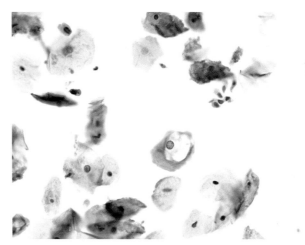

Figure 1.7.10 Low-grade squamous intraepithelial lesion (LSIL). A single koilocyte with a well-defined halo. The nucleus is minimally enlarged and the chromatin is bland. However, the halo is unlikely due to glycogenation because glycogen tends to accumulate primary in intermediate or parabasal cells, which would have cyan cytoplasm.

	Benign Endometrial Cells	Endometrial Adenocarcinoma
Age	Premenopausal women	Middle aged to older women
Location	Endometrium	Endometrium
Signs and symptoms	Exfoliate during menses	Postmenopausal or irregular bleeding
Etiology	Normal physiology	Long-term estrogen stimulation (endometrioid) or early *TP53* mutation (serous, clear cell)
Cytomorphology	• Small fragments of cells forming hyperchromatic crowded groups; rarely single cells *(Figures 1.8.1* and *1.8.2)* • Hobnailed borders to tissue fragments is a characteristic finding *(Figure 1.8.3)* • Cytomorphology may vary depending on the day of menses and the patient's hormonal state • Some fragments may have two layers of cells: glandular cells surrounding stromal cells • Small cells with high N/C ratios and hyperchromasia *(Figure 1.8.4)* • Oval nuclei with relatively smooth nuclear contours and minimal size variation *(Figure 1.8.5)* • Powdery or granular chromatin pattern *(Figure 1.8.3)* • The presence of rare small vacuoles and/or neutrophils is a characteristic feature *(Figure 1.8.3)*	• Usually small fragments cells forming hyperchromatic crowded groups; rarely single cells *(Figure 1.8.6)* • Hobnailed borders consistent with glandular and likely endometrial differentiation *(Figure 1.8.7)* • Usually only one population of malignant cells • Larger cells with high N/C ratios and hyperchromasia *(Figures 1.8.6* and *1.8.8)* • Enlarged nuclei that range from round to pleomorphic and may have irregular nuclear borders *(Figure 1.8.6)* • Chromatin is more coarse and may have nucleoli *(Figures 1.8.6* and *1.8.7)* • Larger and more frequent vacuoles with increased numbers of neutrophils *(Figures 1.8.9* and *1.8.10)*
Special studies	None	None
Molecular alterations	N/A	*TP53* mutations (serous and clear cell); often mutations in *PTEN, KRAS,* or *PAX2* (endometrioid)
Treatment	N/A	Total abdominal hysterectomy with bilateral salpingo-oophorectomy and/or regional node dissection, chemoradiation
Clinical implications	N/A	Varies greatly and depends on stage

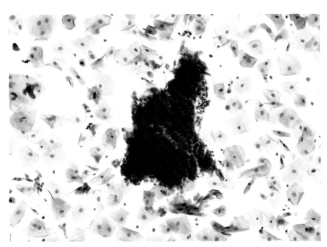

Figure 1.8.1   Benign endometrial cells. A large hyperchromatic crowded group of cells. The nuclei are dark and closer examination will help reveal an endometrial origin. The differential diagnosis primary includes HSIL.

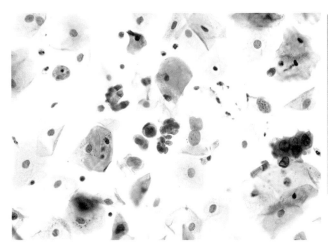

Figure 1.8.2   Benign endometrial cells. Benign endometrial cells are seen as loosely cohesive cells with little cytoplasm, oval-shaped nuclei, and powdery chromatin. Adjacent cells with much larger nuclei and hyperchromasia represent coexisting HSIL in this specimen.

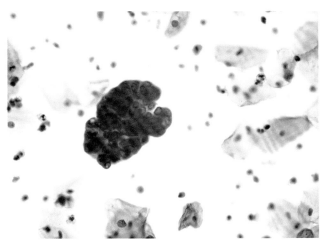

Figure 1.8.3   Benign endometrial cells. This tissue fragment has hobnailed borders, strongly suggesting an endometrial origin. The cells have powdery chromatin, dark nuclei, and slight variations in nuclear contours and size. Only rare neutrophils can be seen, along with a few small cytoplasm vacuoles.

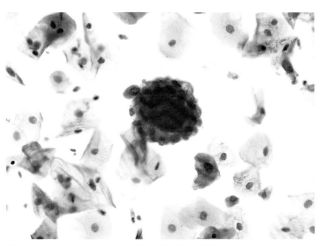

Figure 1.8.4   Benign endometrial cells. A small fragment of endometrial cells in a "double contour" configuration, caused by endometrial cells surrounding stromal cells. Note the hobnailed edge to the tissue fragment. The double contour is not seen in endometrial carcinoma.

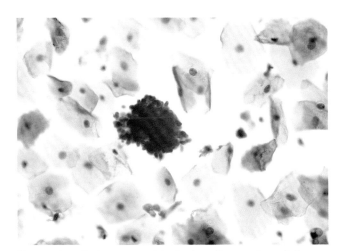

Figure 1.8.5   Benign endometrial cells. A small group of crowded, hyperchromatic benign endometrial cells. The cells have elongated nuclei and minimal cytoplasm. Some nuclei project from the tissue fragment edges, creating a "feathering" effect that may cause concern for AIS.

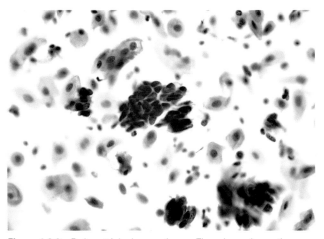

Figure 1.8.6   Endometrial adenocarcinoma. These hyperchromatic adenocarcinoma cells are much larger than benign endometrial cells and demonstrate greater variation in nuclear shape, size, and border irregularity. The differential diagnosis include AIS and HSIL.

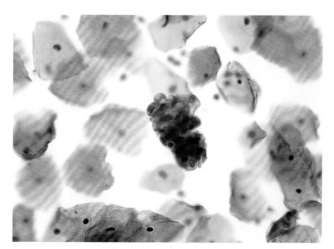

Figure 1.8.7　Endometrial adenocarcinoma. A group of endometrial adenocarcinoma cells with enlarged hyperchromatic nuclei with nuclear border variation and prominent cytoplasmic vacuolization.

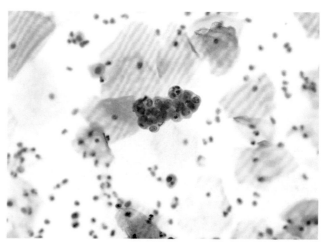

Figure 1.8.8　Endometrial adenocarcinoma. A small group of endometrial adenocarcinoma cells, some with coarse chromatin or small nucleoli. There is an increased number intracytoplasmic neutrophils. These cells may be difficult to distinguish from benign endometrial cells, resulting in a diagnosis of atypical glandular cells.

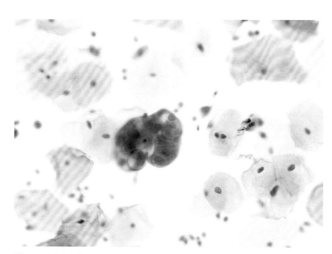

Figure 1.8.9　Endometrial adenocarcinoma. These cells have prominent vacuolization, a feature that should cause concern for an endometrial adenocarcinoma. The nuclei otherwise have bland chromatin and some variation in nuclear size.

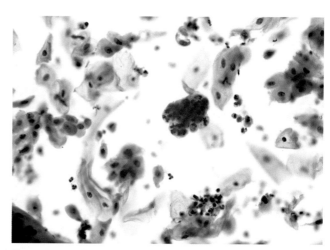

Figure 1.8.10　Endometrial adenocarcinoma. The number of neutrophils associated with these endometrial cells is concerning, as they obscure the nuclei and cause difficulty in cytomorphologic assessment. These large cells are known as "bags of polyps" and are suspicious for adenocarcinoma

	Endometrial Adenocarcinoma	Metastatic Adenocarcinoma
Age	Middle aged to older women	Primarily older adults
Location	Endometrium	Most gynecologic tract with subsequent exfoliation into the cervical canal
Signs and symptoms	Postmenopausal or irregular bleeding	Often none from the metastatic tumor; usually patient has a history of an aggressive carcinoma, which may have recurred
Etiology	Long-term estrogen stimulation (endometrioid) or early *TP53* mutation (serous, clear cell)	Metastatic malignancy
Cytomorphology	• Usually small fragments cells forming hyperchromatic crowded groups; rarely single cells *(Figure 1.9.1)* • Hobnailed borders consistent with glandular and likely endometrial differentiation *(Figure 1.9.2)* • Usually only one population of malignant cells • Larger cells with high N/C ratios and hyperchromasia *(Figure 1.9.2)* • Enlarged nuclei that range from round to pleomorphic and may have irregular nuclear borders *(Figure 1.9.3)* • Chromatin is more coarse and may have nucleoli *(Figures 1.9.4 and 1.9.5)* • Larger and more frequent vacuoles with increased numbers of neutrophils *(Figure 1.9.3)* • Tumor diathesis may be present and suggest against a metastasis *(Figure 1.9.5)*	• Morphology depends on the site of origin, but typically forms three-dimensional tissue fragments with smooth edges and/or single atypical cells *(Figures 1.9.6 and 1.9.7)* • Gland formation and/or cytoplasmic vacuolization may be present • Large cells with high N/C ratios and hyperchromasia *(Figure 1.9.8)* • Marked anisnucleosis and nuclear border irregularities *(Figure 1.9.9)* • Prominent nucleoli and/or coarse chromatin are common *(Figures 1.9.9 and 1.9.10)* • Intracytoplasmic neutrophils are not a common feature • Clean background (absent tumor diathesis) *(Figures 1.9.6-1.9.10)*
Special studies	None on an exfoliative specimen	None on an exfoliative specimen
Molecular alterations	*TP53* mutations (serous and clear cell); often mutations in *PTEN, KRAS,* or *PAX2* (endometrioid)	Depends on neoplasm type
Treatment	Total abdominal hysterectomy with bilateral salpingo-oophorectomy and/or regional node dissection, chemoradiation	Depends on neoplasm type
Clinical implications	Varies greatly and depends on stage	Depends on neoplasm type

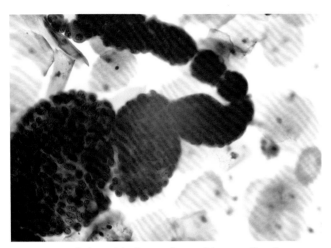

Figure 1.9.1   Endometrial adenocarcinoma. A large papillary fragment containing crowded hyperchromatic cells. The cells have elongated nuclei with moderate size variation and nuclear border irregularity. Some edges are hobnailed (suggesting an endometrial origin), whereas others are smooth (suggesting glandular differentiation).

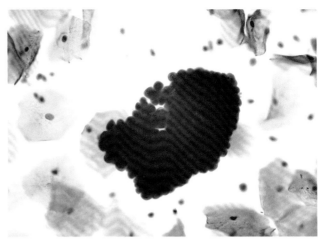

Figure 1.9.2   Endometrial adenocarcinoma. A fragment of cells with dark, crowded nuclei with prominent hobnailed edges. Metastatic serous neoplasms may also have fragments with hobnailed edges.

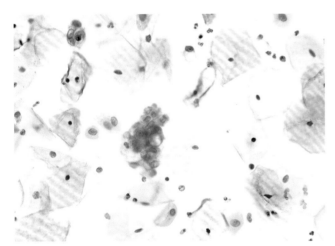

Figure 1.9.3   Endometrial adenocarcinoma. Vacuolization is commonly seen in endometrial carcinoma, but metastatic adenocarcinomas may contain vacuoles as well.

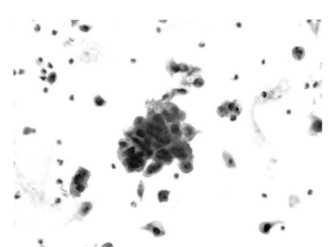

Figure 1.9.4   Enlarge cells with big, irregularly shaped nuclei containing coarse chromatin. The cells are overtly malignant. The foamy cytoplasm and hobnailed borders favor glandular differentiation and an endometrial rather than endocervical origin. The background contains faint granular debris, likely representing tumor diathesis and suggesting a primary malignancy rather than a metastasis.

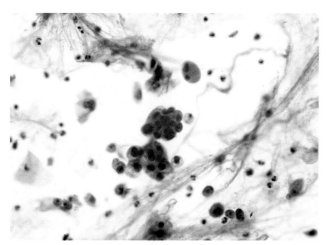

Figure 1.9.5   Endometrial adenocarcinoma. Small groups of malignant cells with prominent nucleoli in a background of tumor diathesis, which favor an cervical squamous carcinoma, endocervical adenocarcinoma, or endometrial adenocarcinoma. Of these three, the associated neutrophils and hobnailed configuration favor an endometrial adenocarcinoma.

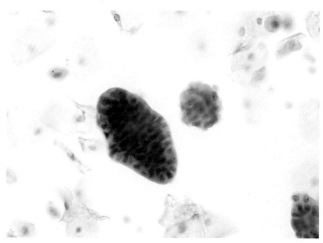

Figure 1.9.6   Metastatic breast ductal carcinoma. This fragment has smooth edges and prominent nucleoli, favoring an adenocarcinoma over a squamous cell carcinoma. The columnar nature could be consistent with an endocervical adenocarcinoma, but this patient had widely metastatic breast ductal carcinoma. The background is clean, whereas cervical adenocarcinomas are usually associated with diathesis.

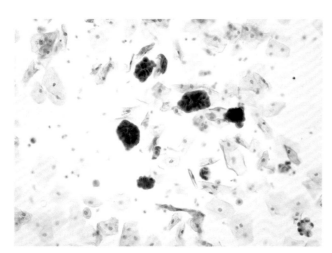

Figure 1.9.7   Metastatic breast ductal carcinoma. Several groups of metastatic breast ductal carcinoma in a clean background. The groups are three-dimensional and contain cells with prominent nucleoli, hyperchromasia, and unusual nuclear shapes.

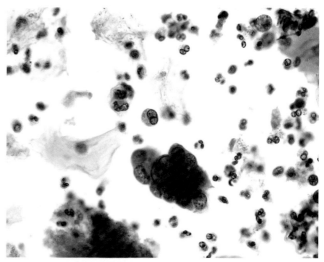

Figure 1.9.8   Metastatic ovarian carcinoma. A three-dimensional glandular structure containing enlarged nuclei of varying sizes and coarse chromatin. The N/C ratios are highly elevated. The background is strangely clean and suggests against a localized invasive carcinoma. This patient had ovarian carcinoma.

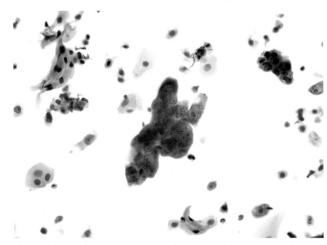

Figure 1.9.9   Metastatic lobular breast carcinoma. Numerous loosely cohesive cells containing enlarged nuclei with coarse chromatin and marked nuclear contour irregularities. The background is free of necrotic debris. The patient had a history of widely invasive lobular breast carcinoma.

Figure 1.9.10   Metastatic adenocarcinoma of unknown primary site. Overtly malignant cells with anisonucleosis and prominent nucleoli. The features are nonspecific for any site of origin, but the clean background favors a metastatic process.

1.10 ADENOCARCINOMA IN SITU (AIS) VERSUS ENDOCERVICAL ADENOCARCINOMA

	Adenocarcinoma in Situ	Endocervical Adenocarcinoma
Age	Younger, reproductive age women	Any age
Location	Cervix	Cervix
Signs and symptoms	Usually asymptomatic	Dyspareunia; bleeding; vaginal discharge; mass on colposcopy may be asymptomatic
Etiology	HPV infection, most commonly HPV 16 and/or 18	HPV infection, most commonly HPV 16 and/or 18; may be associated with adenocarcinoma in situ
Cytomorphology	• Primarily cellular fragments and occasionally single cells *(Figure 1.10.1)* • Monotonous columnar-shaped cells *(Figure 1.10.2)* • Oval-shaped nuclei with minimal cytoplasm *(Figure 1.10.3)* • Hyperchromasia, powdery chromatin, and smooth nuclear borders *(Figure 1.10.4)* • Nuclei may palisade and project from the tissue edge, causing a "feathering" effect *(Figure 1.10.5)*	• Malignant cells in fragments or present singly *(Figures 1.10.6 and 1.10.7)* • Three-dimensional fragments with columnar cells *(Figure 1.10.7)* • Enlarged cells with large nuclei and high N/C ratios *(Figure 1.10.8)* • Nuclear contour irregularities *(Figure 1.10.1)* • Anisonucleosis *(Figure 1.10.8)* • Prominent nucleoli *(Figures 1.10.9 and 1.10.10)* • Necrosis may be present
Special studies	None; a cytomorphologic diagnosis	None; a cytomorphologic diagnosis
Molecular alterations	Under investigation	Under investigation
Treatment	Conization or hysterectomy	Depends on stage; conization, hysterectomy, pelvic lymph node dissection, and/or chemoradiation
Clinical implications	May progress if incompletely excised	Depends on stage; best if complete surgical removal is possible

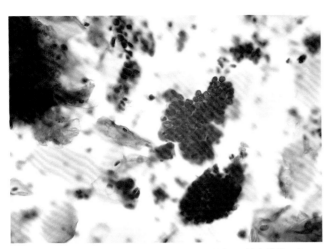

Figure 1.10.1 Adenocarcinoma in situ. The cells have high N/C ratios, hyperchromasia, irregular nuclear borders, and powdery chromatin. There is mild variation in nuclear size, making the cells appear somewhat monotonous.

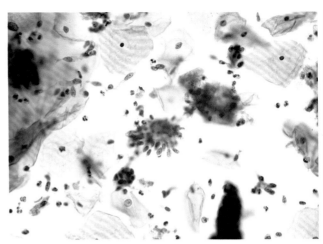

Figure 1.10.2 Adenocarcinoma in situ. These AIS cells demonstrate "feathering", in which bare nuclei appear to project out from a tissue fragment.

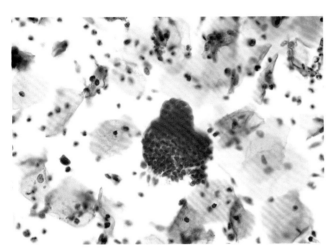

Figure 1.10.3 Adenocarcinoma in situ. This fragment has a smooth edge and bulbous projections, consistent with glandular differentiation. The cells are predominantly in a monolayer and their nuclei are round-to-oval, hyperchromatic, and all around the same size.

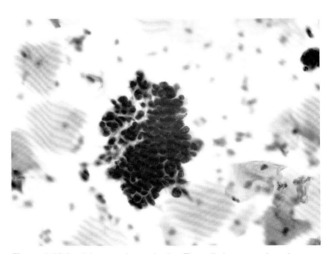

Figure 1.10.4 Adenocarcinoma in situ. The cells have powdery chromatin, hyperchromasia, and only mild nuclear contour irregularities.

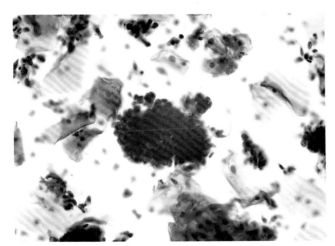

Figure 1.10.5 Adenocarcinoma in situ. The cells at the edge of this fragment have columnar shapes and irregularly arranged nuclei. The nuclei project away from the tissue fragment, giving the appearance of feathers ("feathering").

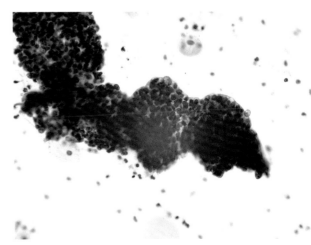

Figure 1.10.6 Endocervical adenocarcinoma. A three-dimensional tissue fragment forms a papillary configuration. The fragment has some smooth edges; these features suggest a glandular differentiation. The cells have crowded, dark nuclei with powdery chromatin. Nuclear size variation is much greater than seen in the previous examples of AIS.

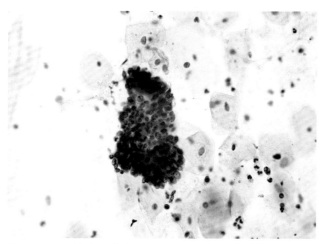

Figure 1.10.7 Endocervical adenocarcinoma. A hyperchromatic crowded group containing columnar cells, which palisade around the edges. The nuclei project outward, mimicking the "feathering" seen in AIS. There is prominent anisonucleosis, suggesting this may be an invasive adenocarcinoma rather than simply AIS.

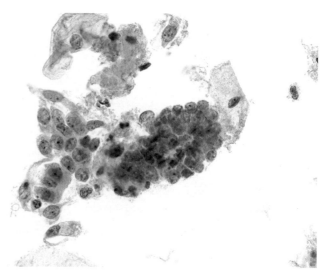

Figure 1.10.8 Endocervical adenocarcinoma. The columnar shape of these malignant cells is best seen on the left side of the field, more compatible with endocervical adenocarcinoma than endometrial adenocarcinoma. The nuclei are varied in size and are greatly enlarged.

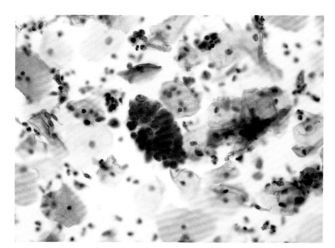

Figure 1.10.9 Endocervical adenocarcinoma. These malignant cells form a morule, which suggests a glandular differentiation. The cells have prominent nucleoli (not a feature of AIS) and great variation in nuclear size. The differential diagnosis includes both endocervical adenocarcinoma and endometrial adenocarcinoma.

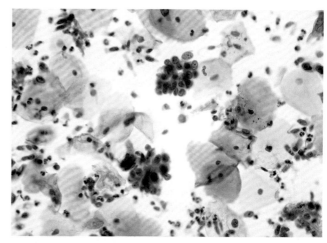

Figure 1.10.10 Endocervical adenocarcinoma. Two small fragments of endocervical adenocarcinoma contain cells with high N/C ratios, irregular nuclear borders, coarse chromatin (not a feature of AIS), and prominent anisonucleosis (also not a feature of AIS).

	Endocervical Adenocarcinoma	Endometrial Carcinoma
Age	Any age	Middle aged to older women
Location	Cervix	Endometrium
Signs and symptoms	Dyspareunia; bleeding; vaginal discharge; mass on colposcopy; may be asymptomatic	Postmenopausal or irregular bleeding
Etiology	HPV infection, most commonly HPV 16 and/or 18; may be associated with adenocarcinoma in situ	Long-term estrogen stimulation (endometrioid) or early *TP53* mutation (serous, clear cell)
Cytomorphology	• Malignant cells in fragments or present singly *(Figure 1.11.1)* • Three-dimensional fragments with columnar cells *(Figure 1.11.2)* • Enlarged cells with large nuclei and high N/C ratios *(Figure 1.11.3)* • Nuclear contour irregularities *(Figure 1.11.1)* • Anisonucleosis *(Figure 1.11.4)* • Prominent nucleoli *(Figure 1.11.5)* • Necrosis may be present	• Usually small fragments of cells forming hyperchromatic crowded groups; rarely single cells *(Figure 1.11.6)* • Hobnailed borders consistent with glandular and likely endometrial differentiation *(Figures 1.11.7 and 1.11.8)* • Usually only one population of malignant cells • Larger cells with high N/C ratios and hyperchromasia *(Figure 1.11.9)* • Enlarged nuclei that range from round to pleomorphic and may have irregular nuclear borders *(Figure 1.11.9)* • Chromatin is more coarse and may have nucleoli *(Figure 1.11.9)* • Larger and more frequent vacuoles with increased numbers of neutrophils *(Figure 1.11.10)*
Special studies	None; a cytomorphologic diagnosis	None
Molecular alterations	Under investigation	*TP53* mutations (serous and clear cell); often mutations in *PTEN, KRAS,* or *PAX2* (endometrioid)
Treatment	Depends on stage; conization, hysterectomy, pelvic lymph node dissection, and/or chemoradiation	Total abdominal hysterectomy with bilateral salpingo-oophorectomy and/or regional node dissection, chemoradiation
Clinical implications	Depends on stage; best if complete surgical removal is possible	Varies greatly and depends on disease stage

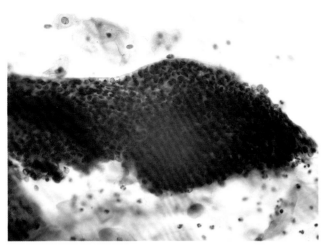

Figure 1.11.1   Endocervical adenocarcinoma. This fragment contains malignant cells with large, dark, overlapping nuclei. The fragment has a smooth edge, indicating glandular differentiation. In contrast, endometrial carcinoma usually does not form large fragments and its fragments have hobnailed edges.

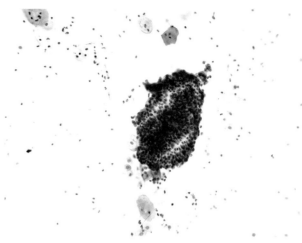

Figure 1.11.2   Endocervical adenocarcinoma. A three-dimensional fragment of cells with, dark oval-shaped nuclei. In some planes, the cells have a columnar shape, which favors an endocervical origin.

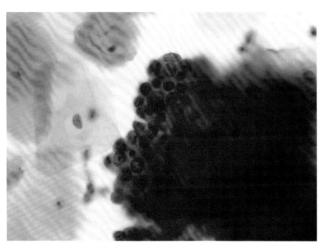

Figure 1.11.3   Endocervical adenocarcinoma. The malignant cells have enlarged nuclei, anisonucleosis, and coarse chromatin. The cells have a glandular appearance, but it is difficult to definitively distinguish between an endometrial and endocervical origin.

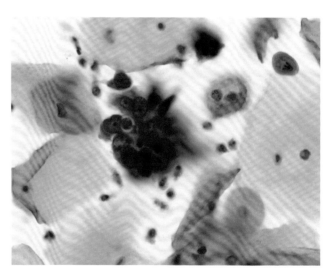

Figure 1.11.4   Endocervical adenocarcinoma. A small group of cells, some with columnar morphology. The cells have large nuclei and granular cytoplasm, as well as coarse chromatin or prominent nucleoli. The columnar shapes favor an endocervical adenocarcinoma, but it is difficult to completely exclude an endometrial origin based on these few cells alone.

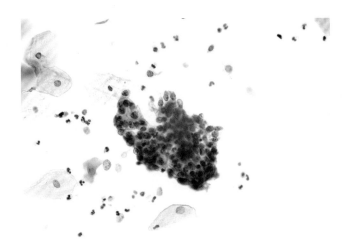

Figure 1.11.5   Endocervical adenocarcinoma. A three-dimensional fragment of malignant cells with enlarged nuclei, irregular nuclear borders, anisonucleosis, and coarse chromatin. Several cells at the fragment edges have a columnar shape, favoring an endocervical rather than endometrial adenocarcinoma.

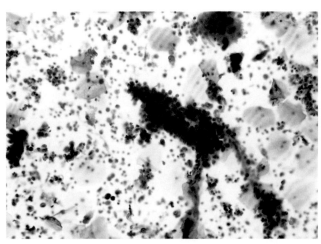

Figure 1.11.6   Endometrial adenocarcinoma. The field is cellular and contains malignant cells both in fragments as well as singly dispersed in the background. The cells are small and have enlarged dark nuclei with minimal cytoplasm. The tissue fragment has hobnailed edges, commonly seen in endometrial adenocarcinomas.

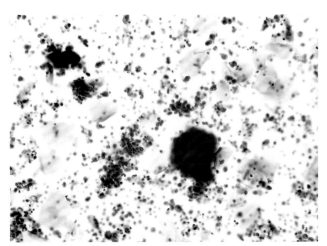

Figure 1.11.7   Endometrial adenocarcinoma. Numerous malignant cells present as discohesive clusters as well as single cells. Many of the cells are admixed with granular debris, likely necrosis secondary to invasion. The cells have minimal cytoplasm and some groups are associated with neutrophils. The differential diagnosis include small cell carcinoma.

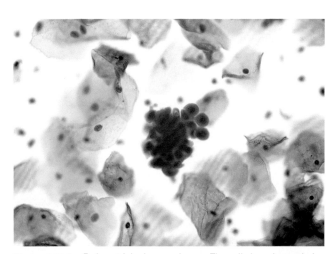

Figure 1.11.8   Endometrial adenocarcinoma. The cells have large, dark nuclei. Because the cytoplasm appears dense, the differential diagnosis includes HSIL and squamous cell carcinoma. However, the presence of small vacuoles favors a glandular differentiation.

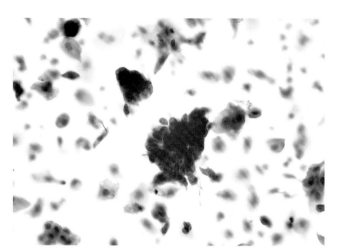

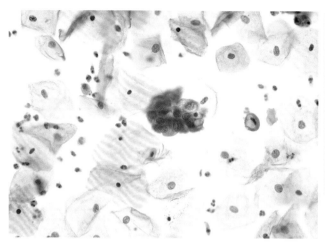

Figure 1.11.9   Endometrial adenocarcinoma. These malignant cells have elongated, enlarged nuclei with coarse chromatin. This elongation may cause one to suspect an AIS or endocervical adenocarcinoma. Thus, while the cells are overtly malignant, identifying a site of origin can sometimes be challenging using cytomorphology alone.

Figure 1.11.10   Endometrial adenocarcinoma. A small group of cells with enlarged nuclei and abundant, foamy cytoplasm. One cell contains a prominent vacuole. These are atypical glandular cells of indeterminate origin, and the patient had an endometrial carcinoma on follow-up.

	Intrauterine Device Change	Endometrial Adenocarcinoma
Age	Any age	Middle aged to older women
Location	Uterus	Endometrium
Signs and symptoms	Usually asymptomatic	Postmenopausal or irregular bleeding
Etiology	Reactive endometrial changes related to IUD	Long-term estrogen stimulation (endometrioid) or early *TP53* mutation (serous, clear cell)
Cytomorphology	• Rare single cells that may cluster together *(Figures 1.12.1* and *1.12.2)* • Enlarged cells with large nuclei and low N/C ratios *(Figure 1.12.3)* • Hyperchromasia with regular nuclear borders or mild border irregularities *(Figures 1.12.4* and *1.12.5)* • Cells may be vacuolated, with vacuoles that compress the nucleus	• Usually small fragments of cells forming hyperchromatic crowded groups; rarely single cells *(Figures 1.12.6* and *1.12.7)* • Hobnailed borders consistent with glandular and likely endometrial differentiation *(Figure 1.12.8)* • Usually only one population of malignant cells • Larger cells with high N/C ratios and hyperchromasia *(Figure 1.12.8)* • Enlarged nuclei that range from round to pleomorphic and may have irregular nuclear borders *(Figure 1.12.8)* • Chromatin is more coarse and may have nucleoli *(Figure 1.12.9)* • Larger and more frequent vacuoles with increased numbers of neutrophils *(Figure 1.12.10)*
Special studies	None	None
Molecular alterations	N/A	*TP53* mutations (serous and clear cell); often mutations in *PTEN, KRAS,* or *PAX2* (endometrioid)
Treatment	N/A	Total abdominal hysterectomy with bilateral salpingo-oophorectomy and/or regional node dissection, chemoradiation
Clinical implications	N/A	Varies greatly and depends on stage

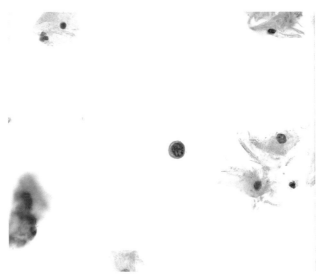

Figure 1.12.1   IUD cell. A single small cell with an enlarged, dark nucleus with regular nuclear borders and minimal cytoplasm. One may consider a diagnosis of ASC-H if a history of IUD placement is not known.

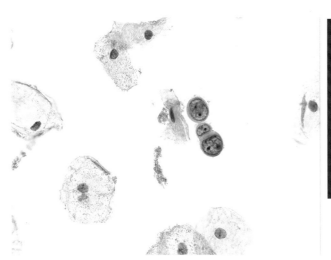

Figure 1.12.2   IUD cells. A loose aggregate of several atypical cells with enlarged nuclei and coarse chromatin. The cytoplasm is minimal and the N/C ratios are elevated, but the cells are small compared with adjacent intermediate cells.

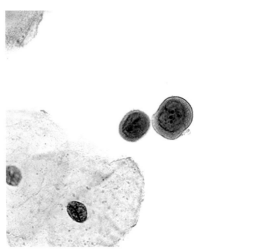

Figure 1.12.3   IUD cells. Two small cells with high N/C ratios and dark chromatin. They are very small compared with the adjacent intermediate cells.

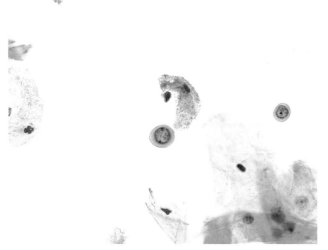

Figure 1.12.4   IUD cells. Two rare cells with centrally placed round nuclei and minimal cytoplasm, found in a patient with an IUD.

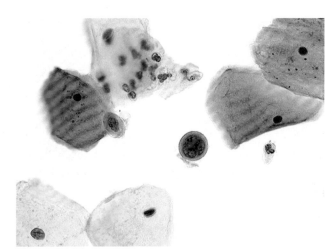

Figure 1.12.5 IUD cells. Two small cells with similar characteristics as the previous figures. The cells lack any of the associated neutrophils typically found in benign and neoplastic endometrial cells.

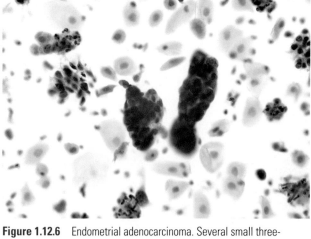

Figure 1.12.6 Endometrial adenocarcinoma. Several small three-dimensional fragments containing cells with crowded dark nuclei. The nuclei are varied in size and have irregular contours. The three-dimensional nature of these fragments favors a glandular differentiation, but features definitive of an endometrial origin are not seen.

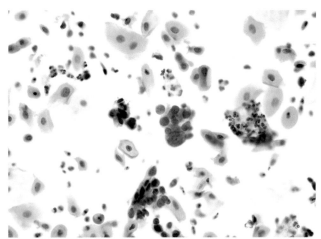

Figure 1.12.7 Endometrial adenocarcinoma. Small three-dimensional fragments of cells with dark nuclei and anisonucleosis. The cells are glandular and malignant in nature, but do not have features specific for an endometrial origin.

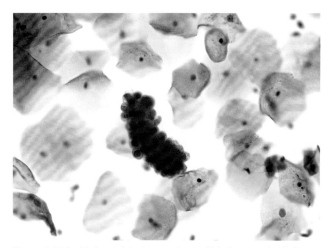

Figure 1.12.8 Endometrial adenocarcinoma. This fragment has hob-nailed edges, consistent with an endometrial origin. The nuclei are large and dark, raising suspicion for an adenocarcinoma.

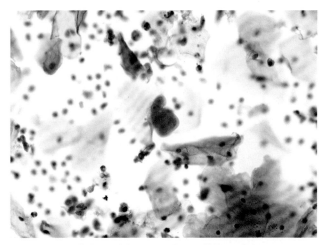

Figure 1.12.9 Endometrial adenocarcinoma. This small three-dimensional group of cells has prominent nucleoli, minimal cytoplasm, and anisonucleosis. It is diagnostic of adenocarcinoma.

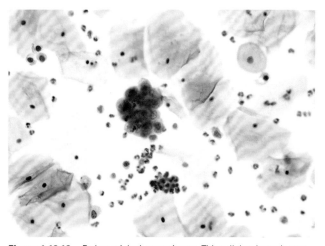

Figure 1.12.10 Endometrial adenocarcinoma. This cellular cluster is associated with numerous neutrophils and has hobnailed edges. The nuclei are enlarged and the diagnosis is at least atypical glandular cells of endometrial origin. Follow up biopsy demonstrated an endometrial adenocarcinoma.

	Reparative Change	High-Grade Squamous Intraepithelial Lesion (HSIL)
Age	Any age	Any age
Location	Cervix	Cervix (also vagina, anus, and vulva)
Signs and symptoms	Asymptomatic	None; detected on routine screening or on colposcopy
Etiology	Reactive changes of cervical epithelial cells (squamous, squamous metaplastic, and glandular) in response to various types of microinjury	Premalignant lesion more commonly associated with high-risk HPV types
Cytomorphology	• Monolayer sheets of monotonous cells *(Figures 1.13.1 and 1.13.2)* • Parallel nuclear orientation *(Figure 1.13.3)* • Cells "stream" within the fragment and have a "school of fish" appearance *(Figure 1.13.3)* • Enlarged, uniform nuclei *(Figure 1.13.4)* • Prominent nucleoli and/or chromocenters *(Figure 1.13.5)*	• Cellular fragments and dispersed single cells *(Figure 1.13.6)* • High N/C ratio due to increased nuclear size and decreased amounts of cytoplasm *(Figure 1.13.7)* • Hyperchromatic nuclei without nucleoli *(Figure 1.13.8)* • Markedly irregular nuclear borders *(Figure 1.13.8)* • Anisonucleosis may be present • Dense, opaque cytoplasm in individual cells
Special studies	None; a cytomorphologic diagnosis	HPV studies
Molecular alterations	N/A	Under investigation; mostly driven by HPV oncogenes
Treatment	N/A	Complete excision
Clinical implications	N/A	May progress to squamous cell carcinoma if incompletely excised

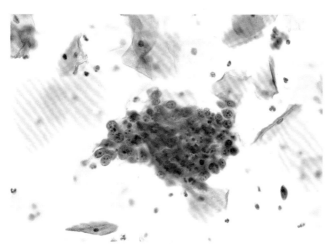

Figure 1.13.1   Reparative change. A small monolayer fragment of cells with enlarged nuclei and little cytoplasm. The nuclei do not demonstrate the "streaming" pattern seen in typical repair, but the nuclei are uniform and have regular borders, and the chromatin pattern is not compatible with HSIL.

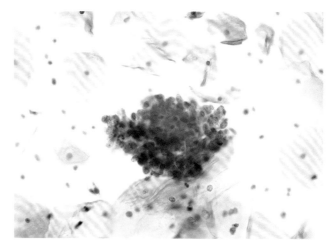

Figure 1.13.2   Reparative change. A similar fragment of cells present in a monolayer with enlarged nuclei. Some cells have small nucleoli, a feature not seen in HSIL. The differential includes endometrial cells, given the high N/C ratio and uniform nuclei seen in these cells.

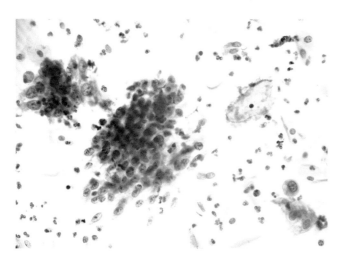

Figure 1.13.3   Reparative change. The nuclei in these fragments are enlarged and are organized in a "streaming" (directional) fashion, giving the appearance of a school of fish swimming together.

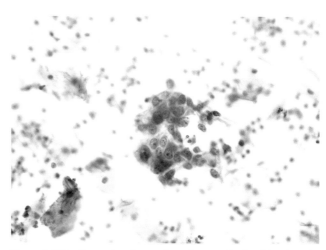

Figure 1.13.4   Reparative change. A small group of cells with enlarged nuclei, uniform nuclear sizes, regular nuclear contours, and distinct nucleoli.

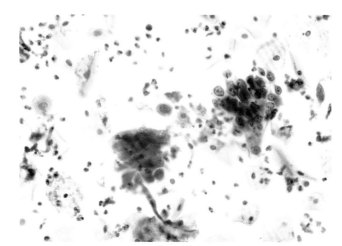

Figure 1.13.5   Reparative change. Two small groups of cells with distinct nucleoli. In small fragments, it can be difficult to appreciate the "school of fish" arrangement seen in reparative change.

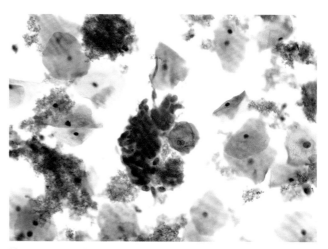

Figure 1.13.6   High-grade squamous intraepithelial lesion (HSIL). A fragment of cells with crowded, hyperchromatic nuclei. The nuclei are arranged in a disorderly fashion within the fragment. The presence of degenerated blood in the background may be due to recent menses, or be indicative of an invasive component.

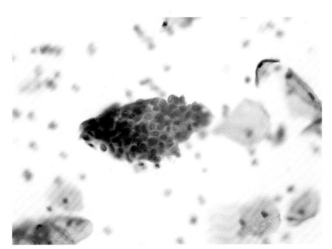

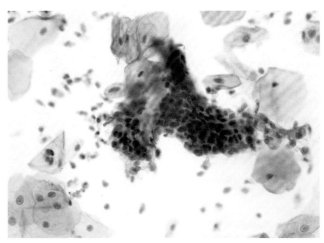

Figure 1.13.7   High-grade squamous intraepithelial lesion (HSIL). This small group of HSIL cells has some nuclei arranged in a "streaming" fashion, emulating reparative change. The cells lack nucleoli and very little cytoplasm. Careful examination of other fields may provide additional evidence for a diagnosis of HSIL.

Figure 1.13.8   High-grade squamous intraepithelial lesion (HSIL). The nuclei are very dark and have variation in size and irregular contours. The nuclei are disorganized within the fragment and do not demonstrate a "school of fish" arrangement.

	Tubal Metaplasia	High-Grade Squamous Intraepithelial Lesion (HSIL)
Age	Any age	Any age
Location	Cervix	Cervix (also vagina, anus, and vulva)
Signs and symptoms	Asymptomatic	None; detected on routine screening or on colposcopy
Etiology	Metaplastic change of endocervical cells in response to injury	Premalignant lesion more commonly associated with high-risk HPV types
Cytomorphology	• Fragments of cuboidal and/or columnar cells; rarely single cells *(Figures 1.14.1 and 1.14.2)* • Cells may demonstrate terminal bars and/or cilia *(Figure 1.14.3)* • Small cells with high N/C ratios and hyperchromasia *(Figure 1.14.1)* • Uniform, round-to-oval shaped nuclei with regular borders *(Figure 1.14.4)* • Multinucleation may be seen *(Figures 1.14.4 and 1.14.5)*	• Cellular fragments and dispersed single cells *(Figures 1.14.6 and 1.14.7)* • High N/C ratio due to increased nuclear size and decreased amounts of cytoplasm *(Figure 1.14.8)* • Hyperchromatic nuclei without nucleoli *(Figures 1.14.8 and 1.14.9)* • Markedly irregular nuclear borders *(Figure 1.14.10)* • Anisonucleosis may be present *(Figure 1.14.10)* • Dense, opaque cytoplasm in individual cells
Special studies	None; a cytomorphologic diagnosis	HPV studies
Molecular alterations	N/A	Under investigation; mostly driven by HPV oncogenes
Treatment	N/A	Complete excision
Clinical implications	N/A	May progress to squamous cell carcinoma if incompletely excised

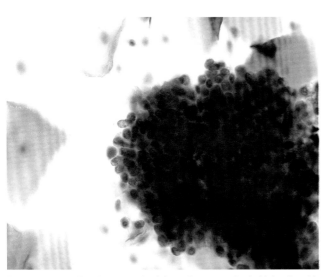

Figure 1.14.1　Tubal metaplasia. A large fragment of cuboidal cells with enlarged, dark nuclei. The nuclei are round, uniform, and have regular contours. At one edge, the fragment has a flat edge representing a terminal bar, which has a few cilia.

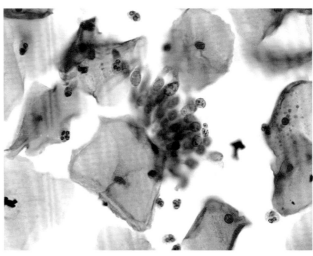

Figure 1.14.2　Tubal metaplasia. These cells appear more columnar and have enlarged, dark nuclei. Cilia are not seen.

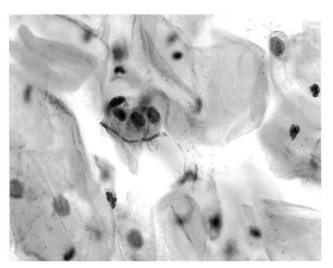

Figure 1.14.3　Tubal metaplasia. Classically, tubal metaplasia cells are cuboidal and ciliated. The nuclei are dark but round and uniform. This small strip of metaplastic cells has a flat border, forming a terminal bar.

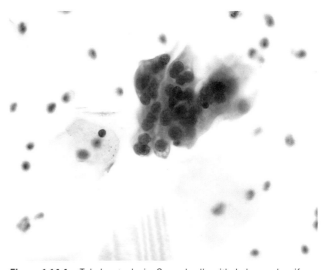

Figure 1.14.4　Tubal metaplasia. Several cells with dark, round, uniform nuclei. The cells are multinucleated and cilia can be seen on the bottom right edge of the fragment.

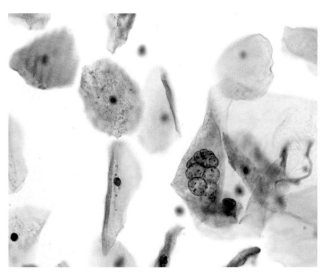

Figure 1.14.5   Tubal metaplasia. A single cell containing numerous enlarged nuclei. The differential diagnosis includes LSIL, which may merit a diagnosis of ASC-US based on the assessment of this cell alone.

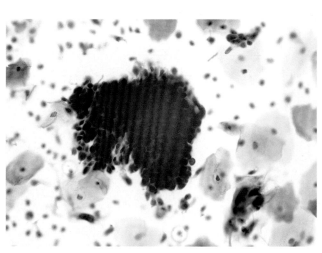

Figure 1.14.6   High-grade squamous intraepithelial lesion (HSIL). This fragment contains cells with enlarged, dark, crowded nuclei. The nuclei have irregular contours and vary in size. The edges of the tissue fragment are not flat, indicating the absence of a terminal bar.

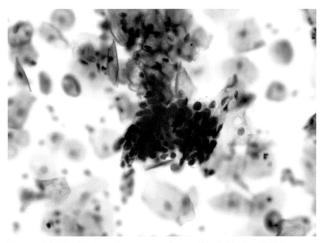

Figure 1.14.7   High-grade squamous intraepithelial lesion (HSIL). A group of cells with enlarged, dark, crowded nuclei. The variation is nuclear size seen here is not compatible with tubal metaplasia.

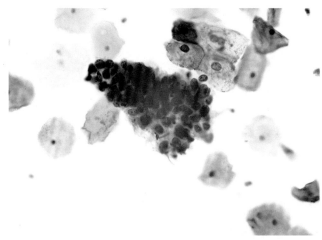

Figure 1.14.8   High-grade squamous intraepithelial lesion (HSIL). The nuclei in this fragment are round and somewhat uniform. However, some cells have irregular nuclear contours and there is no evidence of terminal bars or cilia.

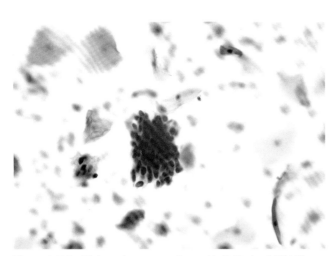

Figure 1.14.9   High-grade squamous intraepithelial lesion (HSIL). The cells in this fragment of HSIL are elongated and appear very dark. By contrast, tubal metaplasia cells usually contain round nucei.

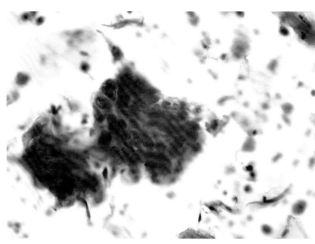

Figure 1.14.10   High-grade squamous intraepithelial lesion (HSIL). These HSIL cells have enlarged nuclei with irregular borders and size variation. The fragment appears to be keratinized, a feature not seen in tubal metaplasia.

	Benign Endometrial Cells	High-Grade Squamous Intraepithelial Lesion (HSIL)
Age	Premenopausal women	Any age
Location	Endometrium	Cervix (also vagina, anus, and vulva)
Signs and symptoms	Exfoliate during menses	None; detected on routine screening or on colposcopy
Etiology	Normal physiology	Premalignant lesion more commonly associated with high-risk HPV types
Cytomorphology	• Small fragments of cells forming hyperchromatic crowded groups; rarely single cells *(Figures 1.15.1 and 1.15.2)* • Hobnailed borders to tissue fragments is a characteristic finding *(Figure 1.15.3)* • Cytomorphology may vary depending on the day of menses and the patient's hormonal state • Some fragments may have two layers of cells: glandular cells surrounding stromal cells • Small cells with high N/C ratios and hyperchromasia *(Figure 1.15.4)* • Oval nuclei with relatively smooth nuclear contours and minimal size variation *(Figure 1.15.5)* • Powdery or granular chromatin pattern *(Figure 1.15.5)* • The presence of rare small vacuoles and/or neutrophils is a characteristic feature	• Cellular fragments and dispersed single cells *(Figures 1.15.6 and 1.15.7)* • High N/C ratio due to increased nuclear size and decreased amounts of cytoplasm *(Figure 1.15.8)* • Hyperchromatic nuclei without nucleoli *(Figures 1.15.8 and 1.15.9)* • Irregular nuclear borders *(Figure 1.15.6)* • Anisonucleosis may be present *(Figure 1.15.10)* • Dense, opaque cytoplasm in individual cells
Special studies	None	HPV studies
Molecular alterations	N/A	Under investigation; mostly driven by HPV oncogenes
Treatment	N/A	Complete excision
Clinical implications	N/A	May progress to squamous cell carcinoma if incompletely excised

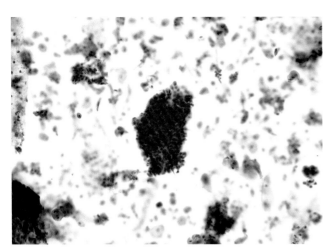

Figure 1.15.1   Benign endometrial cells. A hyperchromatic crowded group of benign endometrial cells. The cells are relatively small and have high N/C ratios; the differential diagnosis includes HSIL and endometrial cells. Examination at closer magnification may help differentiate between the two.

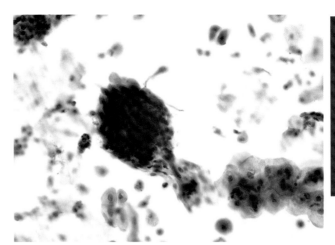

Figure 1.15.2   Benign endometrial cells. A three-dimensional group of endometrial cells. It is difficult to assess the cytomorphology of the central cells, as they are obscured by cellular overlap. This does not favor HSIL, which tends not to form three-dimensional fragments.

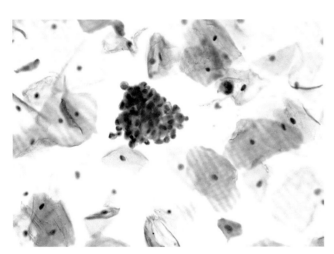

Figure 1.15.3   Benign endometrial cells. This group of cells demonstrates the classic "hobnailed" appearance of cells at the tissue borders and is strongly suggestive of an endometrial origin in a Pap test specimen. The cells have nuclei with smooth borders and little size variation, favoring a benign process.

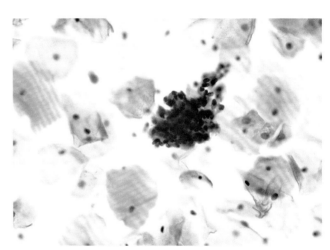

Figure 1.15.4   Benign endometrial cells. The nuclei in this small fragment are oval shaped, dark, and disorganized within the fragment. It is difficult to definitively diagnose them as HSIL or endometrial cells. Other fields in the specimen may contain more clues, although HSIL and endometrial cells can coexist in a specimen.

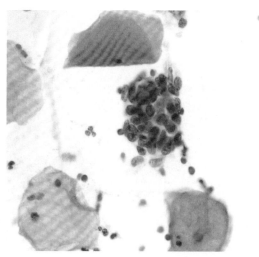

Figure 1.15.5   Benign endometrial cells. These cells have a "histiocytoid" appearance because of their elongated, curved nuclei. This appearance is more commonly associated with endometrial cells than HSIL cells and may represent the stromal component of benign endometrial tissue.

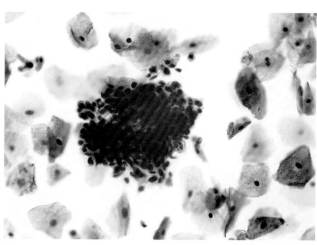

Figure 1.15.6   High-grade squamous intraepithelial lesion (HSIL). This fragment contains cells with very dark nuclei. The nuclei are elongated, and some have nuclear contour irregularities. The nuclei are disorganized within the fragment and also have greater size variation than would be expected in benign endometrial cells, by comparison.

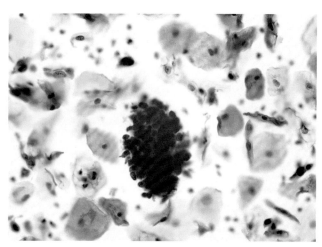

Figure 1.15.7   High-grade squamous intraepithelial lesion (HSIL). These cells have packed nuclei and little cytoplasm can be appreciated. There are few clues to exclude these as endometrial cells, possibly resulting in a diagnosis of ASC-H. The examination of other fields, or a patient history of recent menses, may prove helpful.

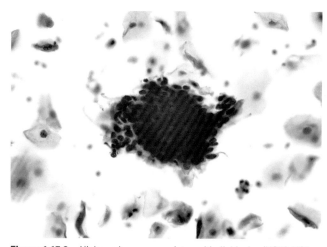

Figure 1.15.8   High-grade squamous intraepithelial lesion (HSIL). HSIL and endometrial cells can both be hyperchromatic. In this case, some of these HSIL cells have nuclear size variation 2:1 compared with neighboring cells, whereas endometrial cell nuclei tend to be more uniform in size.

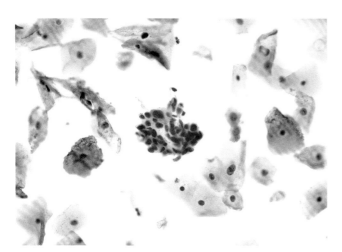

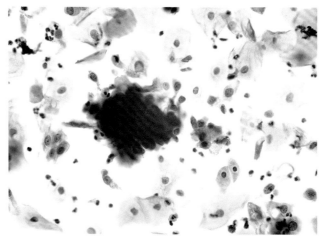

Figure 1.15.9 High-grade squamous intraepithelial lesion (HSIL). The cells in this fragment have significant nuclear size variation, nuclear border irregularities, and nuclear pleomorphism. This favors an HSIL over benign endometrial cells. Other fields should contain similar findings to help confirm the diagnosis.

Figure 1.15.10 High-grade squamous intraepithelial lesion (HSIL). This group of cells has a misleading glandular appearance, as some cells appear columnar at the edges of the fragment. Given the enlarged atypical nuclei with size variation and nuclear border irregularities, the differential would include atypical glandular cells or adenocarcinoma rather than benign endometrial cells.

	Adenocarcinoma in Situ	Benign Endometrial Cells
Age	Younger, reproductive age women	Premenopausal women
Location	Cervix	Endometrium
Signs and symptoms	Usually asymptomatic	Exfoliate during menses
Etiology	HPV infection, most commonly HPV 16 and/or 18	Normal physiology
Cytomorphology	• Primarily cellular fragments and occasionally single cells *(Figures 1.16.1 and 1.16.2)* • Monotonous columnar shaped cells *(Figure 1.16.3)* • Oval-shaped nuclei with minimal cytoplasm *(Figure 1.16.4)* • Hyperchromasia, powdery chromatin, and smooth nuclear borders *(Figure 1.16.4)* • Nuclei may palisade and project from the tissue edge, causing a "feathering" effect *(Figure 1.16.5)*	• Small fragments of cells forming hyperchromatic crowded groups; rarely single cells *(Figures 1.16.6 and 1.16.7)* • Hobnailed borders to tissue fragments is a characteristic finding *(Figure 1.16.8)* • Cytomorphology may vary depending on the day of menses and the patient's hormonal state • Some fragments may have two layers of cells: glandular cells surrounding stromal cells • Small cells with high N/C ratios and hyperchromasia *(Figure 1.16.9)* • Oval nuclei with relatively smooth nuclear contours and minimal size variation *(Figure 1.16.10)* • Powdery or granular chromatin pattern *(Figure 1.16.10)* • The presence of rare small vacuoles and/or neutrophils is a characteristic feature *(Figure 1.16.10)*
Special studies	None; a cytomorphologic diagnosis	None
Molecular alterations	Under investigation	N/A
Treatment	Conization or hysterectomy	N/A
Prognosis	May progress if incompletely excised	N/A

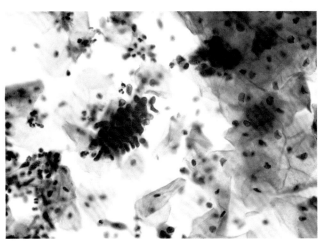

Figure 1.16.1   Adenocarcinoma in situ (AIS). The cells in this fragment have minimal cytoplasm and dark, elongated nuclei. The nuclei project out from the fragment, creating a "feathered" appearance.

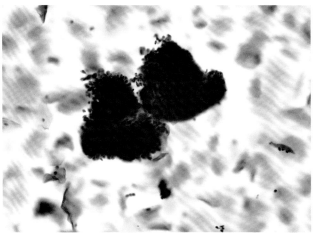

Figure 1.16.2   Adenocarcinoma in situ (AIS). Two three-dimensional fragments contain dark, crowded nuclei. The smooth edge to the fragment on the right suggests a glandular rather than squamous nature. The differential at this magnification includes endometrial cells, adenocarcinoma, and AIS.

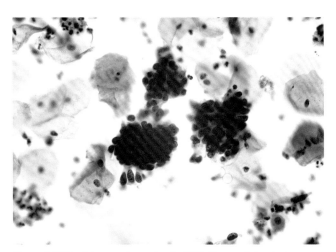

Figure 1.16.3   Adenocarcinoma in situ (AIS). Three cellular clusters containing plump, oval-shaped nuclei with powdery chromatin. Three columnar cells have elongated nuclei, which project away from the fragment (bottom center field) as "feathers".

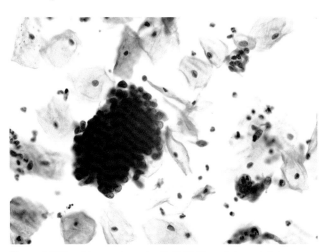

Figure 1.16.4   Adenocarcinoma in situ (AIS). The cells have dark, large, overlapping nuclei. The nuclei are oval shaped and have smooth nuclear contours. The chromatin has a powdery appearance, which should suggest AIS.

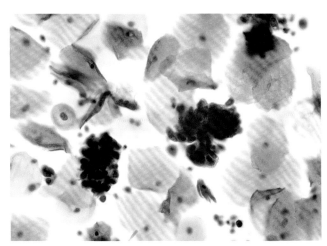

Figure 1.16.5   Adenocarcinoma in situ (AIS). These tissue fragments contain features of glandular differentiation: a smooth border can be seen, as well as one with the "feathering" of elongated nuclei arranged in parallel projecting away from the fragment.

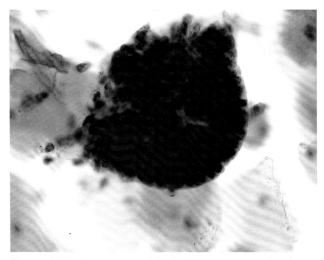

Figure 1.16.6   Benign endometrial cells. This fragment contains glandular cells, as evidenced by its smooth edge and the columnar shape of cells that can be seen through the dark fragment. However, the nuclei are basally arranged and do not project out and away from the fragment as is seen in AIS.

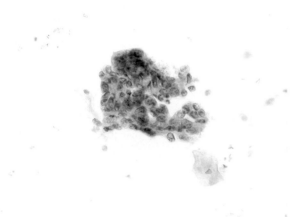

Figure 1.16.7 Benign endometrial cells. The nuclei in this fragment of endometrial cells do not have the powdery chromatin seen in AIS, and several nuclei are gently curved, causing a "histiocytoid" appearance not seen in AIS.

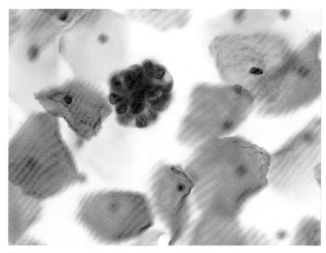

Figure 1.16.8 Benign endometrial cells. This tissue fragment has scalloped edges, suggesting an endometrial origin. The cells have dark nuclei, but they do not have the powdery chromatin of AIS. The nuclei are also predominantly round-to-oval shaped and do not "feather" as in AIS. The cells also have more cytoplasm than is seen in AIS, although this will depend on the patient's hormonal state in other specimens.

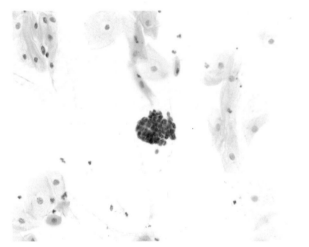

Figure 1.16.9 Benign endometrial cells. A small group of endometrial cells with high N/C ratios and minimal cytoplasm. The nuclei are oval shaped and should be examined at higher magnification. The differential includes endometrial cells as well as AIS.

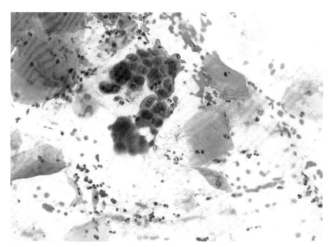

Figure 1.16.10 Benign endometrial cells. Although their nuclei are enlarged, these cells are uniform in size and the cells have more cytoplasm than is seen in AIS. Some nuclei are curved and have a "histiocytoid" appearance.

	Trichomonas vaginalis Changes	Low-Grade Squamous Intraepithelial Lesion (LSIL)
Age	Any age, usually younger women	Any age but more likely to be transient infection in younger women
Location	Cervix	Cervix (also vagina, anus, and vulva)
Signs and symptoms	Frothy, foul-smelling vaginal discharge; vaginal itching	None; detected on routine screening or on colposcopy
Etiology	Sexually transmitted infection	Premalignant lesion associated with both low- and high-risk HPV
Cytomorphology	• *Trichomonas* organisms are the size of neutrophils, cyanophilic, pear-to-round shaped, and contain eosinophilic granules and an eccentric nucleus *(Figure 1.17.1)*. Flagella are not usually visualized. • Background of increased acute inflammation *(Figure 1.17.2)* • Balls of neutrophils are sometimes seen • Superficial and intermediate squamous cells with large hypochromatic and uniform, round, small perinuclear halos *(Figures 1.17.3* and *1.17.4)*	• Squamous cells with enlarged nuclei *(Figure 1.17.5)* • Irregular nuclear borders and/or "raisinoid" nucleus *(Figures 1.17.6* and *1.17.7)* • Occasional binucleation *(Figure 1.17.8)* • Koilocytes have, in addition to the above features, a well-defined polygonal perinuclear halo with sharp edges and central clearing *(Figure 1.17.9)*
Special studies	Ancillary molecular tests available	HPV studies
Molecular alterations	N/A	Under investigation; mostly driven by HPV oncogenes
Treatment	Single dose of metronidazole, or other antibiotic agent	Colposcopy to exclude the presence of HSIL
Clinical implications	N/A	Often regresses, especially in young women

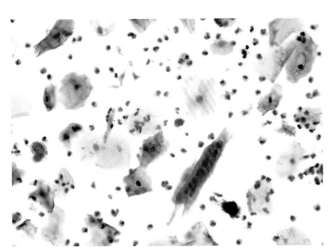

Figure 1.17.1   Trichomonas changes. A *Trichomonas* organism (center) in a background of acute inflammation and reactive squamous cells. Several squamous cells have a thin perinuclear clearing (halo), which is pathognomonic of *Trichomonas* infection and should not be mistaken for a koilocytes.

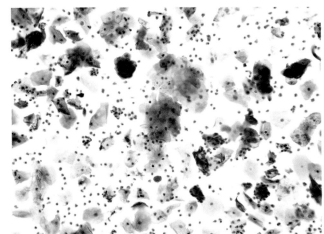

Figure 1.17.2   Trichomonas changes. The field contains numerous neutrophils and mature squamous cells. In the center of the field, a group of superficial squamous cells have small, uniform "trich" halos. A search at high magnification will likely identify the organisms.

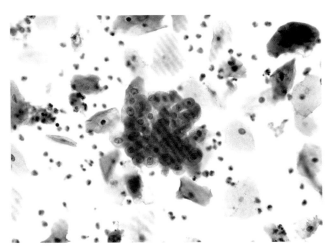

Figure 1.17.3   Trichomonas changes. This group of reactive squamous cells has enlarged nuclei but is hypochromatic. The "trich" halos appear as ill-defined lightened areas around the nuclei.

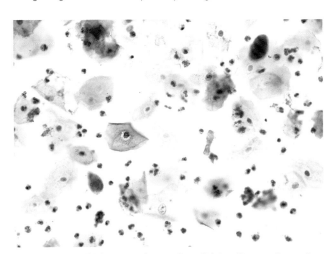

Figure 1.17.4   Trichomonas changes. Superficial and intermediate cells, many with the small, uniform halos consistent with *Trichomonas*. The presence of increased acute inflammatory cells suggests an active infection.

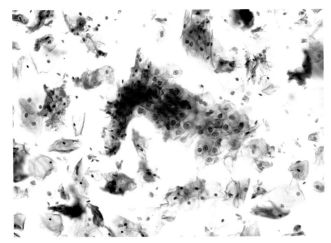

Figure 1.17.5   Trichomonas changes. The cells in this fragment have enlarged nuclei and some are binucleate. The nuclei are more than three times the size of adjacent intermediate cells and thus these cells are diagnostic if LSIL. The poorly defined koilocytic halos in these cells may resemble those seen in *Trichomonas* infection.

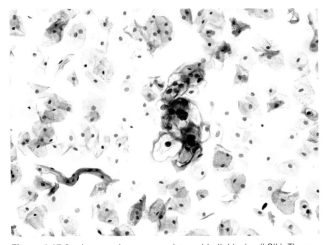

Figure 1.17.6   Low-grade squamous intraepithelial lesion (LSIL). These nuclei are too dark, large, and irregularly shaped for a reactive process and are diagnostic of LSIL. The cells also have large halos that have irregular shapes, unlike the small round halos seen in *Trichomonas* infection.

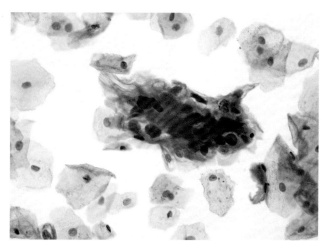

Figure 1.17.7 Low-grade squamous intraepithelial lesion (LSIL). LSIL often has nuclei that look like rocks or raisins, due to their irregular nuclear contours and shapes. These nuclei are much too dark and large to be reactive.

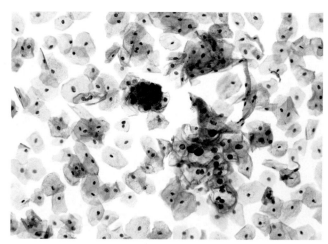

Figure 1.17.8 Low-grade squamous intraepithelial lesion (LSIL). These LSIL cells have dark nuclei and anisonucleosis. Several cells are binucleated. The amount of nuclear enlargement in these cells with ample cytoplasm is diagnostic of LSIL.

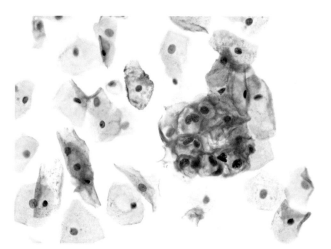

Figure 1.17.9 Low-grade squamous intraepithelial lesion (LSIL). Classic koilocytes, with well-defined, polygonal-shaped halos and atypical nuclei (hyperchromasia, binucleation, enlargement).

	High-Grade Squamous Intraepithelial Lesion (HSIL)	Atrophy
Age	Any age	Usually postmenopausal or postpartum women
Location	Cervix (also vagina, anus, and vulva)	Cervix
Signs and symptoms	None; detected on routine screening or on colposcopy	Usually asymptomatic
Etiology	Premalignant lesion more commonly associated with high-risk HPV types	Decreased levels of estrogen (postmenopausal women) or relatively increased levels of progesterone (postpartum women)
Cytomorphology	• Cellular fragments and dispersed single cells *(Figures 1.18.1* and *1.18.2)* • High N/C ratio due to increased nuclear size and decreased amounts of cytoplasm *(Figure 1.18.3)* • Hyperchromatic nuclei without nucleoli *(Figure 1.18.4)* • Irregular nuclear borders *(Figure 1.18.5)* • Anisonucleosis may be present • Dense, opaque cytoplasm in individual cells	• Parabasal cells present in small groups and present singly *(Figures 1.18.6* and *1.18.7)* • Cells are hyperchromatic and have increased N/C ratios but usually less than seen in HSIL cells *(Figure 1.18.8)* • Nuclei are oval, elongated, and may have mild nuclear border irregularities *(Figures 1.18.9* and *1.18.10)*
Special studies	HPV studies	None; a cytomorphologic diagnosis
Molecular alterations	Under investigation; mostly driven by HPV oncogenes	N/A
Treatment	Complete excision	Topical estrogen
Clinical implications	May progress to squamous cell carcinoma if incompletely excised	N/A

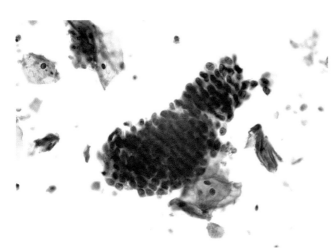

Figure 1.18.1   High-grade squamous intraepithelial lesion (HSIL). A fragment of HSIL containing cells with enlarged, dark, crowded nuclei. The nuclei have nuclear border irregularities and some size variation. The amount of cytoplasm is minimal.

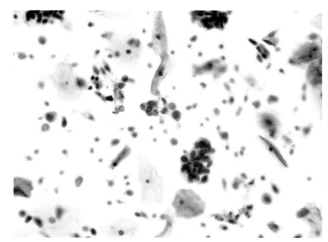

Figure 1.18.2   High-grade squamous intraepithelial lesion (HSIL). The group of cells in the lower center has dark, oval-shaped nuclei and high N/C ratios. The nuclei do not vary much in size and the nuclear borders appear regular. This could represent atrophy, but other atypical groups are seen in the field, as are intermediate and superficial cells, all of which favor HSIL rather than atrophy.

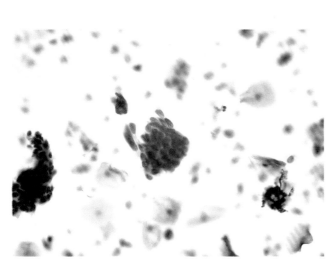

Figure 1.18.3   High-grade squamous intraepithelial lesion (HSIL). Two fragments of HSIL with dark, crowded nuclei and very little cytoplasm. Atrophic cells usually do not appear so hyperchromatic and have more cytoplasm.

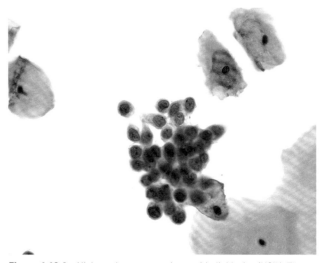

Figure 1.18.4   High-grade squamous intraepithelial lesion (HSIL). The nuclei of these cells appear deceiving small and uniform. Despite their small size, the cells have very little cytoplasm and have nuclear border irregularities. The differential diagnosis includes endometrial cells; atrophic cells usually contain more cytoplasm.

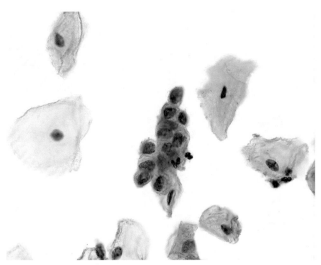

Figure 1.18.5   High-grade squamous intraepithelial lesion (HSIL). A fragment of cells that have dark nuclei and markedly irregular nuclear contours. The high N/C ratio favors HSIL over LSIL, and the nuclear atypia is too severe to represent atrophy.

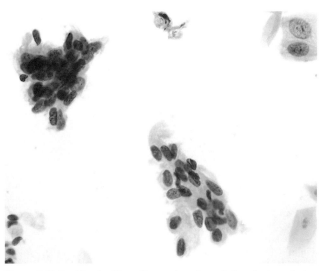

Figure 1.18.6   Atrophy. The cells seen here have dark and enlongated nuclei. They have only mild nuclear border irregularities, and their N/C ratios are not as high as is seen in HSIL. Atrophic changes are often found throughout a specimen, whereas HSIL is usually a more focal finding.

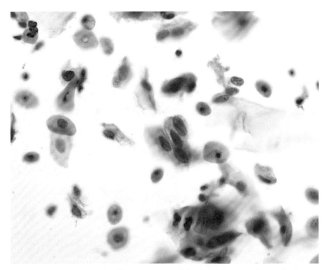

Figure 1.18.7   Atrophy. Numerous parabasal cells; some in small clusters and others present singly. The nuclei are dark, but not as hyperchromatic as most HSIL nuclei. The nuclei have size variation, but some cells only have slightly elevated N/C ratios.

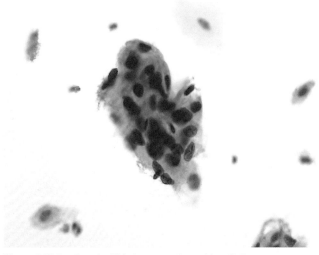

Figure 1.18.8   Atrophy. This fragment of atrophic cells is concerning because of the amount of hyperchromasia seen. The nuclei are of different sizes and have some irregular contours. While this may be called ASC-US in a background of atrophic changes, the cells have more cytoplasm than what is typically seen in HSIL.

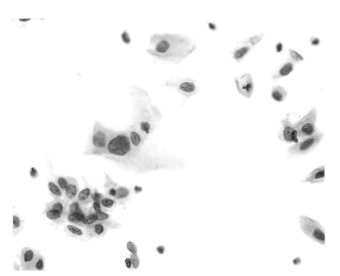

Figure 1.18.9   Atrophy. Various benign atrophic cells with slightly dark nuclei and anisonucleosis. Most cells have regular nuclear contours. The N/C ratios are not concerning.

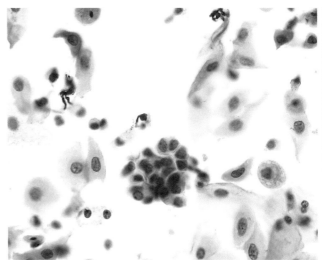

Figure 1.18.10   Atrophy. A similar field containing predominant atrophic parabasal cells. The absence of maturation indicates atrophy and should cause a higher threshold for making a diagnosis of atypia or HSIL.

	Small Cell Carcinoma	**Follicular Cervicitis**
Age	Adult women	Younger, reproductive age women
Location	Cervix (also vagina, anus, and vulva)	Cervix
Signs and symptoms	Vaginal bleeding; cervical mass; may be associated with paraneoplastic sydnromes	Usually asymptomatic; mucopurulent discharge
Etiology	Aggressive carcinoma associated with HPV infection	HPV infection, most commonly HPV 16 and/or 18
Cytomorphology	• Cellular specimen with loosely cohesive and single carcinoma cells *(Figure 1.19.1)* • May have an associated squamous cell carcinoma or adenocarcinoma component • Small cells, slightly larger than lymphocytes *(Figure 1.19.2)* • Little appreciable cytoplasm *(Figure 1.19.3)* • Less monotonous than lymphocytes *(Figure 1.19.3)* • Nuclear molding, which may be less apparent on liquid-based preparations *(Figure 1.19.4)* • "Salt and pepper" (neuroendocrine) chromatin *(Figure 1.19.5)* • Cellular necrosis with intact, dead cyanophilic tumor cells *(Figures 1.19.3 and 1.19.4)* • Increased mitotic activity; apoptotic bodies	• Increased cellularity with dispersed polymorphous lymphocytes *(Figures 1.19.6 and 1.19.7)* • Small lymphocytes admixed with larger lymphocytes *(Figure 1.19.8)* • Lymphocytes may loosely aggregate into pseudofragments *(Figures 1.19.6 and 1.19.9)* • Lymphocytes have a thin rim of blue cytoplasm unlike small cell carcinoma cells *(Figure 1.19.8)* • Coarse/clumpy chromatin *(Figure 1.19.8)* • Tingible body macrophages may be seen *(Figure 1.19.10)*
Special studies	HPV studies	None; a cytomorphologic diagnosis
Molecular alterations	Loss of heterozygosity (3p and 11p)	N/A
Treatment	Hysterectomy, lymphadenectomy, and chemoradiation	Treatment of underlying infection, if present
Clinical implications	May progress to squamous cell carcinoma if incompletely excised	Untreated infection may result in pelvic inflammatory disease and infertility

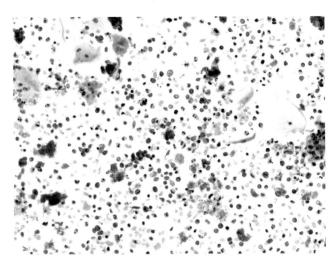

Figure 1.19.1 Small cell carcinoma. The field is cellular and contains numerous small cells with little cytoplasm and size variation beyond that seen in a reactive lymphoid population. The field also contains numerous cyanophilic necrotic cells interspersed between viable cells.

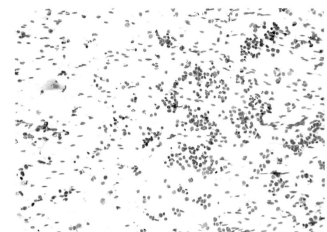

Figure 1.19.2 Small cell carcinoma. Small cell carcinoma present in loose clusters as well as individual cells. In liquid-based preparations (as opposed to conventional smears), small cell carcinoma cells tend to be more discohesive and do not demonstrate as many cellular clusters in which nuclear molding might be seen.

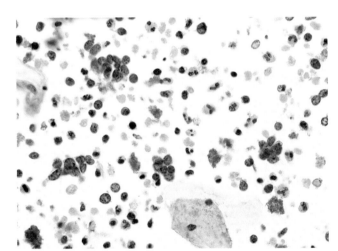

Figure 1.19.3 Small cell carcinoma. Small cell carcinoma cells are larger than lymphocytes, do not contain a thin rim of cytoplasm, and demonstrate anisonucleosis. The nuclei here have "salt and pepper" (both granular and coarse) chromatin, consistent with a neuroendocrine differentiation.

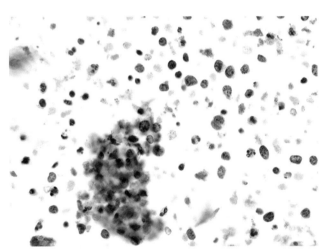

Figure 1.19.4 Small cell carcinoma. Small cell carcinoma cells present in a fragment as well as singly in the background. Within the larger fragment, viable tumor cells alternate with cyanophilic necrotic cells.

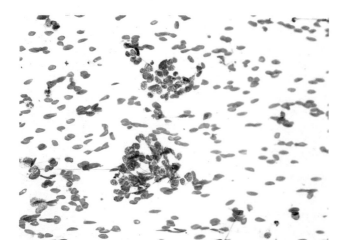

Figure 1.19.5 Small cell carcinoma. The small cell carcinoma cells seen here have no visible cytoplasm. The chromatin pattern is speckled. Some nuclei mold together, and in some cases the chromatin has "streaked" away from the nucleus. This nuclear streaking artifact is minimally seen in liquid-based preparations but is usually prominent on conventional smears.

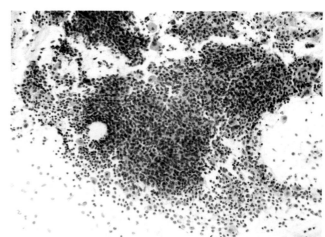

Figure 1.19.6 Follicular cervicitis. A conventional smear in which numerous lymphocytes have aggregated together into a pseudofragment. At this low magnification, the lymphocytes look monotonous but are more easily identifiable as polymorphous at higher magnification. By forming a hyperchromatic fragment, follicular cervicitis has been noted to emulate HSIL on conventional smears.

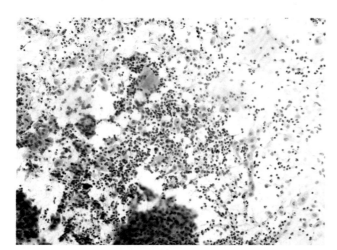

Figure 1.19.7 Follicular cervicitis. Numerous lymphocytes are dispersed throughout the field and obscure other findings. Examination at higher magnification will help exclude the possibility of a small cell carcinoma.

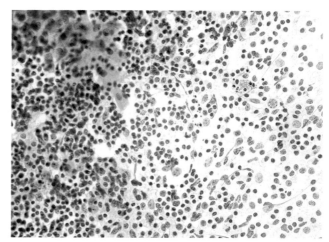

Figure 1.19.8 Follicular cervicitis. The field is cellular with lymphocytes of different sizes. Predominantly seen are small lymphocytes and medium-sized lymphocytes; at this power some of the medium-sized lymphocytes contain nucleoli. Some chromatin streaking artifact is seen, a shared feature between small cell carcinoma and lymphoid cells on conventional smears.

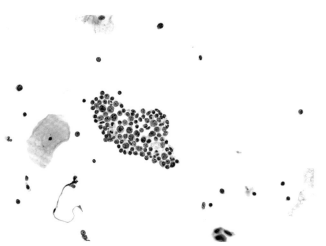
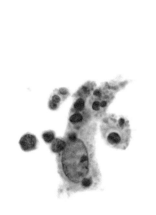
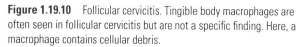

Figure 1.19.9   Follicular cervicitis. Medium-sized and small lymphocytes loosely aggregate as a pseudofragment in this liquid based preparation. A thin rim of blue cytoplasm can be seen in some of the cells. The chromatin pattern is coarse and not of a neuroendocrine nature.

Figure 1.19.10   Follicular cervicitis. Tingible body macrophages are often seen in follicular cervicitis but are not a specific finding. Here, a macrophage contains cellular debris.

2

Pulmonary

	Benign Respiratory Epithelium	Well-Differentiated Adenocarcinoma
Age	Any age	Older adults
Location	Lung	Lung
Signs and symptoms	Inadvertently sampled in patients with radiologic lesions of the lung	Fatigue, weight loss, cough, dyspnea, hemoptysis, chest pain, and/or lesion seen on imaging studies of the lung
Etiology	Not applicable	Classically associated with tobacco smoking; never-smokers are more likely to be younger, female, and/or Asian
Cytomorphology	• Fragments and single cells, which may be numerous in brushing specimens *(Figure 2.1.1)* • Columnar or round-shaped cells with oval nuclei, regular nuclear contours, and bland chromatin *(Figures 2.1.1 and 2.1.2)* • Fragments form a ciliated terminal bar *(Figure 2.1.2)* • Cilia may not be readily identified in every cell or at all in a particular preparation *(Figure 2.1.3)* • Low N/C ratio *(Figures 2.1.1-2.1.3)* • Little nuclear size variation *(Figures 2.1.1-2.1.3)*	• Fragments and/or single cells *(Figures 2.1.4 and 2.1.5)* • Slightly enlarged nuclear size and slightly increased N/C ratio *(Figures 2.1.6 and 2.1.7)* • Mild to moderate nuclear border irregularities *(Figures 2.1.6 and 2.1.7)* • Slight variation in nuclear sizes *(Figures 2.1.6 and 2.1.7)* • Coarse chromatin or prominent nucleoli *(Figures 2.1.6 and 2.1.7)* • Absence of cilia *(Figures 2.1.6 and 2.1.7)*
Special studies	Areas of squamous metaplasia may be positive for markers of squamous differentiation (p40/p63); negative for mesothelial markers. Benign pneumocytes may express TTF-1 and napsin-A.	Usually positive for TTF-1 (nuclear) and napsin-A (cytoplasmic granular); negative for markers of squamous differentiation (p40/p63) unless a squamous component exists; negative for mesothelial markers
Molecular alterations	None	Mutations in EGFR, KRAS, BRAF; ALK, RET, ROS1 translocations; amplification of MET or FGFR1
Treatment	None	Surgical resection +/− chemoradiation for stage I/II tumors; for advanced stage, chemoradiation and/or targeted therapies/immunotherapy
Clinical implications	Reassessment of the lesion seen on imaging studies and possible re-biopsy	Prognosis depends on tumor stage and the presence of targetable molecular alterations/eligibility for immunotherapy

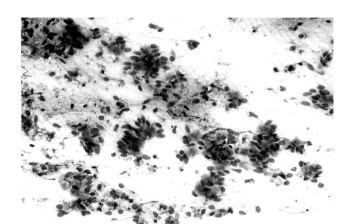

Figure 2.1.1   Benign bronchial respiratory epithelial cells. Numerous benign bronchial epithelial cells forming fragments and present singly in the background.

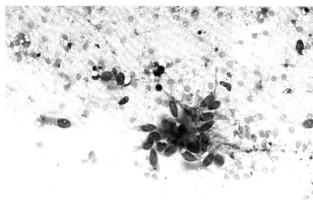

Figure 2.1.2   Benign bronchial respiratory epithelial cells. Benign bronchial cells have a columnar shape and an oval-shaped nucleus with regular contours. The apical portion of the cytoplasm forms a terminal bar upon which cilia can often (but not always) be appreciated.

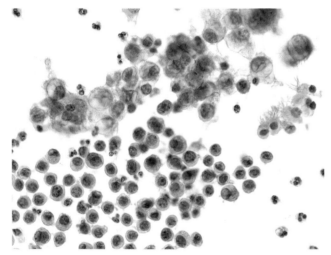

Figure 2.1.3   Benign bronchial respiratory epithelial cells. The benign bronchial cells in the top half of this field have a round shape, and cilia can be difficult to appreciate on some cells. They are intermixed with some goblet cells; pulmonary alveolar macrophages and pneumocytes are seen in the bottom half of the field.

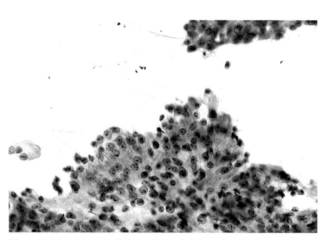

Figure 2.1.4   Adenocarcinoma. This well-differentiated adenocarcinoma forms a cohesive fragment. The cells maintain a fair amount of cytoplasm, but the nuclei are enlarged and have prominent nucleoli.

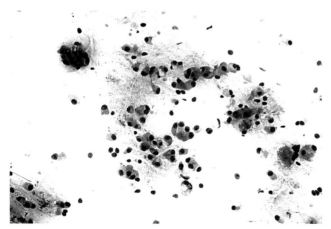

Figure 2.1.5   Adenocarcinoma. These adenocarcinoma cells are deceivingly bland and resemble benign bronchial respiratory epithelial cells. However, the specimen is cellular and cilia are not readily identified, raising suspicion for a well-differentiated adenocarcinoma.

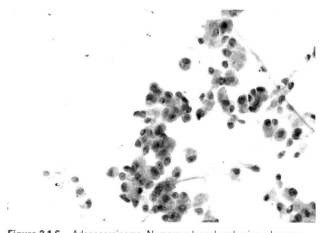

Figure 2.1.6   Adenocarcinoma. Numerous loosely cohesive adenocarcinoma cells can be seen. Pink mucin attaches to some cells, mimicking cilia. The nuclei have irregular nuclear borders and mild size variation; some have prominent nucleoli.

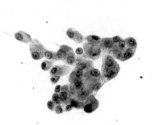

Figure 2.1.7   Adenocarcinoma. A cluster of adenocarcinoma cells with abundant, foamy cytoplasm. Note that the nuclear size variation reaches a ratio beyond 2:1 when comparing some of the cells. The nuclei also have irregular nuclear borders, and the chromatin is clumpy.

	Carcinoid Tumor	Well-Differentiated Adenocarcinoma
Age	Young adults	Older adults
Location	Lung	Lung
Signs and symptoms	Asymptomatic with incidental radiologic detection or chest pain, shortness of breath, diarrhea, flushing, weight gain, cough, and wheezing	Fatigue, weight loss, cough, dyspnea, hemoptysis, chest pain, and/or lesion seen on imaging studies of the lung
Etiology	Unknown. Commonly sporadic and but can be associated with MEN syndrome	Classically associated with tobacco smoking; never-smokers are more likely to be younger, female, and/or Asian
Cytomorphology	• Often cellular, with dispersed single cells without true tissue fragments *(Figure 2.2.1)* • Monotonous population of small epithelioid or spindled cells *(Figure 2.2.2)* • Plasmacytoid configuration (eccentrically placed nucleus) *(Figure 2.2.2)* • Regular nuclear borders *(Figure 2.2.3)* • "Salt-and-pepper" neuroendocrine chromatin pattern, best seen on Pap stained preparations *(Figures 2.2.3 and 2.2.4)*	• Fragments and/or single cells *(Figures 2.2.5-2.2.8)* • Slightly enlarged nuclear size and slightly increased N/C ratio *(Figure 2.2.9)* • Mild to moderate nuclear border irregularities *(Figure 2.2.9)* • Slight variation in nuclear sizes *(Figure 2.2.9)* • Coarse chromatin or prominent nucleoli *(Figure 2.2.6)*
Special studies	Positive for neuroendocrine markers (chromogranin, synaptophysin, INSM1); 50% positive for TTF-1; low Ki-67 index (<2%)	Usually positive for TTF-1 (nuclear) and napsin-A (cytoplasmic granular); negative for markers of squamous differentiation (p40/p63) unless a squamous component exists; negative for mesothelial markers
Molecular alterations	Approximately half of sporadic lung carcinoid tumors have *MEN1* inactivating mutations	Mutations in *EGFR, KRAS, BRAF; ALK, RET, ROS1* translocations; amplification of *MET* or *FGFR1*
Treatment	Surgical resection; when spread to lymph node (atypical carcinoid), may require chemoradiation	Surgical resection +/− chemoradiation for stage I/II tumors; for advanced stage, chemoradiation and/or targeted therapies/immunotherapy
Clinical implications	10-y survival is 50%	Prognosis depends on tumor stage and the presence of targetable molecular alterations/eligibility for immunotherapy

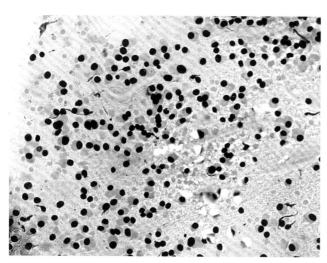

Figure 2.2.1   Carcinoid tumor. Carcinoid tumors often have the general characteristics of other neuroendocrine neoplasms: a cellular population of monotonous, dispersed plasmacytoid cells with regular nuclear contours.

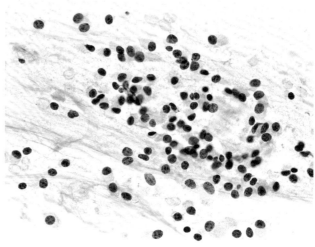

Figure 2.2.2   Carcinoid tumor. The Pap stain reveals the "salt-and-pepper" chromatin pattern found in carcinoid tumors. Carcinoid nuclei are often epithelioid, oval/spindled, or a mixture of both, as seen here.

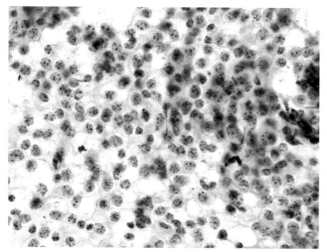

Figure 2.2.3   Carcinoid tumor. These tumor cells possess chromatin with a speckled appearance. The cells are crowded, giving the false impression of a true tissue fragment.

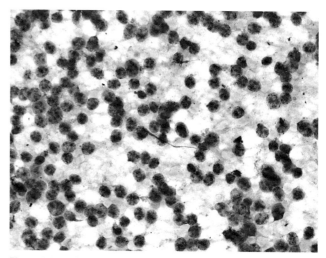

Figure 2.2.4   Carcinoid tumor. This carcinoid tumor has a slightly more concerning appearance, as the nuclei have some irregular nuclear borders and variation in size. The chromatin pattern may be mistaken for the coarse chromatin of an adenocarcinoma, but notice the even distribution of the chromatin within each nucleus.

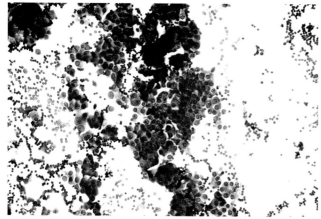

Figure 2.2.5   Adenocarcinoma. These cells form tissue fragments. The cells maintain a moderate amount of cytoplasm, but the nuclei are enlarged and some variation in nuclear size can be seen.

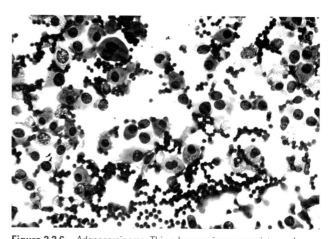

Figure 2.2.6   Adenocarcinoma. This adenocarcinoma consists predominantly of dispersed tumor cells. One binucleate cell (top left) contains prominent nucleoli.

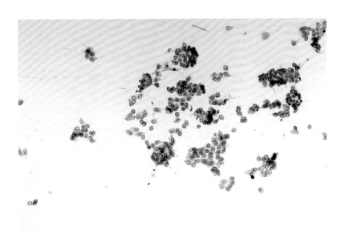

Figure 2.2.7   Adenocarcinoma. These cells have only minimal nuclear size variation and small, pinpoint nucleoli. Well-differentiated adenocarcinomas frequently have eccentrically placed nuclei. Note the absence of a "salt-and-pepper" chromatin appearance.

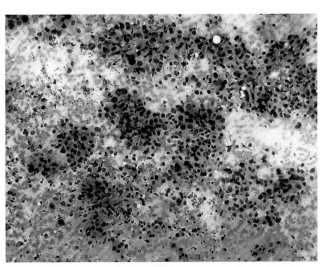

Figure 2.2.8   Adenocarcinoma. Numerous adenocarcinoma cells form tissue fragments and are present singly in the background. While the cells have low N/C ratios, the nuclei have different shapes and sizes, suggesting a malignant process.

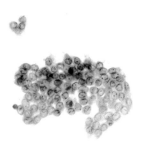

Figure 2.2.9   Adenocarcinoma. At this high magnification, irregularities in the nuclear contours can be appreciated as well as the presence of nuclear grooves.

	Carcinoid Tumor	Small-Cell Carcinoma
Age	Young adults	Older adults
Location	Lung	Lung
Signs and symptoms	Asymptomatic with incidental radiologic detection or chest pain, shortness of breath, diarrhea, flushing, weight gain, and cough, wheezing	Cough, chest pain, shortness of breath, weight loss, fatigue; symptoms associated with para-neoplastic syndromes
Etiology	Unknown. Commonly sporadic and but can be associated with MEN syndrome	Predominantly tobacco smoking; radon exposure
Cytomorphology	• Often cellular, with predominantly dispersed single cells with or without tissue fragments *(Figures 2.3.1-2.3.3)* • Monotonous population of epithelioid or spindled cells *(Figures 2.3.4 and 2.3.5)* • Plasmacytoid configuration (eccentrically placed nucleus) *(Figure 2.3.4)* • Regular nuclear borders *(Figure 2.3.4)* • "Salt-and-pepper" neuroendocrine chromatin pattern, best seen on Pap stained preparations *(Figure 2.3.5)*	• Often cellular with predominantly dispersed single cells with or without tissue fragments *(Figures 2.3.6 and 2.3.7)* • Background of necrosis and/or apoptotic cells *(Figures 2.3.8 and 2.3.9)* • Despite the name, cells are larger than bystanding inflammatory cells and are pleomorphic (more obvious on Diff-Quik preparations) *(Figure 2.3.9)* • Cells have little cytoplasm and nuclei may "mold" together *(Figure 2.3.7)* • "Salt-and-pepper" neuroendocrine chromatin pattern, best seen on Pap stained preparations *(Figure 2.3.10)* • Crush/smearing artifact on smear preparations *(Figure 2.3.6)*
Special studies	Positive for neuroendocrine markers (chromogranin, synaptophysin, INSM1); 50% positive for TTF-1; low Ki-67 index (<2%)	Considered a morphologic diagnosis. May paradoxically lack expression of neuroendocrine markers (chromogranin, synaptophysin, INSM1); dotlike positivity for pan-keratin; 90% positive for TTF-1 (not specific for a lung origin); high Ki-67 index (often >90%)
Molecular alterations	Approximately half of sporadic lung carcinoid tumors have *MEN1* inactivating mutations	Inactivating mutations in *TP53* or *RB*
Treatment	Surgical resection; when spread to lymph node (atypical carcinoid), may require chemoradiation	Primarily chemoradiation
Clinical implications	10-y survival is 50%	Poor prognosis

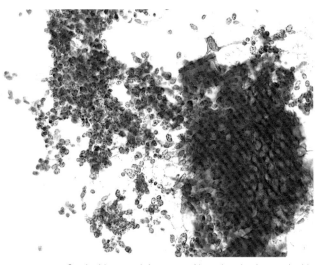

Figure 2.3.1   Carcinoid tumor. A fragment of loosely cohesive carcinoid tumor cells can be appreciated on the left-hand side of the field. Compare with the fragment containing bronchial respiratory epithelium and goblet cells on the right-hand side.

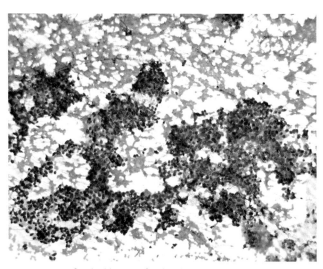

Figure 2.3.2   Carcinoid tumor. Carcinoid tumor cells form a "packeted" architecture in this field. Even at this low magnification, the cells appear small and monomorphic.

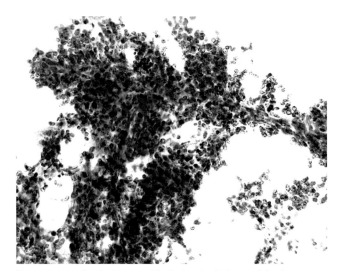

Figure 2.3.3   Carcinoid tumor. The lesional cells have minimal cytoplasm and oval-shaped nuclei. The cells are associated with a fibrovascular core.

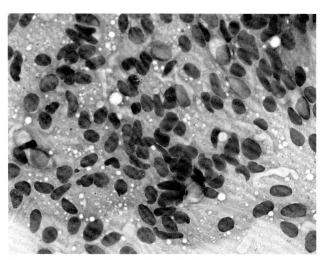

Figure 2.3.4   Carcinoid tumor. These cells have spindled nuclei and cytoplasm that blends with the background. For cells with identifiable cytoplasm in this field, a plamacytoid configuration can be appreciated.

2 PULMONARY

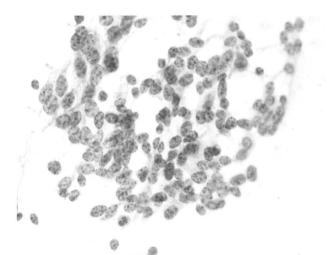

Figure 2.3.5   Carcinoid tumor. At high magnification, a "salt-and-pepper" neuroendocrine chromatin pattern can be seen on this Pap stained preparation.

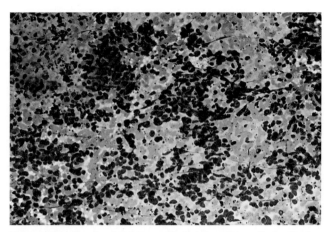

Figure 2.3.6   Small-cell carcinoma. The field is cellular with discohesive small cells, and the background contains necrotic and apoptotic derbris. Note the smearing artifact, in which the nuclear chromatin contained by some of the cells appears to be stretched in a horizontal direction.

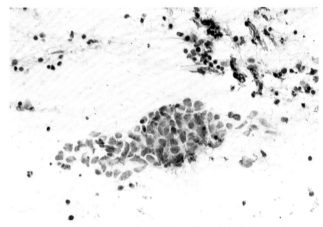

Figure 2.3.7   Small-cell carcinoma. The cells contain little cytoplasm and the nuclei appear to "mold" against each other, causing irregularities in nuclear shapes.

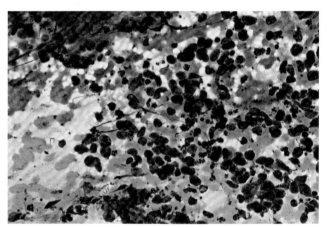

Figure 2.3.8   Small-cell carcinoma. The neuroendocrine chromatin pattern can be difficult to appreciate on Diff-Quik–stained preparations, resulting in homogenous-appearing chromatin. This field also contains chromatin smearing artifact and apoptotic debris.

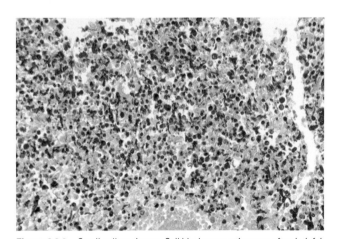

Figure 2.3.9   Small-cell carcinoma. Cell block preparations are often helpful in the cytomorphologic identification of small-cell carcinoma and also allow for the performance of immunohistochemical studies. Here, viable tumor cells are intermixed with intact necrotic cells "blobs" that stain pink. This corresponds with the "geographic necrosis" often seen on tissue specimens.

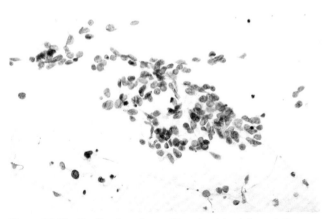

Figure 2.3.10   Small-cell carcinoma. There is minimal size variation between the cells. The chromatin pattern is speckled, suggesting a neuro-endocrine differentiation.

	Small-Cell Carcinoma	Reserve Cell Hyperplasia
Age	Older adults	Any
Location	Lung	Lung
Signs and symptoms	Cough, chest pain, shortness of breath, weight loss, fatigue; symptoms associated with para-neoplastic syndromes	Symptoms associated with processes causing lung injury or with a lung lesion seen on imaging studies
Etiology	Predominantly tobacco smoking; radon exposure	Nonspecific proliferation of bronchial reserve cells in response to lung injury; typically considered a background reactive change
Cytomorphology	• Often cellular with predominantly dispersed single cells with or without tissue fragments *(Figures 2.4.1* and *2.4.2)* • Background of necrosis and/or apoptotic cells • Despite the name, cells are larger than bystanding inflammatory cells and are pleomorphic (more obvious on Diff-Quik preparations) *(Figure 2.4.3)* • Cells have little cytoplasm, and nuclei may "mold" together *(Figures 2.4.4* and *2.4.5)* • "Salt-and-pepper" neuroendocrine chromatin pattern, best seen on Pap stained preparations *(Figures 2.4.4* and *2.4.5)*	• Usually a focal finding in an exfoliative cytology specimen • Cells form loosely cohesive tissue fragments with rare or absent single cells in the background *(Figure 2.4.6)* • Cells are monotonous with round nuclei and regular nuclear contours *(Figures 2.4.7-2.4.10)* • Bland chromatin pattern with small chromocenters *(Figures 2.4.9* and *2.4.10)* • Nuclear molding is absent
Special studies	Considered a morphologic diagnosis. May paradoxically lack expression of neuroendocrine markers (chromogranin, synaptophysin, INSM1); dotlike positivity for pan-keratin; 90% positive for TTF-1 (not specific for a lung origin); high Ki-67 index (often >90%)	Typically seen in exfoliative specimens in which immunohistochemistry cannot be performed due to low cellularity
Molecular alterations	Inactivating mutations in *TP53* or *RB*	None
Treatment	Primarily chemoradiation	None
Clinical implications	Poor prognosis	Nonspecific finding. May require a repeat procedure if neoplastic cells were expected and not seen

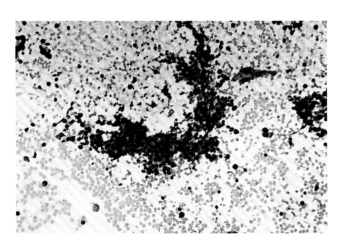

Figure 2.4.1   Small-cell carcinoma. A fragment of loosely cohesive small cells, with additional single cells in the background.

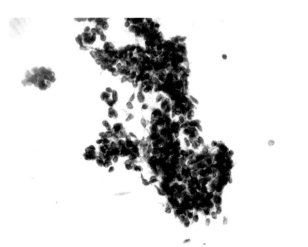

Figure 2.4.2   Small-cell carcinoma. The nuclei are oval shaped, and the cells have no appreciable cytoplasm.

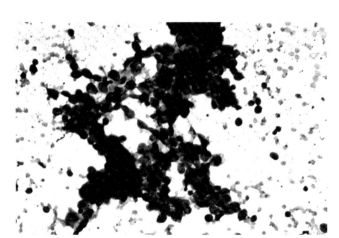

Figure 2.4.3   Small-cell carcinoma. This fragment contains small cells in which the nuclei have an epithelioid appearance. Nuclear border irregularities and anisonucleosis can be appreciated.

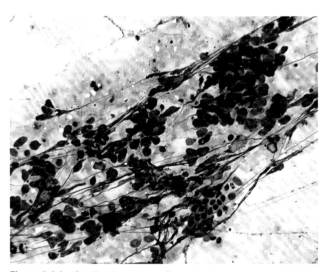

Figure 2.4.4   Small-cell carcinoma. The cells demonstrate a prominent "streak artifact" in which the chromatin of some cells has formed thin threads along the direction of the smearing force.

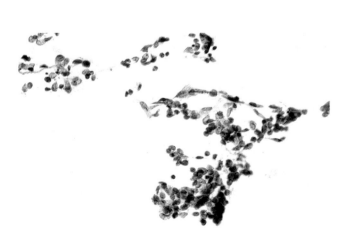

Figure 2.4.5   Small-cell carcinoma. The cells have a "speckled" chromatin appearance suggestive of neuroendocrine differentiation.

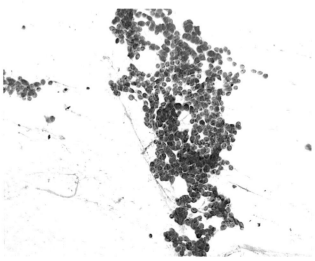

Figure 2.4.6   Reserve cell hyperplasia. This monolayer fragment contains reserve cells which appear monomorphic and possess very little cytoplasm.

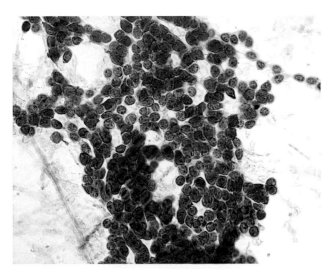

Figure 2.4.7   Reserve cell hyperplasia. Reserve cells have regular nuclear contours, round nuclei, and little variation in nuclear size.

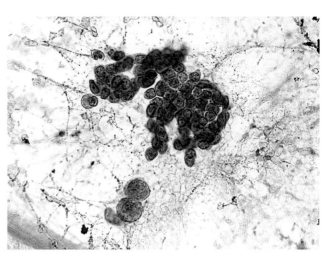

Figure 2.4.8   Reserve cell hyperplasia. While reserve cells can form tight clusters, they retain their round nuclear shape and do not demonstrate the nuclear molding seen in small-cell carcinoma.

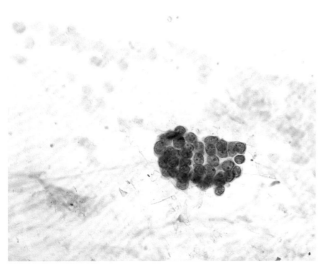

Figure 2.4.9   Reserve cell hyperplasia. The chromatin is bland, and the nuclei contain small chromocenters.

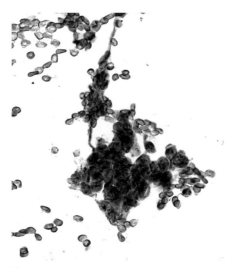

Figure 2.4.10   Reserve cell hyperplasia. Reserve cells can be mistaken for small-cell carcinoma but are not usually present in large numbers.

	Large-Cell Neuroendocrine Carcinoma (LCNEC)	Small-Cell Carcinoma
Age	Older adults	Older adults
Location	Lung	Lung
Signs and symptoms	Cough, chest pain, shortness of breath, weight loss, fatigue; symptoms associated with para-neoplastic syndromes	Cough, chest pain, shortness of breath, weight loss, fatigue; symptoms associated with para-neoplastic syndromes
Etiology	Predominantly tobacco smoking	Predominantly tobacco smoking; radon exposure
Cytomorphology	• Fragments with single cells in the background *(Figures 2.5.1 and 2.5.2)* • Moderate amount of cytoplasm *(Figure 2.5.3)* • Cells are larger than small-cell carcinoma cells *(Figure 2.5.3)* • Vesicular chromatin, often with prominent nucleoli *(Figure 2.5.3)* • May form rosette structures *(Figure 2.5.4)* • Nuclear molding may be present *(Figure 2.5.5)*	• Often cellular with predominantly dispersed single cells with or without tissue fragments *(Figure 2.5.6)* • Background of necrosis and/or apoptotic cells *(Figure 2.5.7)* • Despite the name, cells are larger than bystanding inflammatory cells and are pleomorphic (more obvious on Diff-Quik preparations) *(Figure 2.5.8)* • Cells have little cytoplasm and nuclei may "mold" together *(Figures 2.5.8 and 2.5.9)* • "Salt-and-pepper" neuroendocrine chromatin pattern, best seen on Pap stained preparations *(Figures 2.5.8 and 2.5.10)*
Special studies	Variable positivity for neuroendocrine markers (chromogranin, synaptophysin, INSM1); pan-keratin positive; high Ki-67 (>40%)	Considered a morphologic diagnosis. May paradoxically lack expression of neuroendocrine markers (chromogranin, synaptophysin, INSM1); dotlike positivity for pan-keratin; 90% positive for TTF-1 (not specific for a lung origin); high Ki-67 index (often >90%)
Molecular alterations	Inactivating mutations in *TP53* or *RB*, in a subset	Inactivating mutations in *TP53* or *RB*
Treatment	Surgical resection with chemoradiation for early stage; chemoradiation for late stage	Primarily chemoradiation
Clinical implications	Poor prognosis; worse prognosis than non–small-cell carcinoma of equivalent stage	Poor prognosis

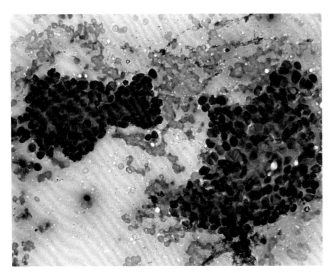

Figure 2.5.1 Large-cell neurendocrine carcinoma. Two large three-dimensional fragments containing cells that are large in size and identifiable cytoplasm despite high N/C ratios.

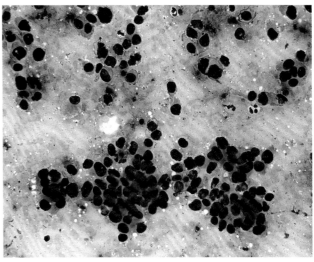

Figure 2.5.2 Large-cell neurendocrine carcinoma. Cells are present in fragments as well as dispersed in the background. Some cells form rosette structures (bottom of the field), which may be mistaken for glandular formations of an adenocarcinoma.

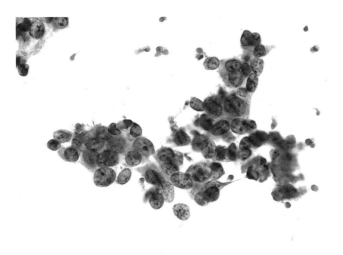

Figure 2.5.3 Large-cell neurendocrine carcinoma. The cells here contain either coarse chromatin or prominent nucleoli. Note the moderate amount of granular cytoplasm, irregular nuclear borders, and variation in nuclear sizes.

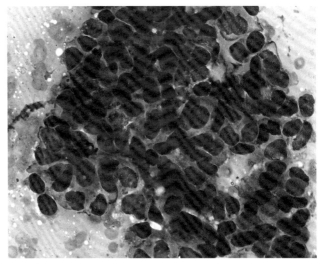

Figure 2.5.4 Large-cell neurendocrine carcinoma. The cells seen here contain a moderate amount of cytoplasm and form a three-dimensional cluster. Many of the cells have a rosette arrangement, in which the nuclei encircle areas of cytoplasm.

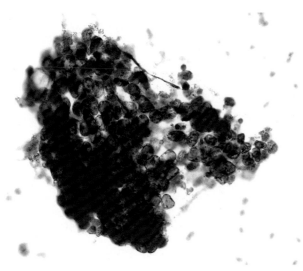

Figure 2.5.5 Large-cell neurendocrine carcinoma. The nuclei appear to "mold" together in some areas, similar to what can be seen in small-cell carcinoma.

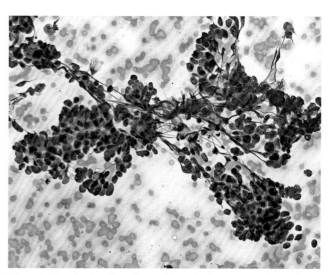

Figure 2.5.6 Small-cell carcinoma. The cells demonstrate chromatin streak artifact and nuclear molding. The cells are present in fragments as well as single in the background.

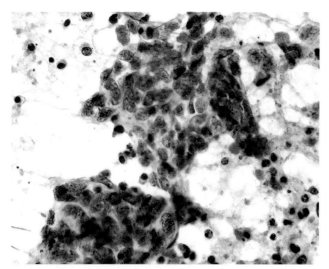

Figure 2.5.7 Small-cell carcinoma. Here, numerous small-cell carcinoma cells cluster together in a background of necrotic debris. The debris is also interspersed between the cells, giving the false appearance of cytoplasm.

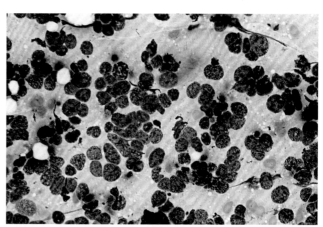

Figure 2.5.8 Small-cell carcinoma. The cells mold against one another, causing compression of adjacent nuclei. A "salt-and-pepper" chromatin pattern can be seen here, although it is usually best appreciated on a Pap stained preparation.

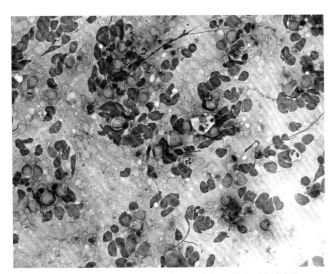

Figure 2.5.9   Small-cell carcinoma. Some of the cells in this field have a thin rim of a cytoplasm, giving them the appearance of leukemic blast cells. However, the majority of cells have indiscernible cytoplasm.

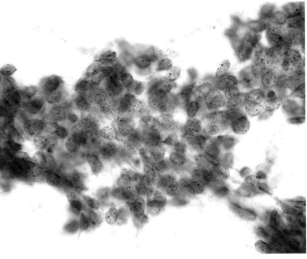

Figure 2.5.10   Small-cell carcinoma. This Pap stained smear demonstrates the "salt-and-pepper" chromatin pattern seen in small-cell carcinoma as well as most other neuroendocrine neoplasms.

	Adenocarcinoma	Squamous Cell Carcinoma
Age	Older adults	Older adults
Location	Lung	Lung
Signs and symptoms	Fatigue, weight loss, cough, dyspnea, hemoptysis, chest pain, and/or lesion seen on imaging studies of the lung	Fatigue, weight loss, cough, dyspnea, hemoptysis, chest pain, and/or lesion seen on imaging studies of the lung
Etiology	Classically associated with tobacco smoking; never-smokers are more likely to be younger, female, and/or Asian	Classically associated with tobacco smoking
Cytomorphology	• Tissue fragments which may form glandular structures or three-dimensional fragments (Figures 2.6.1 and 2.6.2) • Singly dispersed cells in poorly differentiated or necrotic tumors • Usually eccentrically placed nucleus with coarse chromatin and/or prominent nucleoli (Figures 2.6.3 and 2.6.4) • Foamy cytoplasm which may contain mucin vacuoles (Figure 2.6.5) • Anisonucleosis, hyperchromasia, and irregular nuclear borders (Figures 2.6.3-2.6.5)	• Tissue fragments and dispersed single cells, often with a background of necrosis (Figures 2.6.6 and 2.6.7) • Nuclei tend to be centrally placed (Figures 2.6.7 and 2.6.8) • Dense cytoplasm that may form irregular, rigid projections (Figure 2.6.8) • Keratinizing tumor cells which have pink cytoplasm on Pap stained preparations • Pyknotic nuclei are small and hyperchromatic and have markedly irregular borders, or nuclei with coarse chromatin or prominent nucleoli (Figures 2.6.9 and 2.6.10)
Special studies	Usually positive for TTF-1 (nuclear) and napsin-A (cytoplasmic granular); negative for markers of squamous differentiation (p40/p63) unless a squamous component exists; negative for mesothelial markers.	Positive for p40/p63 and negative for TTF-1 and napsin-A. Negative for HPV studies unless metastatic from other sites.
Molecular alterations	Mutations in *EGFR, KRAS, BRAF, ALK, RET, ROS1* translocations; amplification of *MET* or *FGFR1*	Driver mutations have not been well established
Treatment	Surgical resection +/– chemoradiation for stage I/II tumors; for advanced stage, chemoradiation and/or targeted therapies/immunotherapy	Surgical resection +/– chemoradiation for stage I/II tumors; for advanced stage, chemoradiation and/or immunotherapy
Clinical implications	Prognosis depends on tumor stage and the presence of targetable molecular alterations/eligibility for immunotherapy	Prognosis depends on tumor stage and eligibility for immunotherapy

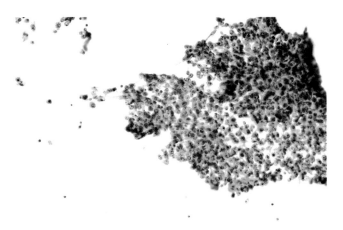

Figure 2.6.1   Adenocarcinoma. A tissue fragment of loosely cohesive cells. The cells lack cilia and have prominent nucleoli.

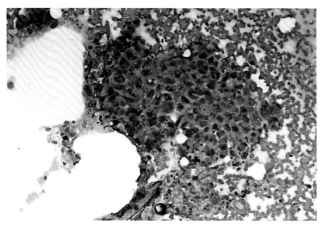

Figure 2.6.2   Adenocarcinoma. Cells containing a moderate amount of cytoplasm and nuclear border irregularities. There is more than a 4:1 variation in size among some adjacent nuclei.

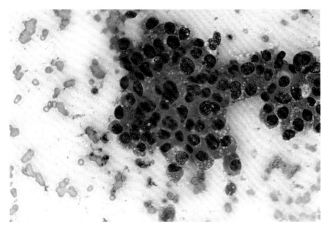

Figure 2.6.3   Adenocarcinoma. These cells have abundant cytoplasm, as well as intranuclear inclusions, a feature sometimes seen in lung adenocarcinomas. Other features of malignancy seen here include aniso-nucleosis, large cell size, and nuclear contour irregularities.

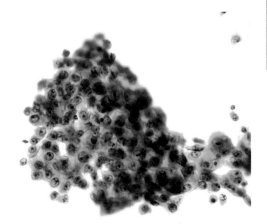

Figure 2.6.4   Adenocarcinoma. The prominent nucleoli seen here are likely not reactive in nature due to their large size. Many of the cells have deceiving regular nuclear borders, but the nuclear size variation strongly suggests a malignant process.

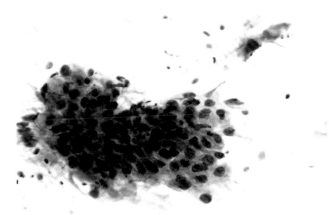

Figure 2.6.5   Adenocarcinoma. The cytoplasm of these cells stains a pink color, indicating the presence of mucin.

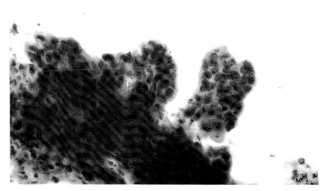

Figure 2.6.6   Squamous cell carcinoma. Squamous cell carcinoma can also have prominent nucleoli. As opposed to adenocarcinoma, squamous cell carcinoma cells often have rigid cytoplasm and centrally placed nuclei and may have concentrically arranged cells in a syncytial architecture (center of fragment).

2 PULMONARY

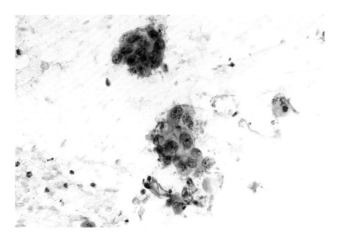

Figure 2.6.7   Squamous cell carcinoma. It can be challenging to determine whether poorly differentiated carcinoma cells represent an adenocarcinoma or squamous cell carcinoma. Many of the cells seen here have centrally placed nuclei, suggesting the possibility of a squamous cell carcinoma.

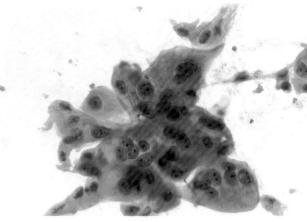

Figure 2.6.8   Squamous cell carcinoma. These cells have vacuolated, bubbly cytoplasm that may resemble an adenocarcinoma. However, the cytoplasm forms polygonal shapes with odd projections, and some nuclei are centrally placed.

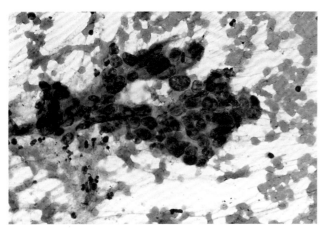

Figure 2.6.9   Squamous cell carcinoma. When poorly differentiated, squamous cell carcinoma often shares features of adenocarcinoma: anisnucleosis, irregular nuclear borders, high N/C ratio, large cell size, and coarse chromatin.

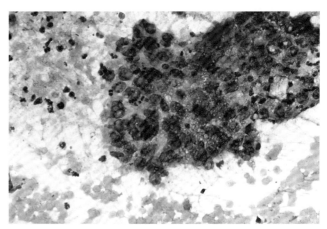

Figure 2.6.10   Squamous cell carcinoma. Squamous cell carcinoma with a background of necrotic granular debris and inflammation (top left corner). Squamous cell carcinomas are often associated with necrosis, although this can also sometimes be seen in adenocarcinoma.

	Malignant Mesothelioma	Squamous Cell Carcinoma
Age	Older adults	Older adults
Location	Lung	Lung
Signs and symptoms	Unilateral chest pain; progressive shortness of breath; cough; weight loss	Fatigue, weight loss, cough, dyspnea, hemoptysis, chest pain, and/or lesion seen on imaging studies of the lung
Etiology	Asbestos exposure; radiation exposure	Classically associated with tobacco smoking
Cytomorphology	• Three-dimensional tissue fragments and/or dispersed single cells *(Figures 2.7.1 and 2.7.2)* • Large cell size *(Figure 2.7.3)* • Abundant cytoplasm with two-toned, granular cytoplasm and cytoplasmic vacuoles *(Figure 2.7.4)* • Spaces ("windows") between cells *(Figure 2.7.4)* • Binucleation *(Figures 2.7.3 and 2.7.5)* • Irregular nuclear contours and anisonucleosis *(Figure 2.7.3)* • Coarse chromatin and/or prominent nucleoli *(Figure 2.7.5)*	• Tissue fragments and dispersed single cells, often with a background of necrosis *(Figures 2.7.6 and 2.7.7)* • Nuclei tend to be centrally placed *(Figures 2.7.7 and 2.7.8)* • Dense cytoplasm that may form irregular, rigid projections *(Figure 2.7.8)* • Keratinizing tumor cells which have pink cytoplasm on Pap stained preparations • Anisnucleosis and irregular nuclear contours *(Figures 2.7.8 and 2.7.9)* • Pyknotic nuclei are small, hyperchromatic and have markedly irregular borders, or nuclei with coarse chromatin or prominent nucleoli *(Figure 2.7.10)*
Special studies	Usually positive for calretinin (cytoplasmic and nuclear), WT-1, and/or D2-40. Rarely positive for p40/p63. Negative for TTF-1 and napsin-A. Loss of BAP-1 (nuclear) expression. FISH to detect homozygous deletion of *p16* on chromosome 9	Positive for p40/p63 and negative for TTF-1 and napsin-A. Usually negative for mesothelial markers such as calretinin, WT-1, and D2-40.
Molecular alterations	Mutations in *BAP1* or *NF2* genes	Driver mutations have not been well established
Treatment	Surgery, chemoradiation, and/or targeted therapies.	Surgical resection +/− chemoradiation for stage I/II tumors; for advanced stage, chemoradiation and/or immunotherapy
Clinical implications	Extremely poor	Prognosis depends on tumor stage and eligibility for immunotherapy

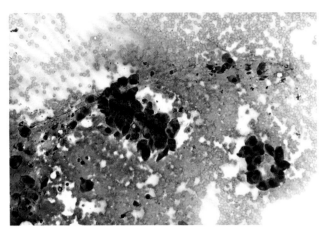

Figure 2.7.1   Mesothelioma. Cells present in both tissue fragments and dispersed single cells.

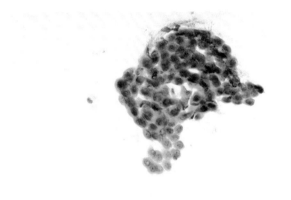

Figure 2.7.2   Mesothelioma. Cells in a three-dimensional fragment. Note the large cell size and the presence of abundant cytoplasm.

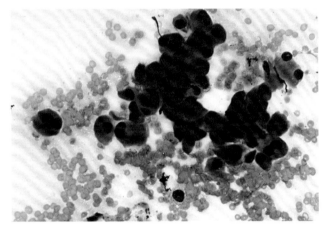

Figure 2.7.3   Mesothelioma. Cells with abundant, "two-toned", granular cytoplasm. Mesothelioma is included under neoplasms that can present with "large pink cells."

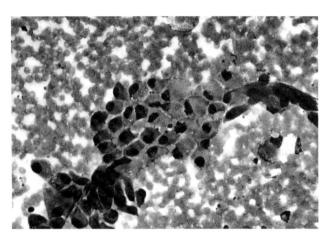

Figure 2.7.4   Mesothelioma. Cells in a monolayer sheet with intercellular spaces ("windows") between many of the cells. Small cytoplasmic vacuoles are present in some of the cells.

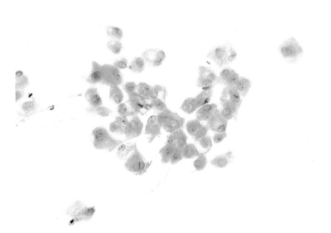

Figure 2.7.5   Mesothelioma. Loosely cohesive cells, some binucleated, with abundant cytoplasm. Many of the cells have polygonally shaped cytoplasm.

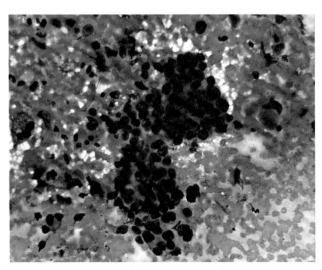

Figure 2.7.6   Squamous cell carcinoma. A tissue fragment of squamous cell carcinoma with single carcinoma cells in the background. Necrosis can be seen, as evidenced by the presence of some granular debris and macrophages.

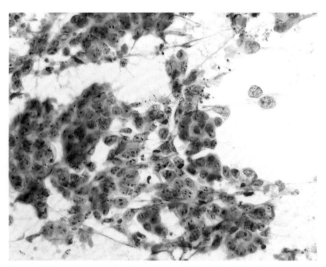

Figure 2.7.7   Squamous cell carcinoma. Cells with minimal cytoplasm, enlarged nuclei, and coarse chromatin. Granular debris is present in the background, an indication of necrosis. The architecture is syncytial.

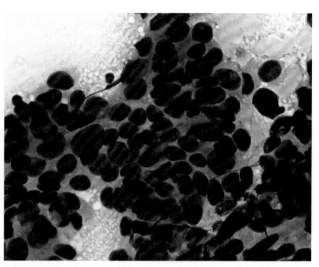

Figure 2.7.8   Squamous cell carcinoma. Cells with high N/C ratios and great variation in nuclear size.

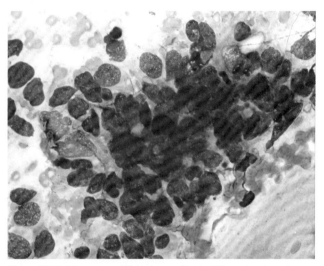

Figure 2.7.9   Squamous cell carcinoma. Poorly differentiated carcinoma, with some single stripped nuclei present in the background. The differential diagnosis includes squamous cell carcinoma, adenocarcinoma, mesothelioma, and other poorly differentiated malignancies.

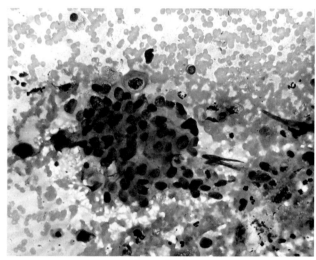

Figure 2.7.10   Squamous cell carcinoma. Some cells in this fragment have centrally placed nuclei and dense, polygonal cytoplasm. The nuclear contours are irregular, and there is variation in nuclear size.

	Malignant Mesothelioma	Adenocarcinoma
Age	Older adults	Older adults
Location	Lung	Lung
Signs and symptoms	Unilateral chest pain; progressive shortness of breath; cough; weight loss	Fatigue, weight loss, cough, dyspnea, hemoptysis, chest pain, and/or lesion seen on imaging studies of the lung
Etiology	Asbestos exposure; radiation exposure	Classically associated with tobacco smoking; never-smokers are more likely to be younger, female, and/or Asian
Cytomorphology	• Three-dimensional tissue fragments and/or dispersed single cells *(Figures 2.8.1 and 2.8.2)* • Large cell size *(Figure 2.8.2)* • Abundant cytoplasm with two-toned, granular cytoplasm and cytoplasmic vacuoles *(Figure 2.8.3)* • Spaces ("windows") between cells *(Figure 2.8.4)* • Binucleation *(Figure 2.8.3)* • Irregular nuclear contours and anisonucleosis *(Figures 2.8.2 and 2.8.5)* • Coarse chromatin and/or prominent nucleoli *(Figure 2.8.4)*	• Tissue fragments which may form glandular structures or three-dimensional fragments *(Figure 2.8.6)* • Singly dispersed cells in poorly differentiated or necrotic tumors • Usually eccentrically placed nucleus with coarse chromatin and/or prominent nucleoli *(Figures 2.8.7 and 2.8.8)* • Foamy cytoplasm which may contain mucin vacuoles *(Figure 2.8.9)* • Anisonucleosis, hyperchromasia, and irregular nuclear borders *(Figure 2.8.10)*
Special studies	Usually positive for calretinin (cytoplasmic and nuclear), WT-1, and/or D2-40. Negative for TTF-1 and napsin-A. Loss of BAP-1 (nuclear) expression. FISH to detect homozygous deletion of *p16* on chromosome 9	Usually positive for TTF-1 (nuclear) and napsin-A (cytoplasmic granular); negative for markers of squamous differentiation (p40/p63) unless a squamous component exists; negative for mesothelial markers
Molecular alterations	Mutations in *BAP1* or *NF2* genes	Mutations in *EGFR, KRAS, BRAF, ALK, RET, ROS1* translocations; amplification of *MET* or *FGFR1*
Treatment	Surgery, chemoradiation, and/or targeted therapies.	Surgical resection +/− chemoradiation for stage I/II tumors; for advanced stage, chemoradiation and/or targeted therapies/immunotherapy
Clinical implications	Extremely poor	Prognosis depends on tumor stage and the presence of targetable molecular alterations/eligibility for immunotherapy

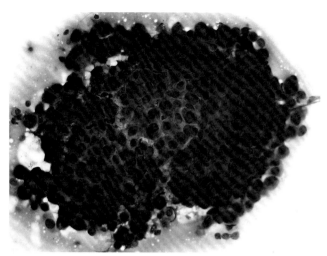

Figure 2.8.1   Mesothelioma. A large fragment of cells, resembling an adenocarcinoma. The cells have abundant cytoplasm; however, this can also occur in adenocarcinomas. The presence of intercytoplasmic gaps between some cells ("windows") may suggest the possibility of mesothelioma in this instance.

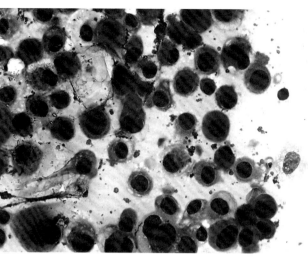

Figure 2.8.2   Mesothelioma. Here, the mesothelioma presents predominantly as a single cell, dispersed population. Some cells are binucleate, and some have intracytoplasmic vacuoles.

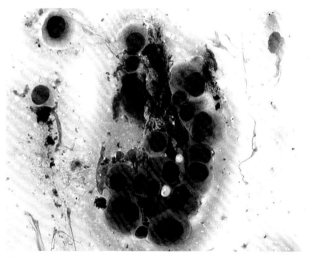

Figure 2.8.3   Mesothelioma. Cells with abundant cytoplasm and some binucleate forms. Some cells have deceiving regular nuclear contours.

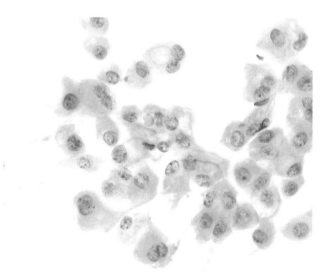

Figure 2.8.4   Mesothelioma. These cells have abundant cytoplasm which provides a polygonal shape to the cells. The chromatin is coarse, and some irregularities in the nuclear borders can be seen.

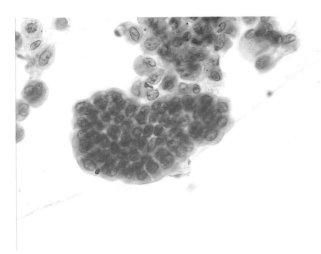

Figure 2.8.5 Mesothelioma. A tight cluster of cells resembling a mor-ule, a finding that can also be seen in adenocarcinoma. The nuclear bor-ders are irregular, and the nuclei appear to overlap due to their increased size and the tissue fragment's three-dimensionality.

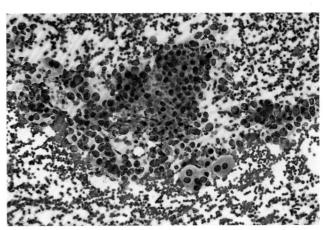

Figure 2.8.6 Adenocarcinoma. These cells are present in a tissue frag-ment as well as single in the background. Most nuclei have very irregular nuclear borders, and prominent nucleoli can be seen in some of the cells.

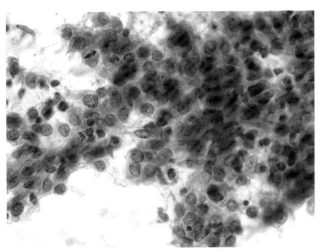

Figure 2.8.7 Adenocarcinoma. These cells form a three-dimensional structure. Their nuclei have many different sizes and shapes. The chroma-tin pattern is coarse, with some cells having distinct nucleoli.

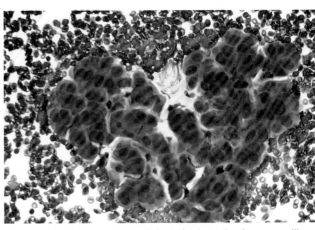

Figure 2.8.8 Adenocarcinoma. A tissue fragment that forms a papillary-like structure, which may distinguish the cells from a squamous cell carci-noma but not a mesothelioma. The cells maintain an abundant amount of granular cytoplasm, which can also be seen in mesothelioma.

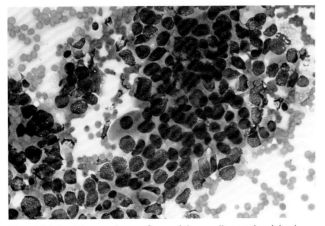

Figure 2.8.9 Adenocarcinoma. Some of these cells contain minimal cytoplasm. The nuclei are large and have irregular shapes and borders.

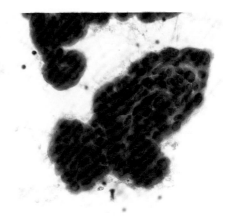

Figure 2.8.10 Adenocarcinoma. The nuclei are dark and have irregular borders. Anisnoculeosis is a prominent feature, with the size of some adjacent nuclei differing by more than 4:1.

	Granuloma	Neoplasm
Age	Any age	Older adults
Location	Lung	Lung
Signs and symptoms	Depends on etiology: shortness of breath, cough, enlarged mediastinal lymph nodes (on imaging), fever, weight loss, fatigue, night sweats, hemoptysis	Fatigue, weight loss, cough, dyspnea, hemoptysis, chest pain, and/or lesion seen on imaging studies of the lung
Etiology	Various; most commonly secondary to sarcoidosis or an infectious process	Primary lung cancer (many are associated with tobacco smoking) or metastasis from secondary sites
Cytomorphology	• A mixture of epithelioid histiocytes and lymphocytes, with or without multinucleated giant cells *(Figure 2.9.1)* • Necrosis may or may not be present *(Figure 2.9.2)* • Epithelioid histiocytes have abundant cytoplasm and often have carrot-shaped or curvilinear nuclei *(Figure 2.9.3)* • Lymphocytes are often associated with the histiocytes *(Figures 2.9.4* and *2.9.5)* and may undergo chromatin smearing artifact radiating away from the cellular groups	• Proliferative process resulting in numerous cells in tissue fragments and/or individually dispersed *(Figures 2.9.6* and *2.9.7)* • Neoplastic cells usually share certain features, such as cytoplasm and chromatin quality and stand out from normal background cells *(Figure 2.9.8)* • Nuclear and cell shapes and sizes vary depending on tumor type and differentiation *(Figures 2.9.6-2.9.8)* • Malignant neoplasms may demonstrate necrosis, irregular nuclear borders, anisnucleosis, high N/C ratios, and either coarse chromatin or prominent nucleoli *(Figures 2.9.9* and *2.9.10)*
Special studies	Generally a morphologic diagnosis; epithelioid histiocytes are highlighted by CD68 immunostain and are keratin negative	Depends on tumor type; most are primary or metastatic carcinomas and will be positive for keratin
Molecular alterations	None	Various; depends on tumor type
Treatment	Treatment of underlying disease	Depends on tumor type
Clinical implications	Surgery is usually unnecessary; thus the recognition of granulomatous inflammation results in faster treatment and prevents unnecessarily surgery and/or additional biopsies	Prognosis depends on tumor type and stage but is generally poor.

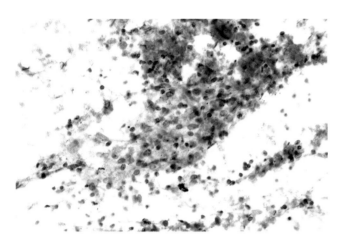

Figure 2.9.1   Granuloma. Granulomatous inflammation consisting of epithelioid histiocytes, lymphocytes, and necrotic debris.

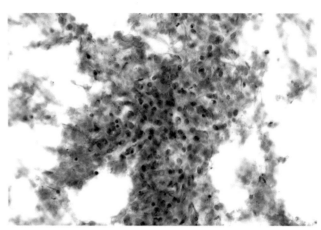

Figure 2.9.2   Granuloma. A granuloma is characterized by the presence of epithelioid histiocytes with closely associated and interspersed lymphocytes. Within a population of epithelioid histiocytes, some cells will have elongated nuclei shaped like carrots or hyphens, a specific feature.

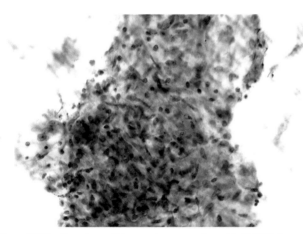

Figure 2.9.3   Granuloma. This granuloma contains epithelioid histiocytes which form a whirling pattern and are dotted with lymphocytes. The histiocytic nuclei range from oval to spindle in shape.

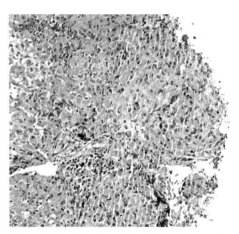

Figure 2.9.4   Granuloma. Granulomas are sometimes more readily appreciated on cell block material, where areas of low cellular density contain histiocytes with abundant cytoplasm.

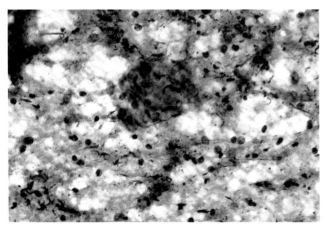

Figure 2.9.5   Granuloma. A granuloma is seen in the center of the field, with scattered background lymphocytes. Some lymphocytes have smeared chromatin, a phenomenon often seen in granulomatous inflammation.

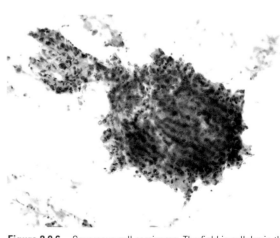

Figure 2.9.6   Squamous cell carcinoma. The field is cellular in this keratinizing squamous cell carcinoma, with cells present in a tissue fragment as well as scattered in the background.

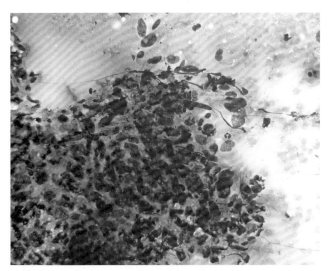

Figure 2.9.7 Synovial sarcoma. These neoplastic spindle cells were aspirated from a sarcoma. Despite variations in nuclear shape and size, one common feature is the spindle shape to the nuclei.

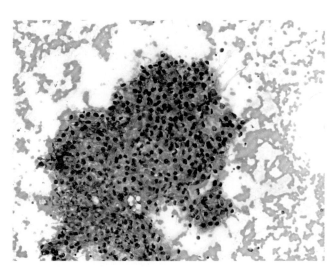

Figure 2.9.8 Metastatic renal cell carcinoma. A monotonous neoplastic population of renal cell carcinoma cells. The neoplastic cells all have similar, vacuolated cytoplasm.

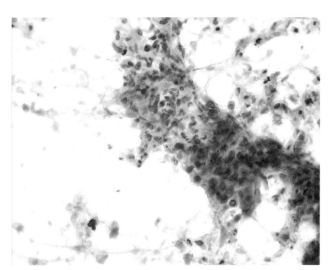

Figure 2.9.9 Squamous cell carcinoma. Some neoplasms can create a granulomatous response. In this case, the squamous cell carcinoma on the bottom right side of the field is adjacent to granulomatous inflammation on the top half of the field. Thus, the presence of necrotizing granulomatous inflammation should raise the possibility of an unsampled or undersampled malignancy.

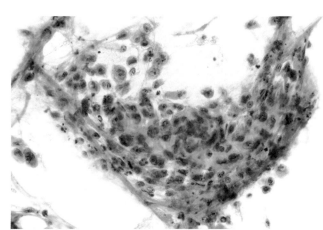

Figure 2.9.10 Squamous cell carcinoma. These neoplastic cells demonstrate many features of malignancy—irregular nuclear borders, coarse chromatin and/or prominent nucleoli, and anisonucleosis.

	Non-Hodgkin Lymphoma (NHL)	Small-Cell Carcinoma
Age	All ages	Older adults
Location	Lung	Lung
Signs and symptoms	Painless lymphadenopathy, fevers, night sweats, fatigue, weight loss	Cough, chest pain, shortness of breath, weight loss, fatigue; symptoms associated with paraneoplastic syndromes
Etiology	Associated with autoimmune diseases, viruses, radiation, chemotherapy, and immunodeficiencies	Predominantly tobacco smoking; radon exposure
Cytomorphology	• Discohesive population of cells *(Figures 2.10.1* and *2.10.2)* • Monotonous or pleomorphic population of cells, depending on lymphoma type • Thin cytoplasmic rim *(Figure 2.10.3)* • Lymphoglandular bodies in background *(Figure 2.10.1)* • Chromatin streaking artifact on conventional smear preparations *(Figure 2.10.4)* • Coarse chromatin or prominent nucleoli *(Figure 2.10.5)*	• Often cellular with predominantly dispersed single cells with or without tissue fragments *(Figure 2.10.6)* • Background of necrosis and/or apoptotic cells *(Figure 2.10.7)* • Despite the name, cells are larger than bystanding inflammatory cells and are pleomorphic (more obvious on Diff-Quik preparations) *(Figure 2.10.8)* • Chromatin streaking artifact on conventional smear preparations *(Figure 2.10.8)* • Cells have little cytoplasm and nuclei may "mold" together *(Figures 2.10.9* and *2.10.10)* • "Salt-and-pepper" neuroendocrine chromatin pattern, best seen on Pap stained preparations *(Figure 2.10.10)*
Special studies	Negative for keratin and usually positive for CD45. Most are of B-cell origin and express B-cell markers (eg, CD20).	Considered a morphologic diagnosis. May paradoxically lack expression of neuroendocrine markers (chromogranin, synaptophysin, INSM1); dotlike positivity for pan-keratin; 90% positive for TTF-1 (not specific for a lung origin); high Ki-67 index (often >90%)
Molecular alterations	Various, depending on subtype	Inactivating mutations in *TP53* or *RB*
Treatment	Varies and may include watchful waiting, chemotherapy, radiation, immunotherapy, and stem cell transplantation	Primarily chemoradiation
Clinical implications	Treatment is significantly different than for carcinoma	Poor prognosis

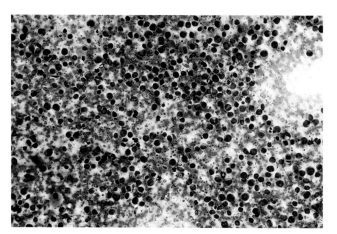

Figure 2.10.1   Non-Hodgkin lymphoma. Numerous lymphoma cells are scattered throughout the field. The background contains small "lymphoglandular bodies," small fragments of cytoplasm often seen in the background of both benign and malignant lymphoid proliferations and absent in small-cell carcinoma.

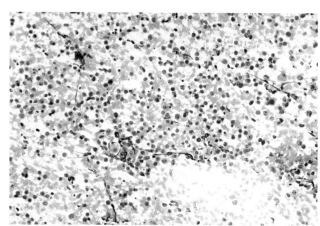

Figure 2.10.2   Non-Hodgkin lymphoma. At this magnification, the lymphoma cells appear monotonous and little cytoplasm can be appreciated. Chromatin streaks, an artifact seen in both small-cell carcinoma and lymphoid populations, are present in several areas.

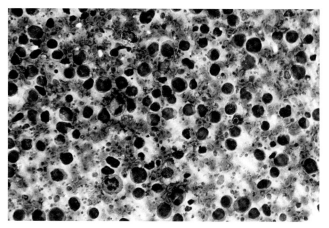

Figure 2.10.3   Non-Hodgkin lymphoma. Lymphoid cells often have a thin rim of blue cytoplasm whereas small-cell carcinoma cells have little appreciable cytoplasm. Note the small purple "lymphoglandular bodies" seen throughout the background.

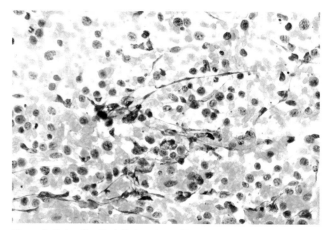

Figure 2.10.4   Non-Hodgkin lymphoma. The cytoplasm of lymphoid cells is more difficult to appreciate on air-dried Pap stain preparations. The chromatin pattern of lymphoid cells can mimic the "salt-and-pepper" chromatin pattern seen in neuroendocrine neoplasms such as small-cell carcinoma.

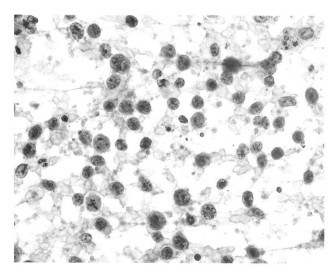

Figure 2.10.5   Non-Hodgkin lymphoma. Lymphoid cells are generally more dispersed than small-cell carcinoma cells, which usually form at least some small fragments in which nuclear molding can be seen.

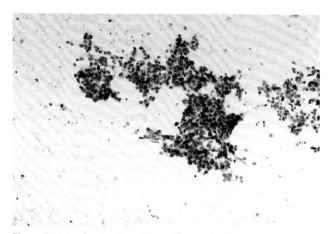

Figure 2.10.6   Small-cell carcinoma. These cells form small, irregularly shaped tissue fragments. The cells are loosely cohesive, and some cells can be seen singly in the background.

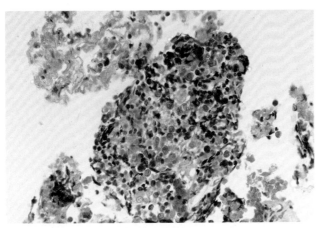

Figure 2.10.7 Small-cell carcinoma. Cell block preparations are helpful in highlighting the "geographic" necrosis seen in small-cell carcinoma—viable cells adjacent to intact necrotic cells.

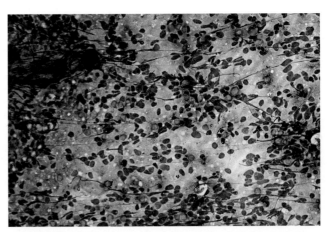

Figure 2.10.8 Small-cell carcinoma. This small-cell carcinoma specimen demonstrates hypercellularity prominent nuclear streaking artifact.

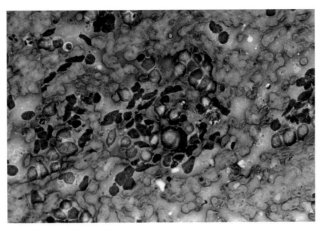

Figure 2.10.9 Small-cell carcinoma. This field contains rare small cells with a thin rim of cytoplasm, which mimics a lymphoid morphology. However, most of the cells have little identifiable cytoplasm and adjacent cells have prominent nuclear molding, features not seen in lymphomas.

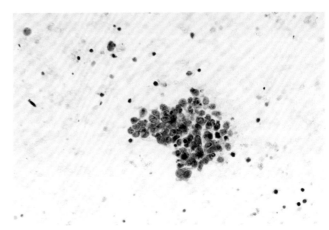

Figure 2.10.10 Small-cell carcinoma. These cells have little cytoplasm, and their nuclei are irregularly shaped due to the nuclear molding often seen in this neoplasm.

	Goblet Cell Hyperplasia	Adenocarcinoma
Age	Any age but more often in adults	Older adults
Location	Lung	Lung
Signs and symptoms	Symptoms related to underlying cause	Fatigue, weight loss, cough, dyspnea, hemoptysis, chest pain, and/or lesion seen on imaging studies of the lung
Etiology	A nonspecific, protective response to chronic injury of the bronchial epithelium	Classically associated with tobacco smoking; never-smokers are more likely to be younger, female, and/or Asian
Cytomorphology	• Tissue fragments containing a mixture of benign bronchial respiratory cells and goblet cells, or rare individually dispersed goblet cells *(Figure 2.11.1)* • Goblet cells may be the predominate cell type *(Figure 2.11.2)* • Goblet cells are columnar cells that usually appear as "punched out" spaces containing mucin in tissue fragments • Goblet cells may undergo reactive changes and have mild nuclear irregularities and small nucleoli *(Figures 2.11.3 and 2.11.4)* • Bronchial respiratory cells may also have reactive atypia, but the presence of cilia is reassuring for a benign process *(Figures 2.11.3 and 2.11.5)*	• Tissue fragments which may form glandular structures or three-dimensional fragments *(Figures 2.11.6 and 2.11.7)* • Singly dispersed cells may predominate *(Figure 2.11.8)* • Usually eccentrically placed nucleus with coarse chromatin and/or prominent nucleoli *(Figures 2.11.7 and 2.11.9)* • Foamy cytoplasm which may contain mucin vacuoles *(Figure 2.11.9)* • Anisonucleosis, hyperchromasia, and irregular nuclear borders *(Figure 2.11.10)*
Special studies	Special stains for mucin (mucicarmine) will be positive in goblet cells	Usually positive for TTF-1 (nuclear) and napsin-A (cytoplasmic granular); negative for markers of squamous differentiation (p40/p63) unless a squamous component exists; negative for mesothelial markers
Molecular alterations	None	Mutations in *EGFR, KRAS, BRAF, ALK, RET, ROS1* translocations; amplification of *MET* or *FGFR1*
Treatment	Treat the underlying cause	Surgical resection +/− chemoradiation for stage I/II tumors; for advanced stage, chemoradiation and/or targeted therapies/immunotherapy
Clinical implications	A background finding in exfoliative lung specimens.	Prognosis depends on tumor stage and the presence of targetable molecular alterations/eligibility for immunotherapy

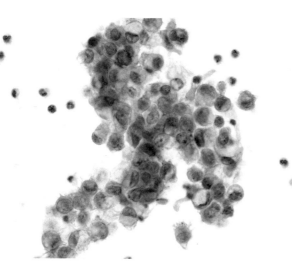

Figure 2.11.1   Goblet cell hyperplasia. A mixture of loosely cohesive goblet cells and bronchial respiratory cells. Most of the cells are round in shape, with goblet cells containing clear-appearing mucin vacuoles and bronchial respiratory cells possessing pink cilia.

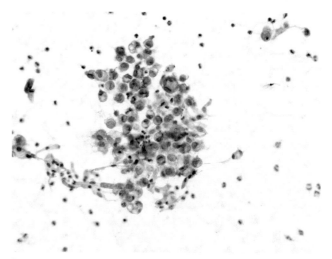

Figure 2.11.2   Goblet cell hyperplasia. A dispersed population of benign goblet cells admixed with bronchial respiratory cells. The goblet cells contain cytoplasmic mucin vacuoles, giving the appearance of a mucinous adenocarcinoma.

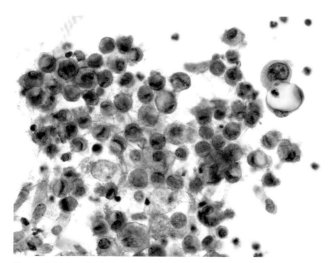

Figure 2.11.3   Goblet cell hyperplasia. A mixture of benign goblet cells and bronchial respiratory cells. Some of the bronchial respiratory cells are columnar shaped, which makes them readily identifiable. Others have a round shape, which may cause them to be mistaken for atypical epithelial cells.

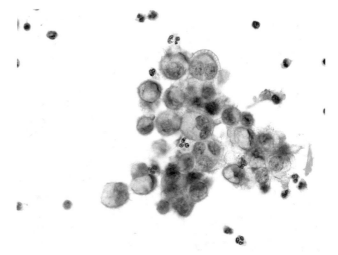

Figure 2.11.4   Goblet cell hyperplasia. Round goblet cells and bronchial respiratory cells. The bronchial respiratory cells are sometimes binucle-ated and contain rare cilia that may be missed.

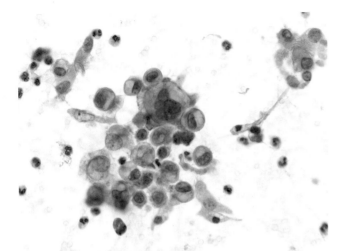

Figure 2.11.5   Goblet cell hyperplasia. Bronchial respiratory cells may have reactive atypia, such as this multinucleated ciliated cell. The presence of benign bronchial respiratory cells provides reassurance that the admixed mucin-containing cells are in fact benign goblet cells.

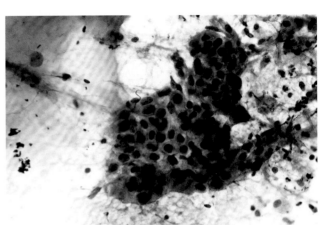

Figure 2.11.6   Adenocarcinoma. The nuclei are dark, vary in size, and have markedly irregular nuclear borders.

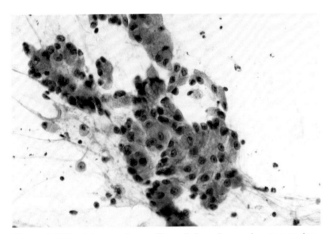

Figure 2.11.7   Adenocarcinoma. The cells have low nuclear to cytoplasmic ratios but have prominent nucleoli and irregular nuclear borders.

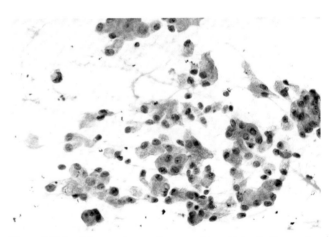

Figure 2.11.8   Adenocarcinoma. As opposed to goblet cells, these cells are more columnar and have foamy cytoplasm rather than a distinct large mucin vacuole.

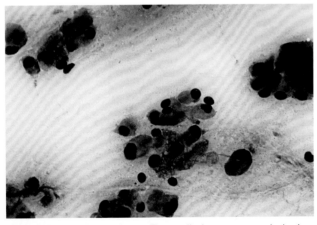

Figure 2.11.9   Adenocarcinoma. These cells demonstrate marked anisonucleosis, a feature lacking in reactive goblet cells.

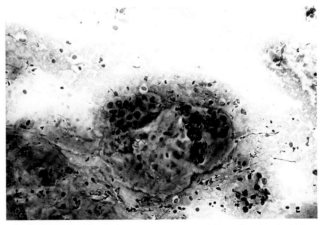

Figure 2.11.10   Adenocarcinoma. The cell nuclei are disordered within the fragment and appear enlarged, with different shapes and sizes.

	Pneumocyte Hyperplasia	Adenocarcinoma
Age	Older adults	Older adults
Location	Lung	Lung
Signs and symptoms	Symptoms associated with underlying cause of acute lung injury, such as shortness of breath and cyanosis	Fatigue, weight loss, cough, dyspnea, hemoptysis, chest pain, and/or lesion seen on imaging studies of the lung
Etiology	Proliferation of type II pneumocytes in response to acute lung injury (secondary to sepsis, pancreatitis, pneumonia, aspiration, etc)	Classically associated with tobacco smoking; never-smokers are more likely to be younger, female, and/or Asian
Cytomorphology	• Shed singly or in groups *(Figures 2.12.1 and 2.12.2)* • Elevated N/C ratios • Mild nuclear membrane irregularities *(Figure 2.12.3)* • May have distinct or prominent nucleoli *(Figures 2.12.4 and 2.12.5)*	• Tissue fragments which may form glandular structures or three-dimensional fragments *(Figures 2.12.6 and 2.12.7)* • Singly dispersed cells in poorly differentiated or necrotic tumors • Usually eccentrically placed nucleus with coarse chromatin and/or prominent nucleoli *(Figure 2.12.8)* • Foamy cytoplasm which may contain mucin vacuoles *(Figure 2.12.9)* • Anisonucleosis, hyperchromasia, and irregular nuclear borders *(Figure 2.12.10)*
Special studies	Usually not performed on exfoliative specimens; positive for TTF-1 and cytokeratin	Usually positive for TTF-1 (nuclear) and napsin-A (cytoplasmic granular); negative for markers of squamous differentiation (p40/p63) unless a squamous component exists; negative for mesothelial markers
Molecular alterations	None	Mutations in *EGFR, KRAS, BRAF, ALK, RET, ROS1* translocations; amplification of *MET* or *FGFR1*
Treatment	Treatment of the underlying cause	Surgical resection +/− chemoradiation for stage I/II tumors; for advanced stage, chemoradiation and/or targeted therapies/immunotherapy
Clinical implications	Pneumocyte hyperplasia is a background reactive change that should not be mistaken for a neoplasm	Prognosis depends on tumor stage and the presence of targetable molecular alterations/eligibility for immunotherapy

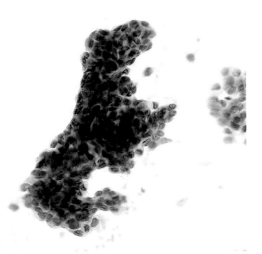

Figure 2.12.1   Pneumocyte hyperplasia. An irregularly shaped fragment of cells with predominantly oval-shaped nuclei with mild nuclear border irregularities. The chromatin is bland in appearance.

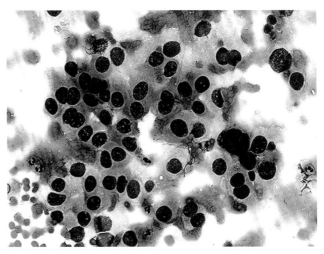

Figure 2.12.2   Pneumocyte hyperplasia. A group of loosely cohesive cells with slight variation in nuclear size and mild nuclear border irregularities.

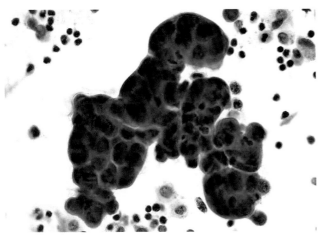

Figure 2.12.3   Pneumocyte hyperplasia. A small branching fragment containing reactive pneumocytes. The cells have high N/C ratios, which may cause concern for an adenocarcinoma.

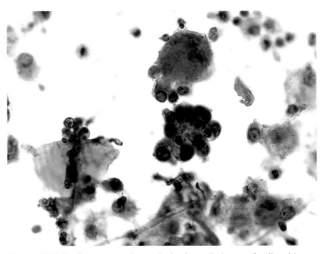

Figure 2.12.4   Pneumocyte hyperplasia. A small cluster of cells with elevated N/C ratios. The nuclei contain small yet distinct nucleoli.

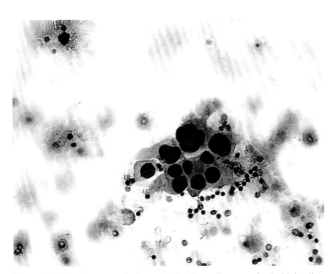

Figure 2.12.5   Pneumocyte hyperplasia. A small group of cuboidal cells with irregularities in their nuclear contours and prominent nucleoli.

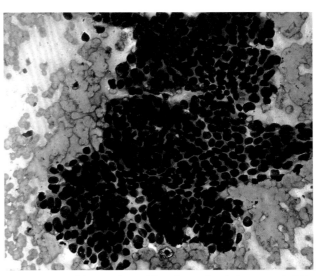

Figure 2.12.6   Adenocarcinoma. The cells are disorderly arranged within the fragment and demonstrate anisonucleosis, nuclear border irregularities, and high N/C ratios.

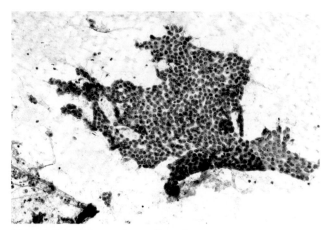

Figure 2.12.7   Adenocarcinoma. The cells are monotonous but have high N/C ratios and prominent nucleoli and are present in large numbers, favoring a neoplastic process.

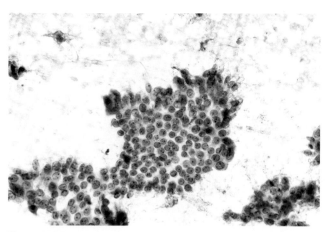

Figure 2.12.8   Adenocarcinoma. Adenocarcinoma cells often have eccentrically placed nuclei with either coarse chromatin or prominent nucleoli (seen here).

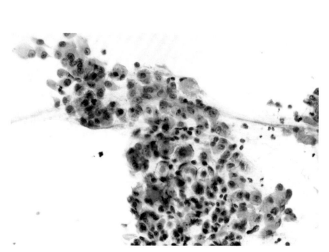

Figure 2.12.9   Adenocarcinoma. Some of these cells contain mucinous vacuoles, which sometimes appear pink on a Pap-stained preparation such as this.

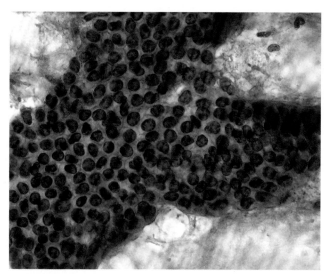

Figure 2.12.10   Adenocarcinoma. The cells have nuclei with markedly irregular contours and great variation in size.

	Postpneumonia Changes	Adenocarcinoma
Age	Any age	Older adults
Location	Lung	Lung
Signs and symptoms	Cough, fever, chills, shortness of breath, fatigue, chest pain, sputum production	Fatigue, weight loss, cough, dyspnea, hemoptysis, chest pain, and/or lesion seen on imaging studies of the lung
Etiology	Pneumonia	Classically associated with tobacco smoking; never-smokers are more likely to be younger, female, and/or Asian
Cytomorphology	• Reactive pneumocytes, respiratory epithelial cells, and macrophages intermixed with inflammatory cells *(Figure 2.13.1)* • Reactive respiratory epithelial cells may form small fragments or be found singly and have increased N/C ratios and prominent nucleoli; cilia may or may not be identified *(Figures 2.13.2 and 2.13.3)* • Hyperplastic pneumocytes may form fragments or be found singly, with polygonal cytoplasm, prominent nucleoli, and irregular nuclear borders *(Figures 2.13.4 and 2.13.5)*	• Tissue fragments which may form glandular structures or three-dimensional fragments *(Figure 2.13.6)* • Singly dispersed cells in poorly differentiated or necrotic tumors *(Figure 2.13.7)* • Necrosis is associated with background acute inflammatory cells *(Figure 2.13.8)* • Usually eccentrically placed nucleus with coarse chromatin and/or prominent nucleoli *(Figure 2.13.9)* • Foamy cytoplasm which may contain mucin vacuoles *(Figure 2.13.9)* • Anisonucleosis, hyperchromasia, and irregular nuclear borders *(Figure 2.13.10)*
Special studies	Usually not performed on exfoliative cytology specimens; pneumocytes are positive for TTF-1 and cytokeratin; macrophages are positive for CD68. Hemosiderin-laden macrophages are positive by iron special stains.	Usually positive for TTF-1 (nuclear) and napsin-A (cytoplasmic granular); negative for markers of squamous differentiation (p40/p63) unless a squamous component exists; negative for mesothelial markers.
Molecular alterations	None	Mutations in *EGFR, KRAS, BRAF, ALK, RET, ROS1* translocations; amplification of *MET* or *FGFR1*
Treatment	Treatment of the underlying pneumonia	Surgical resection +/− chemoradiation for stage I/II tumors; for advanced stage, chemoradiation and/or targeted therapies/immunotherapy
Clinical implications	Background changes that should not be mistaken for a neoplasm	Prognosis depends on tumor stage and the presence of targetable molecular alterations/eligibility for immunotherapy

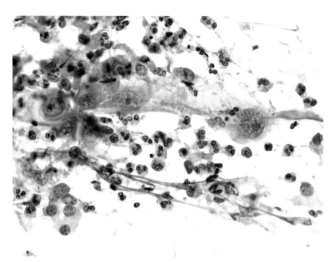

Figure 2.13.1 Postpneumonia changes. A mixture of large, reactive epithelial cells with prominent nucleoli, smaller ciliated bronchial respiratory epithelial cells, and inflammatory cells.

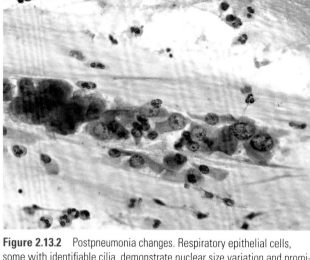

Figure 2.13.2 Postpneumonia changes. Respiratory epithelial cells, some with identifiable cilia, demonstrate nuclear size variation and prominent nucleoli. The nuclear contours remain round and regular.

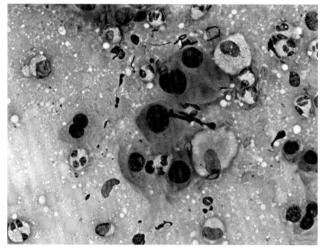

Figure 2.13.3 Postpneumonia changes. High magnification of reactive respiratory epithelial cells, with enlarged nuclei, prominent nucleoli, and rare binucleation. The nuclear contours remain regular. Cilia are present on some cells but are difficult to identify.

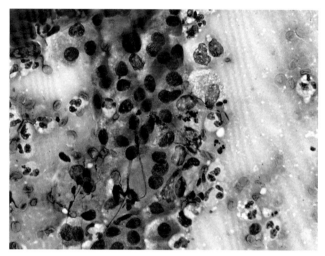

Figure 2.13.4 Postpneumonia changes. Hyperplastic pneumocytes with polygonal cytoplasm, prominent nucleoli, and mild nuclear border irregularities. The cells lack cilia.

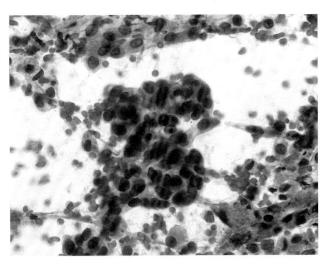

Figure 2.13.5   Postpneumonia changes. Hyperplastic pneumocytes form a three-dimensional structure and can be seen in the background. The nuclei have slight border irregularities and prominent nucleoli.

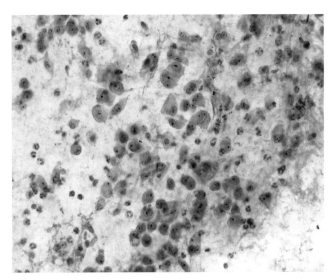

Figure 2.13.6   Adenocarcinoma. A necrotic adenocarcinoma, in which the tumor cells are predominantly individually dispersed in a necrotic background. The nuclei vary greatly in size and have irregular borders and prominent nucleoli.

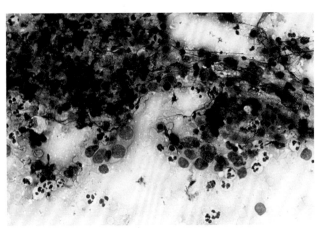

Figure 2.13.7   Adenocarcinoma. A necrotic adenocarcinoma associated with inflammatory cells. The N/C ratios are high, and the nuclei have markedly irregular nuclear borders.

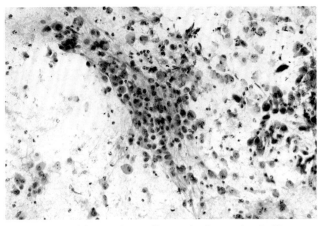

Figure 2.13.8   Adenocarcinoma. Dispersed cells associated with a background of inflammation and necrosis.

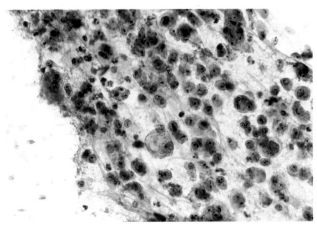

Figure 2.13.9   Adenocarcinoma. Cells demonstrating multinucleation, markedly irregular nuclear borders, coarse chromatin, and anisonucleosis. One cell has abundant, vacuolated cytoplasm.

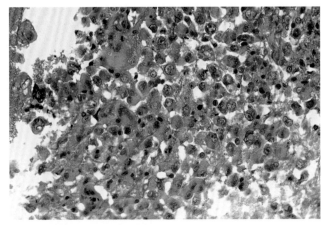

Figure 2.13.10   Adenocarcinoma. The nuclei are eccentrically placed, vary greatly in size, and have markedly irregular nuclear borders.

	Squamous Metaplasia	Squamous Cell Carcinoma
Age	Any, but generally adults	Older adults
Location	Lung	Lung
Signs and symptoms	Depends on the underlying etiology	Fatigue, weight loss, cough, dyspnea, hemoptysis, chest pain, and/or lesion seen on imaging studies of the lung
Etiology	Repetitive injury to the bronchial epithelium (often due to tobacco smoking) in which pseudostratified epithelium is replaced by stratified squamous epithelium	Classically associated with tobacco smoking
Cytomorphology	• Cells present singly or in tissue fragments with thin gaps between cells, creating a "tiling" effect (*Figures 2.14.1* and *2.14.2*) • Cells contain dense cytoplasm which may be keratinized (*Figure 2.14.3*) • Metaplastic cells may be associated with benign ciliated respiratory epithelial cells (*Figure 2.14.4*) • Nuclei contain bland chromatin and/or nucleoli (*Figure 2.14.2*) • Nuclear contours are regular (*Figures 2.14.1* and *2.14.5*)	• Tissue fragments and dispersed single cells, often with a background of necrosis (*Figures 2.14.6* and *2.14.7*) • Nuclei tend to be centrally placed (*Figure 2.14.7*) • Dense cytoplasm that may form irregular, rigid projections (*Figure 2.14.8*) • Keratinizing tumor cells which have pink cytoplasm on Pap stained preparations (*Figure 2.14.8*) • Anisnucleosis and irregular nuclear contours (*Figure 2.14.9*) • Pyknotic nuclei are small and hyperchromatic and have markedly irregular borders, or nuclei with coarse chromatin or prominent nucleoli (*Figure 2.14.10*)
Special studies	Positive for squamous markers (p40/p63) and negative for TTF-1 and napsin-A	Positive for p40/p63 and negative for TTF-1 and napsin-A. Negative for HPV studies unless metastatic from other sites
Molecular alterations	None	Driver mutations have not been well established
Treatment	None	Surgical resection +/− chemoradiation for stage I/II tumors; for advanced stage, chemoradiation and/or immunotherapy
Clinical implications	Benign metaplasia which should not be mistaken for a neoplasm	Prognosis depends on tumor stage and eligibility for immunotherapy

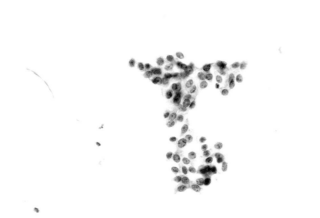

Figure 2.14.1   Squamous metaplasia. A small fragment of metaplastic squamous cells. The cells have regular nuclear borders and bland chromatin.

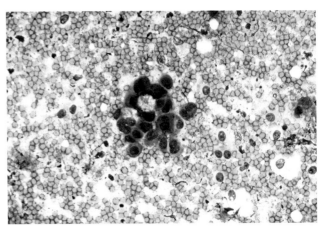

Figure 2.14.2   Squamous metaplasia. Metaplastic squamous cells, each with dense-appearing cytoplasm. Thin gaps can be seen between some cells, causing the cells to emulate tiles from a mosaic.

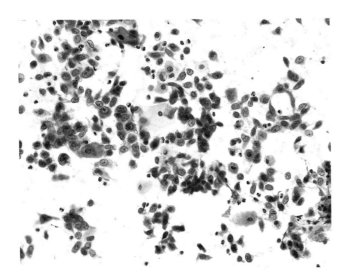

Figure 2.14.3   Squamous metaplasia. Rare keratinized metaplastic cells have pink cytoplasm and are admixed with numerous non-keratinized metaplastic cells.

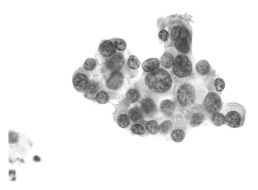

Figure 2.14.4   Squamous metaplasia. In this fragment, metaplastic cells (lacking cilia) are associated with benign ciliated respiratory epithelial cells. This helps identify the presence of squamous metaplasia in a specimen and dismiss metaplastic changes as benign.

2 PULMONARY

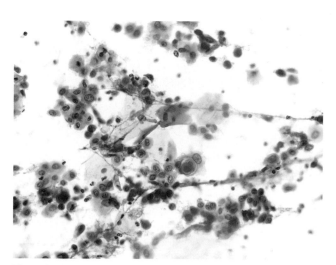

Figure 2.14.5 Squamous metaplasia. Metaplastic squamous cells with regular nuclear contours and small nucleoli. The nuclei are centrally placed, and the cell cytoplasm is dense. A benign squamous pearl has formed in the center of the field.

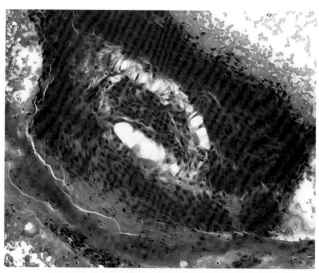

Figure 2.14.6 Squamous cell carcinoma. The cells in the fragment have enlarged nuclei, causing an appearance of overlapping nuclei.

Figure 2.14.7 Squamous cell carcinoma. There are keratinizing, dispersed malignant cells in a background of necrosis. Keratinaceous debris can be seen with "ghost" nuclei in the center of the field.

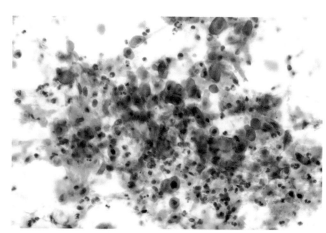

Figure 2.14.8 Squamous cell carcinoma. The malignant cells are keratinizing and have irregular cytoplasmic projections.

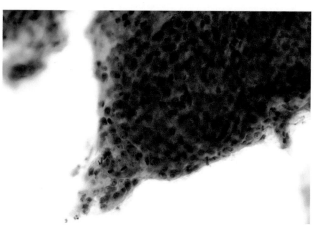

Figure 2.14.9 Squamous cell carcinoma. Cells with high N/C ratios, variation in nuclear size, and irregular nuclear borders. Some cells have enlarged nucleoli.

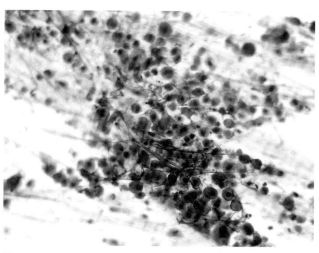

Figure 2.14.10 Squamous cell carcinoma. The field contains numerous malignant cells, many with pyknotic nuclei that appear "coal black" and have markedly irregular nuclear borders.

	Pulmonary Alveolar Proteinosis	*Pneumocystis jirovecii* Infection
Age	Any; average age is 39 y	Any
Location	Lung	Lung
Signs and symptoms	Shortness of breath, fever, cough, weight loss	Atypical interstitial pneumonia; fever; cough; wheezing; fatigue; chest pain
Etiology	Autoimmunity to granulocyte-macrophage colony stimulating factor (GM-CSF), which reduces alveolar macrophage development and function. Can also be caused secondarily to malignancy, infection, and environmental exposures	Opportunistic fungus seen in immunosuppressed patients and historically associated with AIDS patients
Cytomorphology	• Background of dispersed granular debris and acellular crystalloids *(Figures 2.15.1-2.15.3)* • Background pigmented macrophages *(Figures 2.15.1-2.15.3)* • PAS-positive material in macrophages and background *(Figures 2.15.4 and 2.15.5)*	• Scattered cohesive groups of granular debris *(Figures 2.15.6-2.15.8)* • Granular debris contains negative images of organisms *(Figures 2.15.9 and 2.15.10)*
Special studies	Amorphous material is positive by the PAS and PAS-diastase special stains; negative for special silver stains	Organisms are positive for special silver stains (eg, GMS); negative for PAS
Molecular alterations	Not relevant in most cases	Not applicable
Treatment	Whole lung lavage	Pentamidine and treatment of the underlying cause of immunosuppression
Clinical implications	Patients may undergo remission and symptoms may recur. Underlying causes (such as malignancy) should be excluded	Fatal in untreated patients

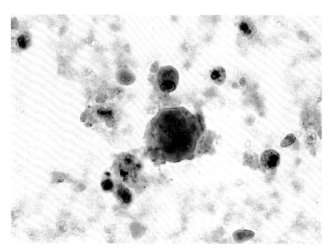

Figure 2.15.1   Pulmonary alveolar proteinosis. Dispersed granular debris, crystalloids, and pigmented macrophages are commonly seen in pulmonary alveolar proteinosis.

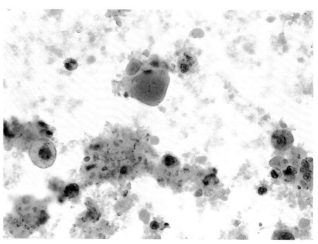

Figure 2.15.2   Pulmonary alveolar proteinosis. The field contains granular debris, crystalloids, and pigmented macrophages.

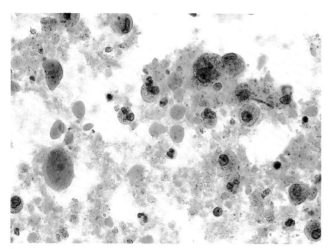

Figure 2.15.3   Pulmonary alveolar proteinosis. In this field, several macrophages contain abundant pigment.

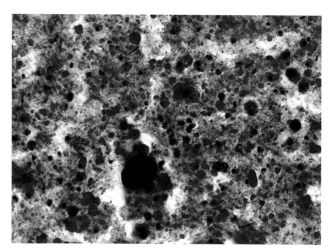

Figure 2.15.4   Pulmonary alveolar proteinosis. The granular and amorphous debris are positive by PAS and PAS-diastase special stains.

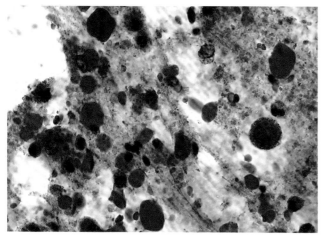

Figure 2.15.5   Pulmonary alveolar proteinosis. This separate field of a PAS special stain demonstrates granular debris, macrophages, and amorphous material.

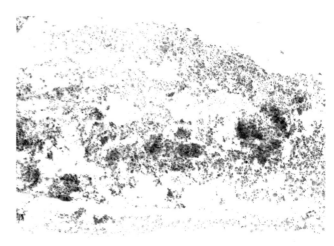

Figure 2.15.6   *Pneumocystis jirovceii.* The organisms form clumps of granular debris (alveolar casts) which appear red in this field. The background contains pulmonary alveolar macrophages and inflammatory cells.

2 PULMONARY

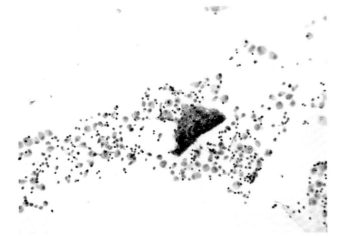

Figure 2.15.7 *Pneumocystis jirovceii.* A higher magnification view of clumped, foamy-appearing debris which is formed from *Pneumocystis* organisms. The organisms do not stain on routine cytologic preparations, providing the "empty spaces" seen within the debris.

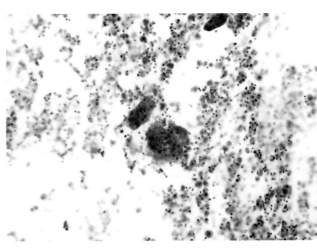

Figure 2.15.8 *Pneumocystis jirovceii.* Separate field demonstrating several clumps of *Pneumocystis* organisms forming "alveolar casts".

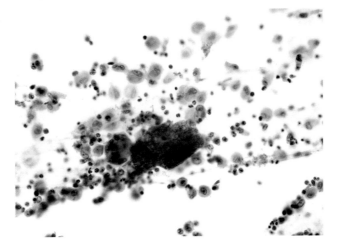

Figure 2.15.9 *Pneumocystis jirovceii.* A high-magnification view of a group of *Pneumocystis* organisms. While the organisms would be positive on a silver stain, this cytomorphologic finding is pathognomonic of *Pneumocystis*.

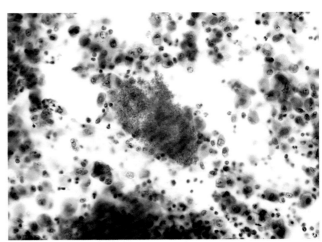

Figure 2.15.10 *Pneumocystis jirovceii.* Examination at high magnification is required to identify the "negative image" appearance of the organisms on routine preparations.

3
Urinary Tract

	Degenerative Atypia	Degenerated High-Grade Urothelial Carcinoma
Age	Any	Usually older adults (>50 y of age)
Location	Urinary tract	Urinary tract
Signs and symptoms	Patients typically submit urine due to hematuria or surveillance for a history of urothelial carcinoma	Asymptomatic or hematuria
Etiology	Benign exfoliated urothelial lining cells that have degenerated within the human body before procurement	Strong association with tobacco smoking; industrial chemical exposures
Cytomorphology	• Predominantly dispersed urothelial cells (Figure 3.1.1) • Degenerated urothelial cells may have vacuolated or granular cytoplasm (Figures 3.1.1 and 3.1.2) • Degenerated urothelial cells with low N/C ratios due to small, pyknotic nuclei (Figure 3.1.3) • The nucleus may be dark and have irregular borders but is generally much smaller and less hyperchromatic than the pyknotic nuclei seen in degenerated HGUC (Figures 3.1.4 and 3.1.5) • Sometimes an indistinct cytoplasmic-nuclear interface • Melamed-Wolinksa bodies are small, round concretions in cytoplasm of degenerated urothelial cells but can also be seen in degenerated HGUC cells (Figure 3.1.3)	• Predominantly single cells but can exist in small fragments (Figure 3.1.6) • Large cells with hyperchromatic nuclei and irregular nuclear borders (Figure 3.1.7) • N/C ratio may not be elevated in degenerated cells due to decreased nuclear size and degenerated cytoplasm (Figure 3.1.7) • Coarse chromatin pattern; in rare instances, cells may have prominent nucleoli instead (Figure 3.1.8) • Some nuclei appear "India ink black" and a chromatin pattern cannot be assessed (Figures 3.1.7 and 3.1.9)
Special studies	FISH to exclude HGUC	FISH to detect chromosomal abnormalities; numerous non–slide-based ancillary tests exist
Molecular alterations	N/A	Aneuploidy; frequently TERT promoter mutations; TP53 mutations
Treatment	N/A	Depending on tumor type and extent of disease (both determined on biopsy), transurethral resection; intravesical BCG; intravesical chemotherapy; cystectomy; and/or chemoradiation
Clinical implications	N/A	Depends on extent of disease and/or responsiveness to intravesical treatment

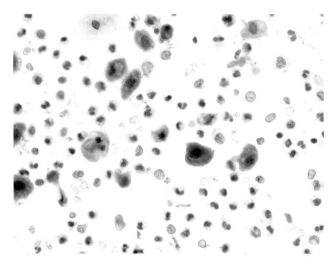

Figure 3.1.1   Degenerative atypia. Several degenerating benign urothelial cells are seen among smaller inflammatory cells. The cytoplasm of the degenerated cells is abundant, vacuolated, and granular. The nuclei are moderately hyperchromatic and have nuclear border irregularities. The N/C ratios are low.

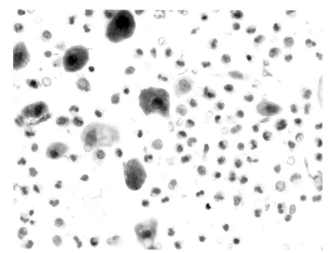

Figure 3.1.2   Degenerative atypia. A field of degenerated benign urothelial cells. The nuclei are relatively uniform in size despite their irregular shapes. The cytoplasm appears bubbly and degenerative.

Figure 3.1.3   Degenerative atypia. Numerous scattered small degenerative benign urothelial cells. The nuclei are small, have irregular border, and are darker than the nuclei of background inflammatory cells. Several cells contain cyanophilic or red-staining round bodies known as Melamed-Wolinska bodies.

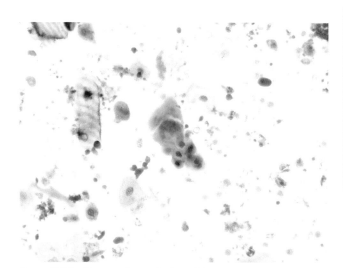

Figure 3.1.4   Degenerative atypia. A small fragment of degenerating benign urothelial cells each containing a small, dark nucleus with irregular borders. The level of hyperchromasia is acceptable for benign cells because their nuclei are not enlarged.

3   URINARY TRACT

Figure 3.1.5 Degenerative atypia. A group of degenerating benign urothelial cells with foamy cytoplasm and irregularly shaped, dark nuclei. The chromatin is not "ink black" as can be seen in degenerated HGUC cells.

Figure 3.1.6 Degenerated high-grade urothelial carcinoma (HGUC). The HGUC cells in this field have very large, dark nuclei. The nuclear borders are highly irregular. Because the cells have degenerating cytoplasm, the N/C ratios are low.

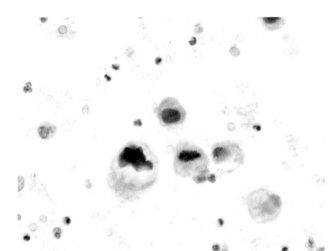

Figure 3.1.7 Degenerated high-grade urothelial carcinoma (HGUC). Large HGUC cells with vacuolated, degenerating cytoplasm. The nuclei are both large and dark, an indication that they possess an abnormal amount of DNA. One nucleus is at least 10 times as large as the nearby red blood cells.

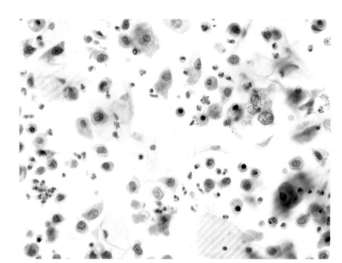

Figure 3.1.8 Degenerated high-grade urothelial carcinoma (HGUC). Numerous degenerating cells, some benign and some malignant, create a busy field. Three cells clustering together at the top right of the field have large nuclei with coarse chromatin, but degenerating cytoplasm. Other cells in the field do not have increased N/C ratios but are suspicious for HGUC, such as the cell in the top right corner, which has engulfed another cell.

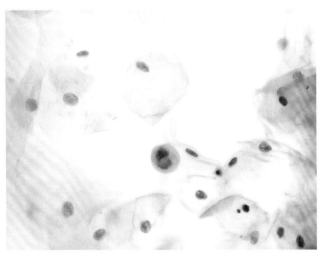

Figure 3.1.9   Degenerated high-grade urothelial carcinoma (HGUC). A single degenerating cell with a pyknotic nucleus. The chromatin is dark and the nucleus is irregularly shaped, almost appearing as two separate nuclei. Such a finding should raise the concern for HGUC, which may appear more convincingly in other fields once examined.

	Renal Tubular Cells	High-Grade Urothelial Carcinoma
Age	Any	Usually older adults (>50 y of age)
Location	Urinary tract	Urinary tract
Signs and symptoms	Asymptomatic; may be exfoliated secondary to renal stones and other causes of hematuria	Asymptomatic or hematuria
Etiology	Benign exfoliated renal tubular cells that have degenerated within the human body before procurement	Strong association with tobacco smoking; industrial chemical exposures
Cytomorphology	• Loosely cohesive clusters of 3-15 small cells with hobnailed edges *(Figure 3.2.1)* • Round nuclei with regular borders *(Figure 3.2.2)* • Low N/C ratios *(Figure 3.2.3)* • Nuclei appear darker than other background cells but are not "ink black" *(Figure 3.2.4)* • At high magnification, cells have slight variation in size but look uniform and smaller than urothelial cells at scanning magnification *(Figure 3.2.5)*	• Predominantly single cells but can exist in small fragments *(Figure 3.2.6)* • Large cells with hyperchromatic nuclei, coarse chromatin, and irregular nuclear borders *(Figure 3.2.7)* • Present in greater numbers than benign renal tubular cells *(Figures 3.2.6 and 3.2.7)* • High N/C ratios in well-preserved HGUC cells *(Figure 3.2.8)*
Special studies	FISH to exclude HGUC	FISH to detect chromosomal abnormalities; numerous non–slide-based ancillary tests exist
Molecular alterations	N/A	Aneuploidy; frequently TERT promoter mutations; TP53 mutations
Treatment	N/A	Depending on tumor type and extent of disease (both determined on biopsy), transurethral resection; intravesical BCG; intravesical chemotherapy; cystectomy; and/or chemoradiation
Clinical implications	N/A	Depends on extent of disease and/or responsiveness to intravesical treatment

Figure 3.2.1   Renal tubular cells. The cells are small and have round nuclei with regular contours and high N/C ratios. Occasional cells have cytoplasmic vacuoles.

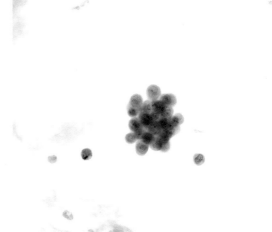

Figure 3.2.2   Renal tubular cells. Renal tubular cells are rarely present as single cells and usually form clusters of less than 20 cells. The clusters have hobnailed edges, causing cytomorphologic overlap with endometrial cells, which can also be seen in the urine.

Figure 3.2.3   Renal tubular cells. The cells appear small and uniform at low magnification, but higher magnification typically demonstrates some variation in nuclear and cellular size.

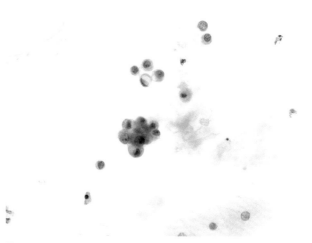

Figure 3.2.4   Renal tubular cells. Scattered renal tubular cells with slight hyperchromasia and vacuolated and/or granular cytoplasm. The nuclei are generally round and regular, and the cells have high N/C ratios.

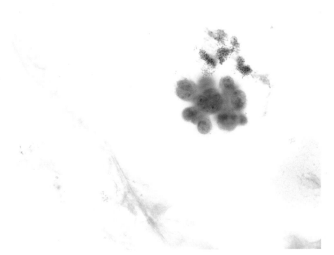

Figure 3.2.5   Renal tubular cells. Occasionally renal tubular cells may be large enough to resemble urothelial cells and their usual features would then cause concern for HGUC. One clue is the typical clustering of the cells in small groups such as this, best identified at low magnification. A second clue is the paucity of renal tubular cells; if there is any doubt, a large number of cells should be required to make a diagnosis of malignancy or suspicious for malignancy.

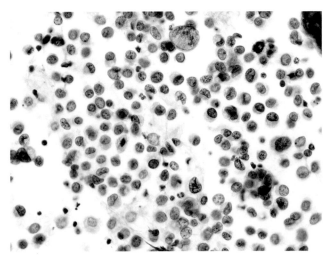

Figure 3.2.6   High-grade urothelial carcinoma (HGUC). The field contains numerous HGUC cells of different sizes. Most cells have high N/C ratios, coarse chromatin, and nuclear contour irregularities; the last two features are not typically seen in renal tubular cells. The cells are mostly individually dispersed, and some cells are much too large to be renal tubular cells.

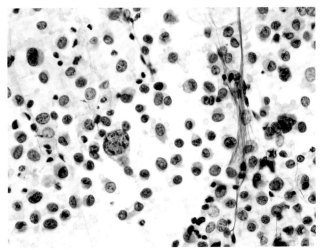

Figure 3.2.7   High-grade urothelial carcinoma (HGUC). A separate field of HGUC cells with high N/C ratios, coarse chromatin, and hyperchromasia. Many of the HGUC cells have regular nuclear borders, while others have irregularly shaped nuclei or nuclear notches.

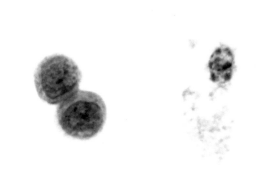

Figure 3.2.8   High-grade urothelial carcinoma (HGUC). Two loosely associated HGUC cells with high N/C ratios, nuclear membrane irregularities, and coarse chromatin. While no intact benign cells are in the background to provide an assessment of cellular size, these cells were much larger than renal tubular cells.

	Umbrella Cells	Degenerated High-Grade Urothelial Carcinoma
Age	Any	Usually older adults (>50 y of age)
Location	Urinary tract	Urinary tract
Signs and symptoms	Asymptomatic	Asymptomatic or hematuria
Etiology	Benign umbrella cells lining the urinary tract that have degenerated within the human body before procurement	Strong association with tobacco smoking; industrial chemical exposures
Cytomorphology	• Individually dispersed cells usually the size of a urothelial cell or larger *(Figure 3.3.1)* • Often abundant, granular and/or vacuolated cytoplasm that may be decreased in degenerating cells, causing an increased N/C ratio *(Figure 3.3.2)* • Usually one or two nuclei; multinucleated cells have identical nuclei *(Figures 3.3.3 and 3.3.4)* • Nuclei are round with regular contours with marginated chromatin and a single small nucleolus *(Figure 3.3.5)*	• Predominantly single cells but can exist in small fragments *(Figure 3.3.6)* • Large cells with hyperchromatic nuclei and irregular nuclear borders *(Figures 3.3.6 and 3.3.7)* • N/C ratio may not be elevated in degenerated cells due to decreased nuclear size and degenerated cytoplasm *(Figures 3.3.6-3.3.8)* • Coarse chromatin pattern; in rare instances, cells may have prominent nucleoli instead • Some nuclei have be "India ink black" and a chromatin pattern cannot be assessed *(Figure 3.3.9)*
Special studies	FISH to exclude HGUC	FISH to detect chromosomal abnormalities; numerous non–slide-based ancillary tests exist
Molecular alterations	N/A	Aneuploidy; frequently TERT promoter mutations; TP53 mutations
Treatment	N/A	Depending on tumor type and extent of disease (both determined on biopsy), transurethral resection; intravesical BCG; intravesical chemotherapy; cystectomy; and/or chemoradiation
Clinical implications	N/A	Depends on extent of disease and/or responsiveness to intravesical treatment

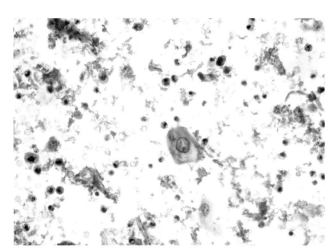

Figure 3.3.1   Umbrella cells. An umbrella cell in the center field is much larger than the surrounding inflammatory cells. The nucleus is seen centrally and the cytoplasm is abundant and granular. The chromatin is condensed along the nuclear membrane.

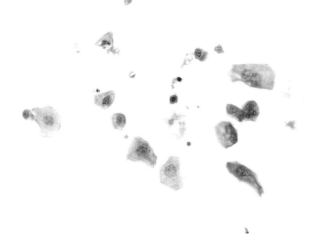

Figure 3.3.2   Umbrella cells. Numerous umbrella cells of different sizes. However, they all have similar-sized nuclei, polygonal cytoplasm, and the same granular cytoplasm. The N/C ratios vary widely.

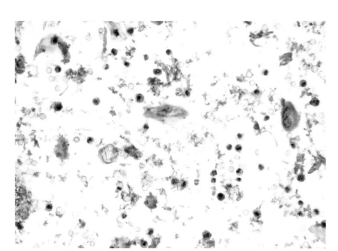

Figure 3.3.3   Two binucleated umbrella cells with abundant, granular cytoplasm in a background of blood and inflammation. The cells have cytoplasm that appears pale around the nuclei.

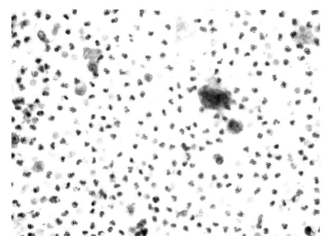

Figure 3.3.4   A large trinucleated umbrella cell can be seen in a background of acute inflammatory cells. The cytoplasm is degenerated and not intact. The three nuclei are uniform and round and have prominent nucleoli.

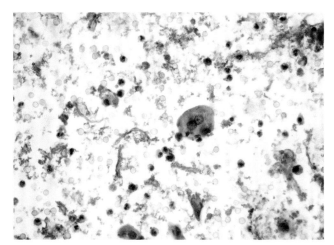

Figure 3.3.5   Umbrella cell. A binucleated umbrella cell in background of degenerated blood and intact red blood cells. The nuclei are identical, each with a single nucleoli and peripherally condensed chromatin.

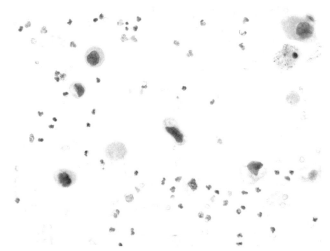

Figure 3.3.6   Degenerated high-grade urothelial carcinoma (HGUC). Degenerated high-grade urothelial cells with low N/C ratios due to the pyknotic nature of their nuclei. The nuclei are dark and have highly irregular nuclear borders. Overall, the cells and their nuclei are very large compared with the background inflammatory cells.

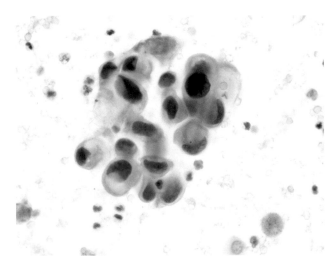

Figure 3.3.7   Degenerated high-grade urothelial carcinoma (HGUC). Despite their low N/C ratios, the cells and their nuclei are quite large. Some cells have "India ink black" nuclei.

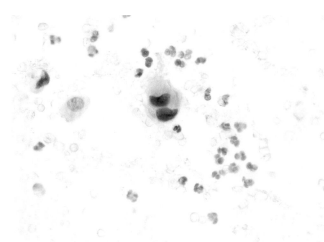

Figure 3.3.8   Degenerated high-grade urothelial carcinoma (HGUC). Two degenerated HGUC cells, one being engulfed by the other. The cells have extremely dark nuclei and highly irregular nuclear contours.

Figure 3.3.9   Degenerated high-grade urothelial carcinoma (HGUC). A single degenerated HGUC cell has dark chromatin and a nucleus that is more than 10 times larger than the nearby red blood cell. The nuclear borders are markedly irregular, and the N/C ratio is elevated.

	Low-Grade Urothelial Neoplasia	Benign Urothelial Tissue Fragments
Age	Any	Any; more often adults
Location	Urinary tract	Urinary tract
Signs and symptoms	Asymptomatic	Asymptomatic or hematuria
Etiology	Associated with cigarette smoking	Most have no known etiology; urolithiasis is the most common known cause
Cytomorphology	• Cellular specimen containing numerous monotonous urothelial cells singly dispersed and/or in tissue fragments (Figures 3.4.1 and 3.4.2) • Predominantly seen in washing/barbotage specimens • Tissue fragments may contain a fibrovascular core lined by the urothelial cells (Figures 3.4.2 and 3.4.3) • The urothelial cells have eccentrically placed nuclei ~1.5 times the size of red blood cells which are round to oval shaped (Figures 3.4.1 and 3.4.4) • Regular nuclear contours (Figure 3.4.1) • Bland chromatin with a small chromocenter (Figure 3.4.1) • The cell cytoplasm is oval, spindled, or columnar shaped and may be tapered (Figures 3.4.1 and 3.4.4)	• Small- to medium-sized fragments of urothelial cells (Figure 3.4.5) • Fragments contain "cytoplasmic collars" in which the cytoplasm faces toward the tissue fragment edges (Figures 3.4.6 and 3.4.7) • The urothelial cells are round, causing a hobnailed appearance to fragment edges (Figures 3.4.6 and 3.4.7) • Nuclei are round and have regular contours (Figures 3.4.6 and 3.4.7) • N/C ratios are usually below 0.5 (Figures 3.4.5-3.4.8) • Tissue fragments lack fibrovascular cores (Figures 3.4.5-3.4.8) • Umbrella cells may be associated with some fragments
Special studies	FISH to detect chromosomal abnormalities; numerous non–slide-based ancillary tests exist	FISH to exclude urothelial carcinoma
Molecular alterations	Aneuploidy; frequently TERT promoter mutations; FGFR mutations	N/A
Treatment	Typically transurethral resection and/or fulguration	N/A
Clinical implications	Generally excellent, but patients have a high risk of lifelong recurrence	N/A

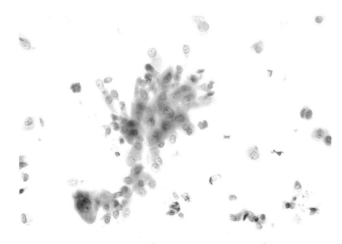

Figure 3.4.1   Low-grade urothelial carcinoma. The fragment does not contain a fibrovascular core, but the cells are monotonous, with uniform, bland nuclei and tapered cytoplasm.

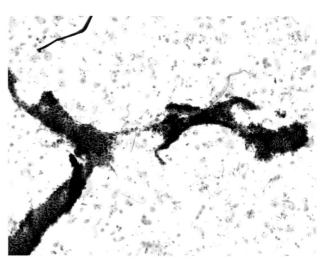

Figure 3.4.2   Low-grade urothelial carcinoma. A large tissue fragment with a true fibrovascular core, representing a papillary urothelial neoplasm. The fragment should be examined at higher magnification to exclude the presence of any high-grade features. In this case, the fragment contained uniform cells with small nuclei and regular nuclear contours and HGUC cells were not seen in the background.

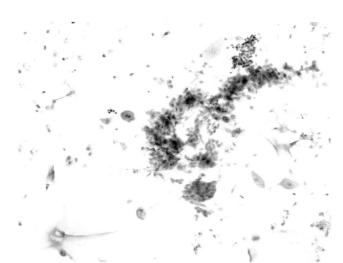

Figure 3.4.3   Low-grade urothelial carcinoma. The field shows a true papillary fragment containing a fibrovascular core. Monotonous urothelial cells are loosely attached to the fragment. These cells have oval-shaped nuclei, regular nuclear contours, and minimal anisonucleosis.

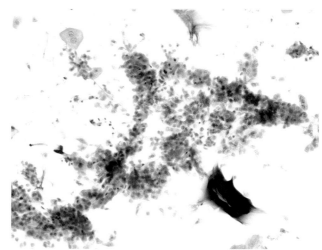

Figure 3.4.4   Low-grade urothelial carcinoma. A true papillary fragment with a fibrovascular core lined by monotonous, bland urothelial cells. The cells have small nuclei and N/C ratios below 0.5. No features of HGUC can be seen (hyperchromasia, high N/C ratios, irregular nuclear contours, or coarse chromatin).

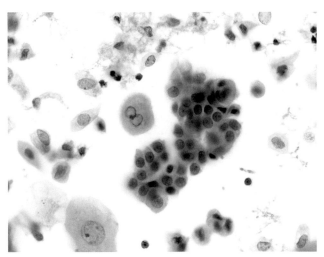

Figure 3.4.5   Benign urothelial tissue fragment. A small tissue fragment representing benign urothelium is seen. The nuclei are round and uniform and have regular contours. The fragment lacks a fibrovascular core, and the cells do not have tapered cytoplasm.

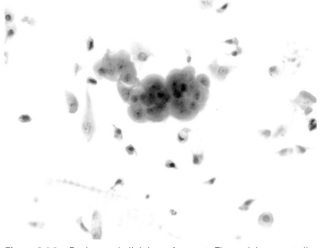

Figure 3.4.6   Benign urothelial tissue fragment. The nuclei are centrally placed, with cytoplasm lining the edge of the fragment, causing a "hob-nailed" effect. These are known as "cytoplasmic collars" and are thought to be associated with benign urothelium and not low-grade urothelial neoplasms.

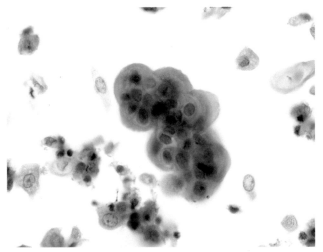

Figure 3.4.7   Benign urothelial tissue fragment. This small fragment of urothelial cells demonstrates cytoplasmic collars; the nuclei are primary seen centrally within the tissue fragment.

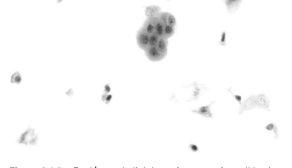

Figure 3.4.8   Benign urothelial tissue fragment. A small benign urothelial tissue fragment with cytoplasmic collars. The fragment is not associated with a fibrovascular core, and the cells do not have tapered cytoplasm.

	High-Grade Urothelial Carcinoma	Low-Grade Urothelial Neoplasia
Age	Usually older adults (>50 y of age)	Any
Location	Urinary tract	Urinary tract
Signs and symptoms	Asymptomatic or hematuria	Asymptomatic
Etiology	Strong association with tobacco smoking; industrial chemical exposures	Associated with cigarette smoking
Cytomorphology	• Predominantly single cells but can exist in small fragments *(Figure 3.5.1)* • Large cells with hyperchromatic nuclei, coarse chromatin, and irregular nuclear borders *(Figures 3.5.2 and 3.5.3)* • High N/C ratios in well-preserved HGUC cells *(Figure 3.5.4)*	• Cellular specimen containing numerous monotonous urothelial cells singly dispersed and/or in tissue fragments *(Figure 3.5.5)* • Predominantly seen in washing/barbotage specimens • Tissue fragments may contain a fibrovascular core lined by the urothelial cells *(Figure 3.5.6)* • The urothelial cells have eccentrically placed nuclei ~1.5 times the size of red blood cells which are round to oval shaped *(Figure 3.5.7)* • Regular nuclear contours *(Figure 3.5.8)* • Bland chromatin with a small chromocenter *(Figure 3.5.6)* • The cell cytoplasm is oval, spindled, or columnar shaped and may be tapered *(Figures 3.5.6 and 3.5.7)*
Special studies	FISH to detect chromosomal abnormalities; numerous non–slide-based ancillary tests exist	FISH to detect chromosomal abnormalities; numerous non–slide-based ancillary tests exist
Molecular alterations	Aneuploidy; frequently TERT promoter mutations; TP53 mutations	Aneuploidy; frequently TERT promoter mutations; FGFR mutations
Treatment	Depending on tumor type and extent of disease (both determined on biopsy), transurethral resection; intravesical BCG; intravesical chemotherapy; cystectomy; and/or chemoradiation	Typically transurethral resection and/or fulguration
Prognosis	Depends on extent of disease and/or responsiveness to intravesical treatment	Generally excellent, but patients have a high risk of lifelong recurrence

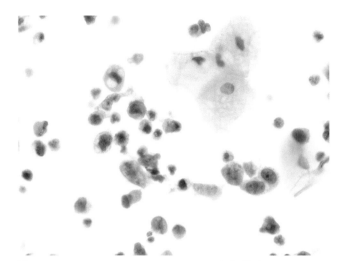

Figure 3.5.1   High-grade urothelial carcinoma (HGUC). Several high-grade urothelial carcinoma cells in various states of preservation. The well-preserved cells have high N/C ratios, while other cells are slightly degenerated and have vacuolated cytoplasm and smaller, darker nuclei with irregular nuclear contours.

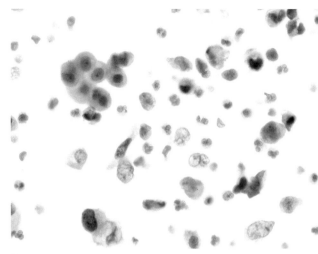

Figure 3.5.2   High-grade urothelial carcinoma (HGUC). High-grade urothelial cells are typically discohesive. Several cells here have high N/C ratios and irregular nuclear contours; many cells have clumpy chromatin which leaves the rest of the nucleus paradoxically hypochromatic.

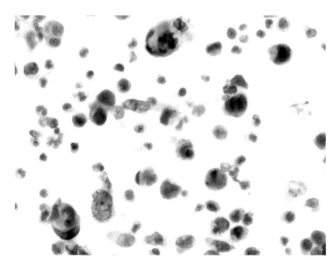

Figure 3.5.3   High-grade urothelial carcinoma (HGUC). Two large carcinoma cells have engulfed other malignant cells, creating a "cell-in-cell" morphology.

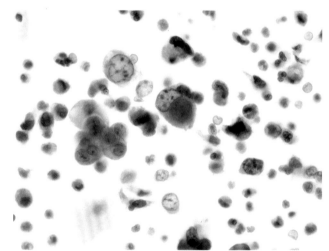

Figure 3.5.4   High-grade urothelial carcinoma (HGUC). The nuclei have highly irregular nuclear contours.

3   URINARY TRACT

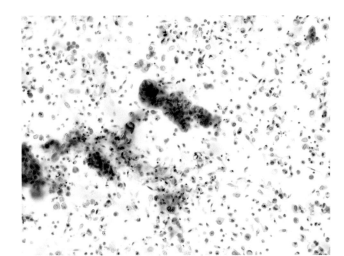

Figure 3.5.5 Low-grade urothelial carcinoma. Small fragments of a low-grade urothelial carcinoma in a background of numerous urothelial cells, many of which are likely to also form the carcinoma. Singly dispersed cells often have elongated cytoplasm.

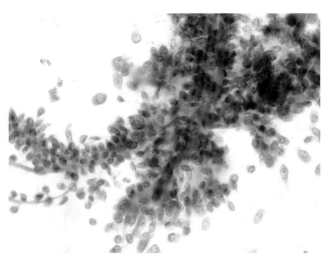

Figure 3.5.6 Low-grade urothelial carcinoma. A fibrovascular stalk lined by numerous monotonous urothelial cells, suggesting a low-grade urothelial neoplasm. The nuclei are uniform and oval-shaped, with regular nuclear borders and small nucleoli.

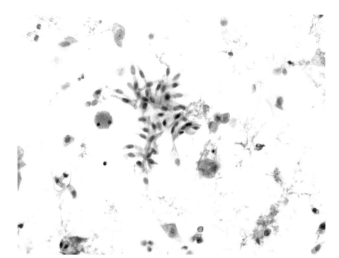

Figure 3.5.7 Low-grade urothelial carcinoma. A small fragment of loosely cohesive spindle cells. Some of these cells are dispersed in the background, where they appear more columnar. The nuclei are oval and very similar in size, compatible with a low-grade urothelial neoplasm.

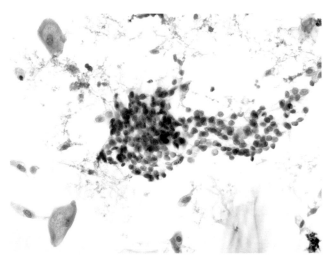

Figure 3.5.8 Low-grade urothelial carcinoma. A fragment of monotonous urothelial cells without a fibrovascular core. The cells are similar in size and oval shaped and have regular nuclear borders. The chromatin is bland and not coarse/clumpy, as is often seen in HGUC.

	Prostate Adenocarcinoma	High-Grade Urothelial Carcinoma
Age	Older men; more common in African Americans	Usually older adults (>50 y of age)
Location	Urinary tract	Urinary tract
Signs and symptoms	Elevated PSA; mass on digital rectal examination; symptoms of metastatic disease as a first presentation in some patients	Asymptomatic or hematuria
Etiology	Environmental factors are under investigation; often associated with a family history; mutations of BRCA1/BRCA2 or Lynch syndrome in some inherited cases	Strong association with tobacco smoking; industrial chemical exposures
Cytomorphology	• Tissue fragments and/or single cells (Figure 3.6.1) • Tissue fragments typically have an underlying acinar architecture • Large cells often with abundant foamy cytoplasm (Figure 3.6.2) • Eccentrically placed round nuclei with regular contours (Figure 3.6.3) • Prominent nucleoli (Figure 3.6.4)	• Predominantly single cells but can exist in small fragments (Figures 3.6.5 and 3.6.6) • Large cells with hyperchromatic nuclei and irregular nuclear borders (Figure 3.6.6) • N/C ratio may not be elevated in degenerated cells due to decreased nuclear size and degenerated cytoplasm (Figure 3.6.7) • Coarse chromatin pattern; in rare instances, cells may have prominent nucleoli instead (Figure 3.6.8)
Special studies	Immunohistochemical studies show the tumor cells are positive for prostate markers such as NKX3.1 and negative for urothelial markers such as GATA-3	Positive for GATA-3 and negative for NKX3.1 by IHC
Molecular alterations	Numerous: telomere shortening, TMPRSS2-ERG rearrangement, GSTP1 promoter hypermethylation, NKX3.1 loss, PTEN loss, AR mutation and/or amplification. Studies ongoing to determine those which are most predictive of aggressive disease	Aneuploidy; frequently TERT promoter mutations; TP53 mutations
Treatment	Surveillance for low-grade disease; otherwise, radical prostatectomy, brachytherapy, hormonal therapy, and/or chemotherapy	Depending on tumor type and extent of disease (both determined on biopsy), transurethral resection; intravesical BCG; intravesical chemotherapy; cystectomy; and/or chemoradiation
Clinical implications	Poor when found in the urine, which indicates advanced disease	Depends on extent of disease and/or responsiveness to intravesical treatment

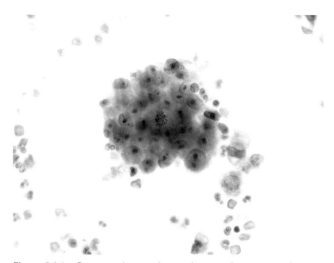

Figure 3.6.1   Prostate adenocarcinoma. A group of prostate carcinoma cells with foamy cytoplasm and large nucleoli. A mitotic figure can be seen in the center of the fragment. Nucleoli this prominent are not usually seen in HGUC and are more suggestive of prostate carcinoma.

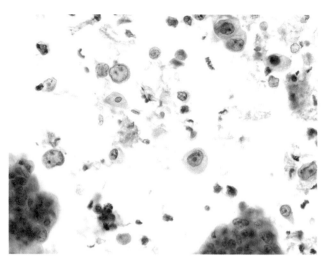

Figure 3.6.2   Prostate adenocarcinoma. A single prostate carcinoma in the center of the field has abundant cytoplasm and a large, prominent nucleolus. Several other malignant cells in the background have high N/C ratios and irregular nuclear borders but lack a prominent nucleolus and could be mistaken for HGUC.

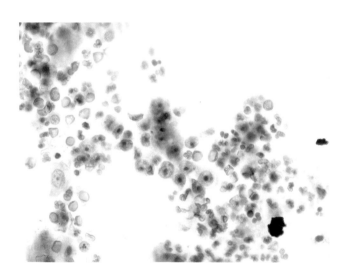

Figure 3.6.3   Prostate adenocarcinoma. Several loosely cohesive prostate carcinoma cells with prominent nucleoli and foamy cytoplasm.

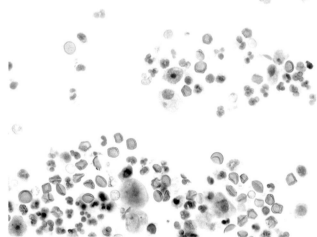

Figure 3.6.4   Prostate adenocarcinoma. A few scattered prostate carcinoma cells can be seen in the field. The cells have prominent nucleoli but minimal cytoplasm. The cells are slightly larger than red blood cells.

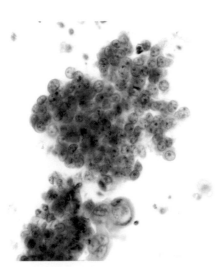

Figure 3.6.5   High-grade urothelial carcinoma (HGUC). The N/C ratios are elevated, and there is significant variation in nuclear size. Many cells have prominent nucleoli which may cause concern for a prostate carcinoma.

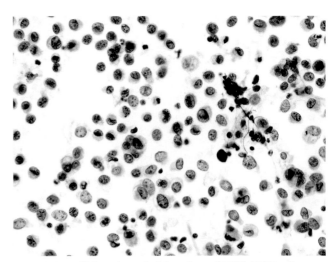

Figure 3.6.6   High-grade urothelial carcinoma (HGUC). HGUC cells are typically discohesive and are seen as individually dispersed cells. The cells have high N/C ratios, anisonucleosis, angulated nuclei, and coarse chromatin.

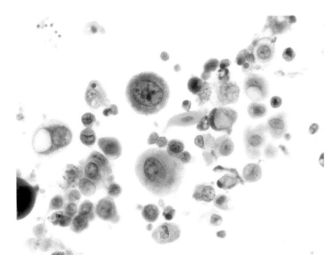

Figure 3.6.7   High-grade urothelial carcinoma (HGUC). Some cells have high N/C ratios while others have more cytoplasm and lower N/C ratios.

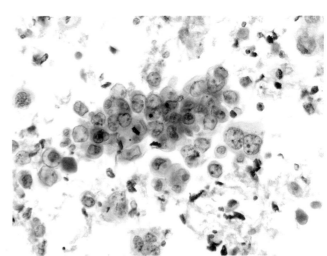

Figure 3.6.8   High-grade urothelial carcinoma (HGUC). A fragment of loosely cohesive HGUC cells with clumped chromatin and paradoxical hypochromasia, a feature that can reportedly be seen in some upper tract carcinomas. The N/C ratios are elevated, and the nuclear borders are irregular.

	Squamous Cell Carcinoma	Degenerated High-Grade Urothelial Carcinoma
Age	Usually older adults	Usually older adults (>50 y of age)
Location	Urinary tract	Urinary tract
Signs and symptoms	Hematuria; dysuria; symptoms at primary site if originating from outside the urinary tract	Asymptomatic or hematuria
Etiology	For primary pure squamous cell carcinoma, classically associated with *S. haematobium* infection in endemic regions; in North America, associated with urinary tract anatomic anomalies and/or chronic cystitis with squamous metaplasia, smoking, bladder stones, chronic indwelling catheters, and cyclophosphamide treatment. HGUC with squamous differentiation is associated with history of HGUC and/or smoking. May be metastatic/invasive from the anus and cervix	Strong association with tobacco smoking; industrial chemical exposures
Cytomorphology	• Predominantly single cells but also small tissue fragments *(Figure 3.7.1)* • Background necrosis may be seen (often reduced in liquid-based preparations) • Dense cytoplasm *(Figure 3.7.2)* • Irregular cytoplasmic projections *(Figures 3.7.1 and 3.7.3)* • Small pyknotic nuclei resulting in low N/C ratios *(Figures 3.7.1 and 3.7.2)* • "India ink black" nuclei with irregular contours *(Figures 3.7.2 and 3.7.3)* • "Ghost" nuclei; cells with poorly staining or absent nuclei *(Figures 3.7.1 and 3.7.3)* • Eosinophilic "keratinizing" cytoplasm on the Pap stain, otherwise may be difficult to distinguish from HGUC *(Figures 3.7.1, 3.7.3, and 3.7.4)*	• Predominantly single cells but can exist in small fragments *(Figure 3.7.5)* • Large cells with hyperchromatic nuclei and irregular nuclear borders *(Figure 3.7.6)* • N/C ratio may not be elevated in degenerated cells due to decreased nuclear size and degenerated cytoplasm *(Figure 3.7.7)* • Coarse chromatin pattern; in rare instances, cells may have prominent nucleoli instead *(Figure 3.7.8)* • Some nuclei may be "India ink black" and a chromatin pattern cannot be assessed *(Figure 3.7.7)*
Special studies	Squamous markers (p40, p63) are positive but cannot prove a urothelial primary site or distinguish pure squamous cell carcinoma from HGUC with squamous differentiation. HPV studies are positive in most squamous cell carcinomas arising from the cervix	Negative for squamous markers by IHC (except for areas of squamous differentiation)
Molecular alterations	Under investigation	Aneuploidy; frequently TERT promoter mutations; TP53 mutations

	Squamous Cell Carcinoma	**Degenerated High-Grade Urothelial Carcinoma**
Treatment	Depends on if primary or metastatic/invasive from secondary site. Radical cystectomy for primary squamous cell carcinoma of the bladder	Depending on tumor type and extent of disease (both determined on biopsy), transurethral resection; intravesical BCG; intravesical chemotherapy; cystectomy; and/or chemoradiation
Clinical implications	Poor for metastatic/invasive from secondary site. For primary squamous cell carcinoma of the bladder, depends on stage and 5-y survival is <50% with treatment	Depends on extent of disease and/or responsiveness to intravesical treatment

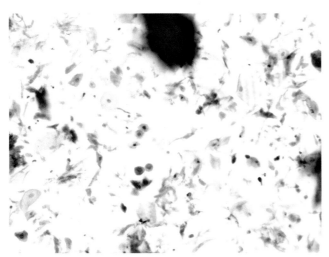

Figure 3.7.1   Squamous cell carcinoma. Scattered pleomorphic cells of keratinizing squamous cell carcinoma, as evidenced by the pink-staining cytoplasm in some atypical cells. While some cells appear more epithelioid and have large nuclei, many cells have irregular-shaped cytoplasm and low N/C ratios.

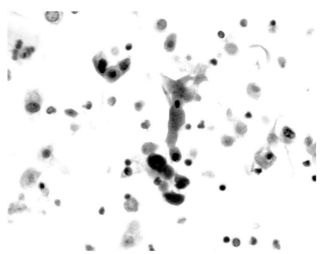

Figure 3.7.2   Keratinizing squamous cell carcinoma. Some cells have pink-orange cytoplasm, while others have cyanophilic cytoplasm. Some nuclei are "India ink black," while others are barely visible ("ghost nuclei").

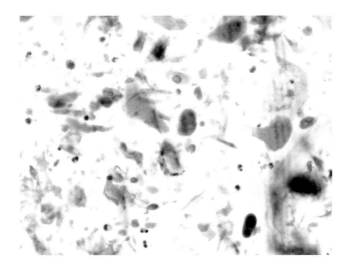

Figure 3.7.3   Squamous cell carcinoma. The field is busy but does not appear overly malignant due to the presence of poor-staining nuclei in many of the cells. However, the field contains numerous cells with irregular and elongated cytoplasm, a finding that strongly suggests atypical squamous cells.

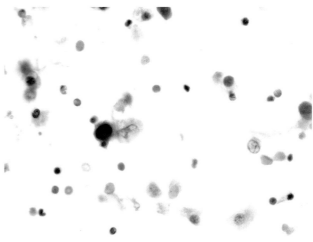

Figure 3.7.4   Squamous cell carcinoma. A single keratinizing squamous cell carcinoma can be seen with dark chromatin and a high N/C ratio. Several other cells in the background have enlarged nuclei with irregular borders and coarse chromatin, likely representing a conventional HGUC component.

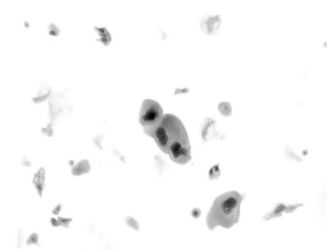

Figure 3.7.5 Degenerated high-grade urothelial carcinoma (HGUC). Degenerated HGUC cells with enlarged, dark nuclei with irregular contours. The N/C ratios are deceiving low.

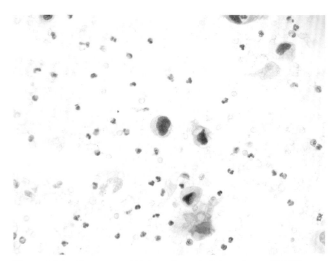

Figure 3.7.6 Degenerated high-grade urothelial carcinoma (HGUC). Several degenerated HGUC cells can be seen in a background of neutrophils. Compared with these benign inflammatory cells, the HGUC nuclei are several times larger. Despite having low N/C ratios, these cells are diagnostic of HGUC.

Figure 3.7.7 Degenerated high-grade urothelial carcinoma (HGUC). Numerous HGUC cells in various states of degeneration. Some cells have extremely high N/C ratios and coarse chromatin, while others have smaller, condensed nuclei that are "India ink black" with an obscured chromatin pattern.

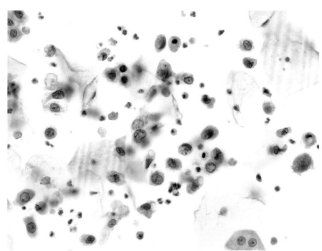

Figure 3.7.8 Degenerated high-grade urothelial carcinoma (HGUC). The field contains well-preserved HGUC cells with high N/C ratios and mild nuclear border irregularities. Other cells have lower N/C ratios and appear bland, while still others have small dark nuclei. The increased number of these atypical cells strongly suggests a neoplastic process.

	Small-Cell Carcinoma	Inflammation
Age	Older adults	Any age
Location	Urinary tract	Urinary tract
Signs and symptoms	Hematuria; dysuria	Hematuria; dysuria
Etiology	Most often arising from the prostate and invading the urinary tract or mixed HGUC-small cell carcinoma; rarely primary small cell carcinoma of the bladder	Nonspecific; often associated with urinary tract infections
Cytomorphology	• Specimens are usually hypercellular, although at low magnification, the dispersed neoplastic cells may be mistaken for inflammation *(Figure 3.8.1)* • Singly dispersed cells with or without tissue fragments/discohesive clusters of cells *(Figure 3.8.2)* • Monotonous population of small cells with high N/C ratios, usually with absent to minimal cytoplasm *(Figure 3.8.3)* • "Salt-and-pepper" chromatin pattern *(Figures 3.8.2 and 3.8.4)* • "Blue blobs" dispersed in the background, indicating cellular necrosis *(Figure 3.8.1)* • Geographic necrosis within tissue fragments, when present *(Figures 3.8.1 and 3.8.4)* • Necrotic debris is often absent or minimal on liquid-based preparations	• Dispersed population of mixed inflammatory cells *(Figure 3.8.5)* • Neutrophils often predominate in urinary tract specimens and can be identified by their multilobated nucleus *(Figure 3.8.6)* • "Blue blobs" in the background representing degenerated neutrophils *(Figures 3.8.6 and 3.8.7)* • Lymphocytes are less commonly seen but more likely to be mistaken for small cell carcinoma due to their mononuclear nature • Lympocytes have angulated nuclei, coarse chromatin, and a thin rim of cytoplasm • Following BCG therapy, epithelioid histiocytes, granulomas, necrotic debris, and multinucleated giant cells may be evident *(Figure 3.8.8)*
Special studies	Generally a morphologic diagnosis. May be positive for neuroendocrine markers (INSM1, chromogranin, synaptophysin); may be positive for NKX3.1 if arising from the prostate (not a sensitive marker for this purpose)	Generally a morphologic diagnosis. Inflammatory cells are negative for neuroendocrine markers by IHC
Molecular alterations	Under investigation	N/A
Treatment	Depends on origin and whether there is a mixed component; often includes radiation therapy	N/A
Clinical implications	Poor	N/A

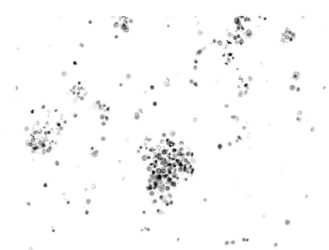

Figure 3.8.1   Small-cell carcinoma. Within the clusters, some cells are viable while others are necrotic and appear as degenerated "blue blobs."

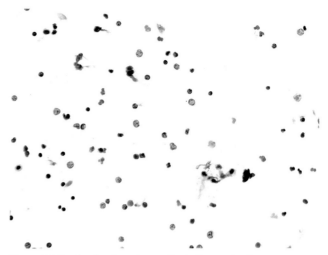

Figure 3.8.2   Small-cell carcinoma. Singly dispersed cells may appear as inflammatory cells (such as mononuclear cells, such as lymphocytes) at low magnification. However, lymphocytes rarely predominate in urinary tract specimens and such a pattern should encourage examination at higher magnification.

Figure 3.8.3   Small-cell carcinoma. The cells are slightly larger than small lymphocytes and may have a thin crescent of cytoplasm or no identifiable cytoplasm.

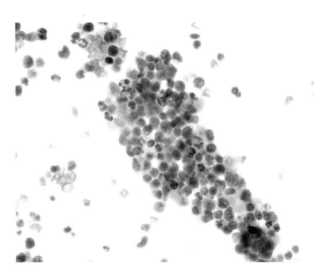

Figure 3.8.4   Small-cell carcinoma. "Geographic necrosis" may be seen in fragments of small-cell carcinoma. Viable cells alternate with necrotic cells that appear as "blue blobs." The chromatin usually has a powdery and/or a "salt-and-pepper" pattern.

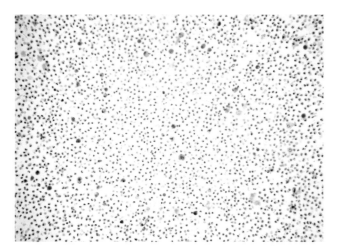

Figure 3.8.5 Inflammation. Numerous dispersed small cells usually indicate the presence of abundant acute inflammation. However, examination at higher power is necessary to exclude the rare small cell carcinoma.

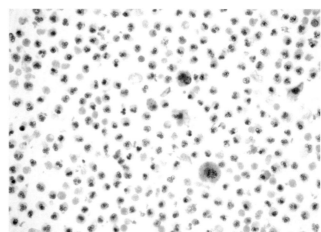

Figure 3.8.6 Inflammation. The presence of numerous acute inflammatory cells is usually accompanied by background "blue blobs" which are degenerated acute inflammatory cells. These can also be seen in small cell carcinomas, in which the neoplastic cells become necrotic.

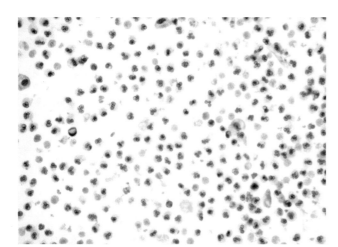

Figure 3.8.7 Inflammation. In inflammatory processes, acute inflammatory cells usually predominate and are not usually confused with small cell carcinoma. Lymphocytosis in urinary tract specimens is rare, as lymphocytes are usually intermixed with other inflammatory cells.

Figure 3.8.8 Inflammation. An epithelioid granuloma is seen in a patient who has recently been treated with BCG instillations. In such patients, lymphocytes, multinucleated giant cells, and necrosis may also be seen.

	Stone Atypia	Degenerated High-Grade Urothelial Carcinoma
Age	Typically adults	Usually older adults (>50 y of age)
Location	Urinary tract	Urinary tract
Signs and symptoms	Hematuria; severe flank pain	Asymptomatic or hematuria
Etiology	Benign urothelial cells lining the urinary tract that have been traumatically exfoliated secondary to stone passage and degenerated within the human body before procurement	Strong association with tobacco smoking; industrial chemical exposures
Cytomorphology	• Small- to medium-sized fragments of urothelial cells *(Figure 3.9.1)* • Increased number of urothelial tissue fragments in voided urine specimens *(Figure 3.9.2)* • N/C ratios at or below 0.5 *(Figures 3.9.1-3.9.4)* • Dark nucleus with mild to moderate nuclear contour irregularities *(Figures 3.9.3 and 3.9.4)* • Small nucleoli *(Figures 3.9.1 and 3.9.2)* • Background blood and/or crystalloids *(Figures 3.9.1, 3.9.2, and 3.9.4)*	• Predominantly single cells but can exist in small fragments *(Figure 3.9.5)* • Large cells with hyperchromatic nuclei and irregular nuclear borders *(Figure 3.9.6)* • N/C ratio may not be elevated in degenerated cells due to decreased nuclear size and degenerated cytoplasm *(Figure 3.9.6)* • Coarse chromatin pattern; in rare instances, cells may have prominent nucleoli instead *(Figures 3.9.7 and 3.9.8)* • Some nuclei may be "India ink black" and a chromatin pattern cannot be assessed
Special studies	FISH to exclude HGUC	FISH to detect chromosomal abnormalities; numerous non–slide-based ancillary tests exist
Molecular alterations	N/A	Aneuploidy; frequently TERT promoter mutations; TP53 mutations
Treatment	N/A	Depending on tumor type and extent of disease (both determined on biopsy), transurethral resection; intravesical BCG; intravesical chemotherapy; cystectomy; and/or chemoradiation
Prognosis	N/A	Depends on extent of disease and/or responsiveness to intravesical treatment

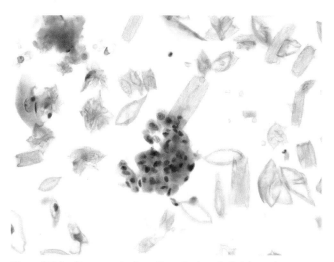

Figure 3.9.1   Stone atypia. A medium-sized urothelial tissue fragment in a background of large crystals and red blood cells. The presence of crystals suggests the possibility of urolithiasis causing hematuria in a patient without a history of urothelial carcinoma. The fragment contains cells with enlarged nuclei, irregular nuclear contour, slight hyperchromasia, and occasional small nucleoli, but the N/C ratios are below 0.5.

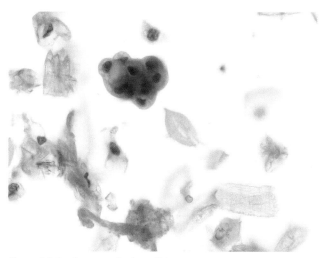

Figure 3.9.2   Stone atypia. A small fragment of urothelial cells with dark nuclei and nuclear border irregularities. The cytoplasm is foamy and abundant, and the cells have low N/C ratios. Crystals can be seen in the background.

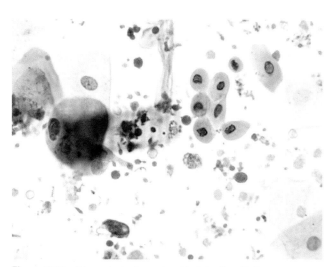

Figure 3.9.3   Stone atypia. Several urothelial cells with the appearance of cells with squamous metaplasia. The nuclei are dark and angulated, but the N/C ratios are low.

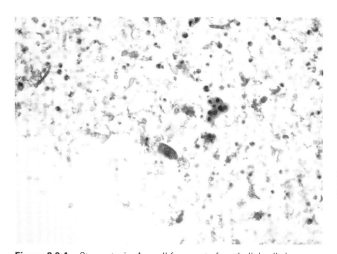

Figure 3.9.4   Stone atypia. A small fragment of urothelial cells in a background of red blood cells and degenerated blood. Despite having dark and angulated nuclei, the cells have low N/C ratios and the nuclei are relatively small.

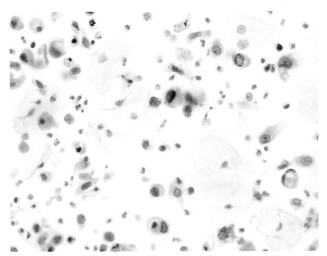

Figure 3.9.5   Degenerated high-grade urothelial carcinoma (HGUC). Numerous degenerated HGUC cells have a deceiving bland appearance. However, the nuclei have markedly irregular borders, and some cells have high N/C ratios. At the bottom center of the field, a "cell-in-cell" pattern can be seen, which should raise suspicion for HGUC.

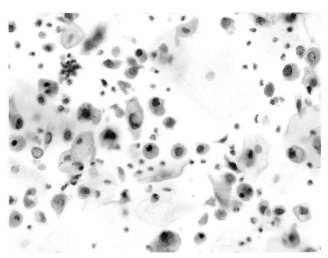

Figure 3.9.6   Degenerated high-grade urothelial carcinoma (HGUC). Degenerated HGUC cells demonstrating various nuclear sizes, cell sizes, and N/C ratios. Some cells have low N/C ratios but have very dark nuclei which are enlarged compared with that of bystander neutrophils.

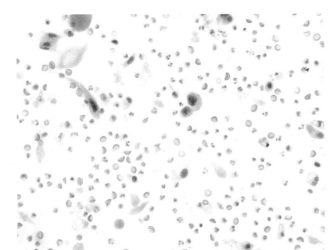

Figure 3.9.7   Degenerated high-grade urothelial carcinoma (HGUC). Two degenerated HGUC cells are loosely associated, and another HGUC cell is elongated and contains large, dark nucleus with irregular borders. As compared with changes in stone atypia, the nuclei are both dark and enlarged in HGUC.

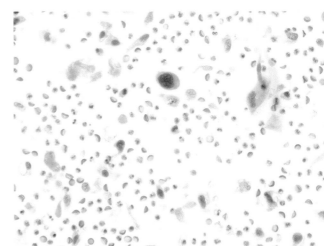

Figure 3.9.8   Degenerated high-grade urothelial carcinoma (HGUC). A very large HGUC cell can be seen in the center of the field. The chromatin pattern is coarse, and the nuclear contours are irregular. Despite having an N/C ratio below 0.7, the amount of chromatin contained within this large, dark nucleus is concerning for HGUC.

	Polyoma (BK) Virus	High-Grade Urothelial Carcinoma
Age	Any; may cause renal failure in AIDS patients; interstitial nephritis; hemorrhagic cystitis	Usually older adults (>50 y of age)
Location	Urinary tract	Urinary tract
Signs and symptoms	Asymptomatic, or with reactivation in immuno-suppressed patients	Asymptomatic or hematuria
Etiology	Reactivation of latent BK polyomavirus infection residing in renal tubular cells and urothelial cells; may be seen more frequently in immuno-suppressed patients	Strong association with tobacco smoking; industrial chemical exposures
Cytomorphology	• Single cells not seen in fragments *(Figure 3.10.1)* • Usually only rare cells in a specimen, but may be increased in immunosuppressed patients • Cells have high N/C ratios with scant degenerated cytoplasm or absent cytoplasm *(Figures 3.10.1 and 3.10.2)* • Nuclei are round with smooth nuclear borders *(Figures 3.10.1 and 3.10.2)* • Marginated chromatin at nuclear borders *(Figure 3.10.3)* • Nuclei have a "ground glass" or "spider web" appearance *(Figure 3.10.4)*	• Predominantly single cells but can exist in small fragments *(Figure 3.10.5)* • Large cells with hyperchromatic nuclei and irregular nuclear borders *(Figure 3.10.6)* • N/C ratio may not be elevated in degenerated cells due to decreased nuclear size and degenerated cytoplasm *(Figure 3.10.6)* • Coarse chromatin pattern; in rare instances, cells may have prominent nucleoli instead *(Figure 3.10.7)*
Special studies	FISH to exclude HGUC; quantitative viral load testing of urine specimens	FISH to detect chromosomal abnormalities; numerous non–slide-based ancillary tests exist
Molecular alterations	N/A	Aneuploidy; frequently TERT promoter mutations; TP53 mutations
Treatment	N/A	Depending on tumor type and extent of disease (both determined on biopsy), transurethral resection; intravesical BCG; intravesical chemotherapy; cystectomy; and/or chemoradiation
Clinical implications	N/A	Depends on extent of disease and/or responsiveness to intravesical treatment

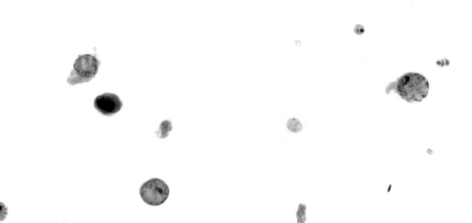

Figure 3.10.1   BK polyomavirus. While the cells have high N/C ratios and dark chromatin, the "ground glass" appearance of the chromatin and condensation of chromatin around the nuclear membrane strongly suggest BK polyomavirus rather than HGUC.

Figure 3.10.2   BK polyomavirus. Note the very round nucleus with regular nuclear contours; rarely do HGUC nuclei appear as such.

Figure 3.10.3   BK polyomavirus. The changes secondary to BK in these cells cause increased concern for HGUC, as the central cell has irregular borders and clumpy chromatin. However, the chromatin is predominantly condensed along the nuclear membrane and has a "ground glass" quality.

Figure 3.10.4   BK polyomavirus. This cell demonstrates changes secondary to BK, creating a homogenous appearance to its chromatin. Despite having an irregular nuclear shape, the chromatin lacks and coarse or clumpy chromatin that would otherwise be concerning for HGUC.

3   URINARY TRACT

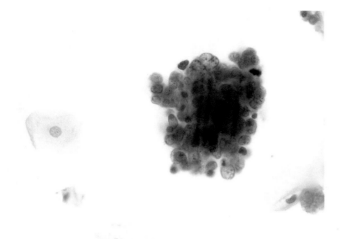

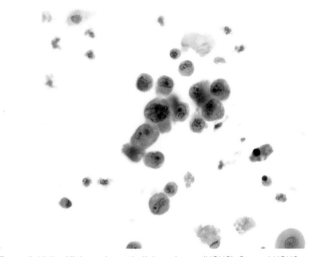

Figure 3.10.5　High-grade urothelial carcinoma (HGUC). A fragment of HGUC. The cells have high N/C ratios, coarse chromatin, and irregular nuclear borders. Cells infected with BK changes are usually seen singly and not in fragments.

Figure 3.10.6　High-grade urothelial carcinoma (HGUC). Several HGUC cells with highly irregular nuclear contours and coarse chromatin. The nuclei vary greatly in shape and size.

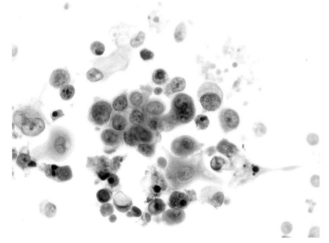

Figure 3.10.7　High-grade urothelial carcinoma (HGUC). Some cells have oval nuclei without contour irregularities, while others have marked irregularities in their nuclear membranes.

4

Thyroid

	Medullary Thyroid Carcinoma (MTC)	Hurthle Cell Neoplasm
Age	Middle-aged adults; younger in familial	Adenomas in young to middle-aged adults, more often female. Carcinomas more common in older men
Location	Thyroid	Thyroid
Signs and symptoms	Painless thyroid mass or cervical lymphadenopathy; flushing and diarrhea in metastatic disease	Usually solitary thyroid nodule; lymphadenopathy if Hurthle cell carcinoma
Etiology	Derived from calcitonin-secreting C cells. Associated with familial syndromes MEN 2A, MEN 2B, familial medullary thyroid carcinoma syndrome, von-Hippel-Lindau disease, and neurofibromatosis	Benign or malignant neoplasm of thyroid follicular cells demonstrating diffuse Hurthle cell change
Cytomorphology	• Loosely cohesive and scattered, monotonous cells (Figure 4.1.1) • Background may contain amorphous amyloid material (Figure 4.1.2). Colloid is absent • Neoplastic cells are epithelioid or spindled with an eccentrically placed nucleus and abundant cytoplasm (Figures 4.1.3 and 4.1.4) • Regular nuclear borders but may demonstrate anisonucleosis (Figure 4.1.5) • Chromatin has a speckled (neuroendocrine) appearance (Figure 4.1.2)	• Loosely cohesive and scattered, monotonous cells (Figures 4.1.6 and 4.1.7) • Transversing capillaries • Scant background colloid and no amyloid • Neoplastic cells have an eccentrically placed nucleus and abundant granular cytoplasm (Figures 4.1.8 and 4.1.9) • Round nuclei with regular borders, sometimes with prominent anisonucleosis and frequent binucleation (Figures 4.1.8 and 4.1.9) • Chromatin is granular and have prominent nucleoli (Figure 4.1.10)
Special studies	Positive for calcitonin, TTF-1, PAX-8, and neuroendocrine markers and negative for thyroglobulin by IHC. Amyloid can be identified by a Congo Red special stain	Positive for TTF-1, PAX-8, and thyroglobulin by IHC; negative for calcitonin and neuroendocrine markers
Molecular alterations	Mutations in RET gene in most familial cases and 50% of sporadic cases. Otherwise, mutations in HRAS or KRAS	Often aneuploidy; Hurthle cell carcinomas appear to follow a different mutational pathway than conventional follicular carcinomas and often have PTEN and/or TP53 mutations
Treatment	Surgical excision	For carcinomas, surgical excision including cervical lymph node dissection
Clinical implications	10-year survival of 75%-85%, worse with distant metastases	Hurthle cell carcinomas are more aggressive than conventional follicular carcinomas

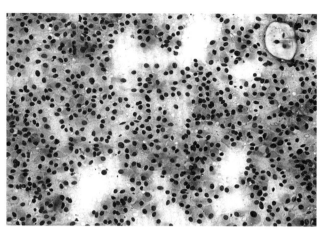

Figure 4.1.1 Medullary thyroid carcinoma. The field contains a dispersed population of plasmacytoid monotonous cells with round nuclei and abundant cytoplasm.

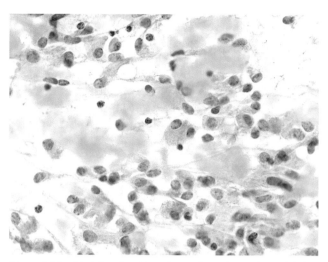

Figure 4.1.2 Medullary thyroid carcinoma. Several amorphous globules of amyloid stain a cyan color on this Pap stained preparation. The neoplastic cells have chromatin with a "salt-and-pepper" appearance, consistent with their neuroendocrine differentiation.

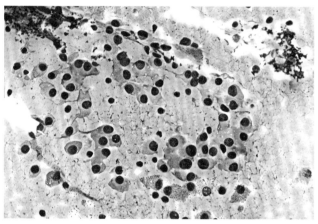

Figure 4.1.3 Medullary thyroid carcinoma. The cells have eccentrically-placed, round nuclei, regular nuclear borders, and mild anisonucleosis.

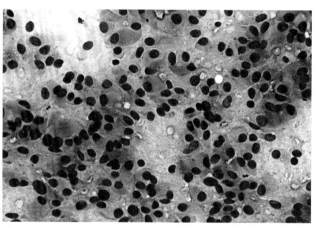

Figure 4.1.4 Medullary thyroid carcinoma. The field contains cells with spindle-shaped nuclei, have abundant cytoplasm and are predominantly in a plasmacytoid configuration.

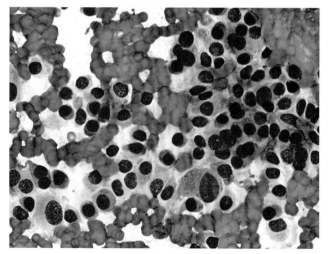

Figure 4.1.5 Medullary thyroid carcinoma. Medullary thyroid carcinoma may produce cells that are binucleate. It is not uncommon to identify some cells with greatly enlarged nuclei, although the nuclear borders remain relatively regular.

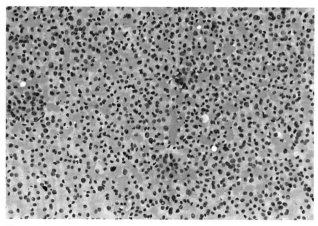

Figure 4.1.6 Hurthle cell neoplasm. A cellular field of monotonous, discohesive thyroid follicular cells with prominent Hurthle cell change.

4 THYROID

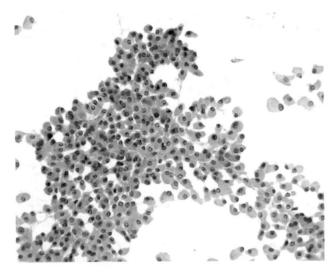

Figure 4.1.7   Hurthle cell neoplasm. Hurthle cells have abundant cyto-plasm and eccentrically placed nucleus. Prominent nucleoli, as seen here, are commonly seen and help exclude medullary thyroid carcinoma.

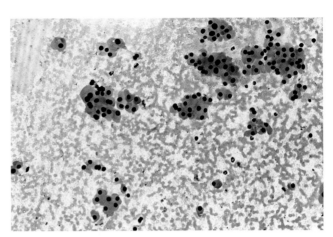

Figure 4.1.8   Hurthle cell neoplasm. Hurthle cells typically have round nuclei with very regular borders, although some variation in nuclear size may be seen between cells.

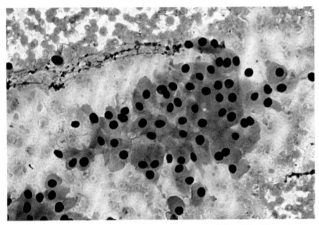

Figure 4.1.9   Hurthle cell neoplasm. A separate field of Hurthle cells that contain abundant cytoplasm and round nuclei with regular contours.

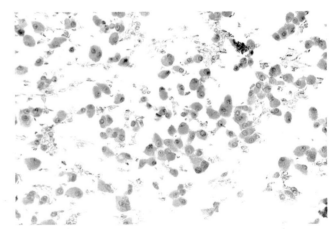

Figure 4.1.10   Hurthle cell neoplasm. This Pap stained preparation demonstates the chromatin pattern seen in Hurthle cells: distinctive or prominent nucleoli, and an absence of the neuroendocrine chromatin pattern as seen in medullary thyroid carcinoma.

	Hurthle Cell Neoplasm	Oncocytic Papillary Thyroid Carcinoma
Age	Adenomas in young to middle aged adults, more often female. Carcinomas more common in older men	Adults; mostly women
Location	Thyroid	Thyroid
Signs and symptoms	Usually solitary thyroid nodule; lymphadenopathy if Hurthle cell carcinoma	Usually solitary thyroid nodule; lymphadenopathy
Etiology	Benign or malignant neoplasm of thyroid follicular cells demonstrating diffuse Hurthle cell change	May be associated with lymphocytic thyroiditis
Cytomorphology	• Loosely cohesive and scattered, monotonous cells (Figures 4.2.1-4.2.3) • Branching capillaries • Rare background colloid and no amyloid • Neoplastic cells have an eccentrically placed nucleus and abundant granular cytoplasm (Figures 4.2.4 and 4.2.5) • Round nuclei with regular borders, sometimes with prominent anisonucleosis and frequent binucleation (Figures 4.2.4 and 4.2.5) • Chromatin is granular and have prominent nucleoli (Figures 4.2.4 and 4.2.5)	• Predominantly cohesive tissue fragments in papillary and/or monolayer sheet configurations (Figures 4.2.6 and 4.2.7) • Usually minimal or absent colloid • Low to nuclear to cytoplasmic ratios due to increased cytoplasm (Figure 4.2.8) • Enlarged oval nuclei with powdery chromatin (Figures 4.2.8-4.2.10) • Irregular nuclear contours (Figures 4.2.8-4.2.10) • Nuclear grooves (Figure 4.2.10) • Intranuclear pseudoinclusions may be present (Figure 4.2.10)
Special studies	Positive for TTF-1, PAX-8, and thyroglobulin by IHC	Positive for TTF-1, PAX-8, and thyroglobulin by IHC
Molecular alterations	Often aneuploidy; Hurthle cell carcinomas appear to follow a different mutational pathway than conventional follicular carcinomas and often have PTEN and/or TP53 mutations	BRAF mutations
Treatment	For carcinomas, surgical excision including cervical lymph node dissection	Surgical excision including cervical lymph node dissection with or without radioactive iodine
Clinical implications	Hurthle cell carcinomas are more aggressive than conventional follicular carcinomas	Generally good but distantly metastatic disease may persist

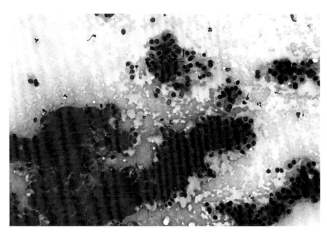

Figure 4.2.1 Hurthle cell neoplasm. A papillary fragment of loosely cohesive Hurthle cells. The cells have round nuclei and abundant cytoplasm. Rare stripped nuclei can also be seen in the background.

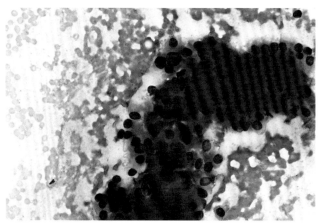

Figure 4.2.2 Hurthle cell neoplasm. Variation in nuclear size is commonly seen in Hurthle cell neoplasms, but the nuclear borders remain regular.

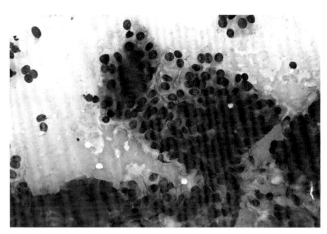

Figure 4.2.3 Hurthle cell neoplasm. Some of the neoplastic cells have oval-shaped nuclei, but nuclear grooves, nuclear border irregularities, and intranuclear pseudoinclusions, all features of papillary thyroid carcinoma, are absent.

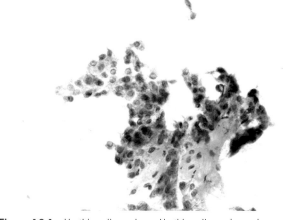

Figure 4.2.4 Hurthle cell neoplasm. Hurthle cell neoplasms have granular cytoplasm and may have small or even prominent nucleoli, as compared with the powdery chromatin of papillary thyroid carcinoma.

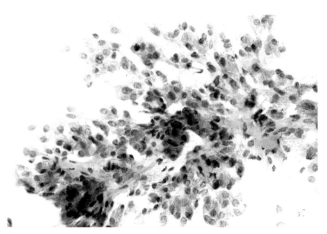

Figure 4.2.5 Hurthle cell neoplasm. The cells in this field possess granular cytoplasm, a feature not typically seen in papillary thyroid carcinoma

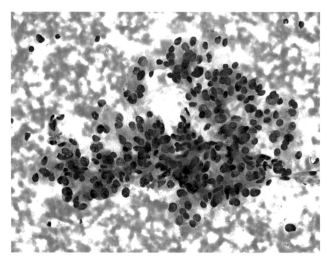

Figure 4.2.6 Oncocytic papillary thyroid carcinoma (PTC). Oncocytic PTC often demonstrates architectural abnormalities, such as the papillary growth pattern seen here.

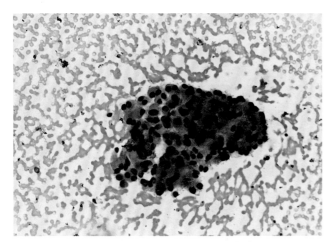

Figure 4.2.7   Oncocytic papillary thyroid carcinoma (PTC). The cells seen here are present in a tissue fragment and cells are not dispersed in the background. This contrasts with most Hurthle cell neoplasms, which often have dispersed single cells.

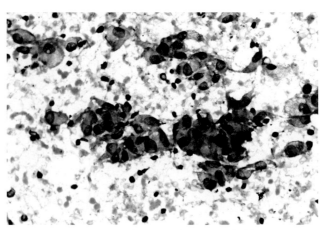

Figure 4.2.8   Oncocytic papillary thyroid carcinoma (PTC). The nuclei here have irregular shapes and nuclear contour irregularities. The cytoplasm is vacuolated but not granular as would be seen in a Hurthle cell neoplasm.

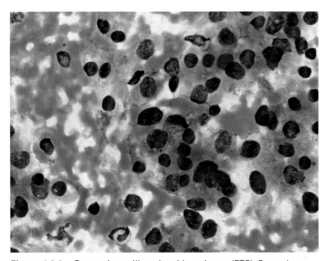

Figure 4.2.9   Oncocytic papillary thyroid carcinoma (PTC). Several nuclei in this field are enlarged, and many contain marked nuclear border irregularities.

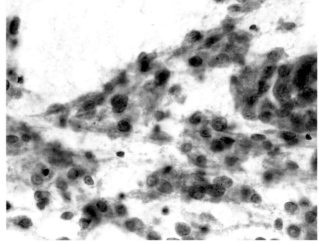

Figure 4.2.10   Oncocytic papillary thyroid carcinoma (PTC). Several intranuclear cytoplasmic pseudoinclusions, a relatively specific feature for PTC, can be seen in this field. Several cells also have nuclear grooves.

	Hashimoto Thyroiditis	Papillary Thyroid Carcinoma
Age	Middle-aged women	Mostly young adult and middle-aged women
Location	Thyroid	Thyroid
Signs and symptoms	Gradual hypothyroidism; may form multinodular goiter	Usually solitary thyroid nodule; lymphadenopathy
Etiology	Autoimmune disease of the thyroid gland; associated with anti-TSH antibodies that block the TSH receptor	Radiation exposure, Hashimoto thyroiditis, familial adenomatous polyposis
Cytomorphology	• Predominantly cohesive tissue fragments that may form three-dimensional fragments and lack papillary architecture *(Figure 4.3.1)* • Colloid may be minimal or absent • Background lymphocytes, which may be associated with tissue fragments *(Figures 4.3.1 and 4.3.2)* • Enlarged nuclei and increased cytoplasm *(Figures 4.3.3 and 4.3.4)* • Nuclear are round to oval with regular contours *(Figure 4.3.5)* • Nucleoli may be seen and can be prominent • Rare nuclear grooves and very rare intranuclear cytoplasmic pseudoinclusions	• Predominantly cohesive tissue fragments in papillary and/or monolayer sheet configurations *(Figures 4.3.6 and 4.3.7)* • Usually minimal or absent colloid • Elevated nuclear to cytoplasmic ratios *(Figure 4.3.8)* • Enlarged oval nuclei with powdery chromatin *(Figure 4.3.9)* • Irregular nuclear contours *(Figures 4.3.8 and 4.3.9)* • Nuclear grooves *(Figure 4.3.10)* • Intranuclear pseudoinclusions may be present *(Figure 4.3.10)*
Special studies	Atypical follicular cells are positive for TTF-1, PAX-8, and thyroglobulin by IHC. Flow cytometry demonstrates polyclonal lymphocytes	Carcinoma cells are usually positive for TTF-1, PAX-8, and thyroglobulin by IHC, but may be lost in anaplastic areas if present
Molecular alterations	None	*BRAF* or *RAS* mutations; *RET-PTC* rearrangements
Treatment	Synthetic hormone replacement	Surgical excision including cervical lymph node dissection with or without radioactive iodine
Clinical implications	Generally good with hormone replacement	Generally good but distantly metastatic disease may persist

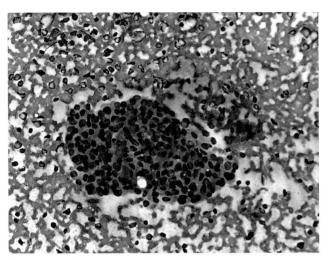

Figure 4.3.1 Hashimoto thyroiditis. A tissue fragment containing thyroid follicular cells with enlarged nuclei. The background contains abundant lymphocytes, which should raise the threshold for making a diagnosis of PTC.

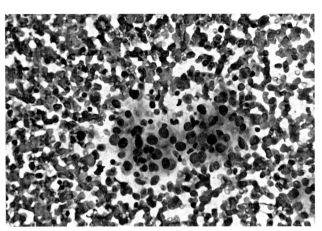

Figure 4.3.2 Hashimoto thyroiditis. A fragment of thyroid follicular cells which have undergone Hurthle cell metaplasia secondary to lymphocytic thyroiditis. Lymphocytes can be seen in the background as well as in association with the thyroid follicular cells.

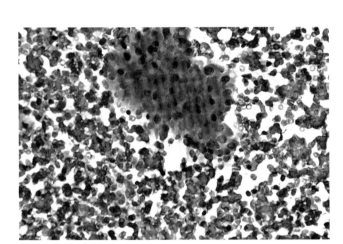

Figure 4.3.3 Hashimoto thyroiditis. While the follicular cells seen here have enlarged nuclei due to Hurthle cell change, the nuclei have regular nuclear borders and are predominantly round in shape.

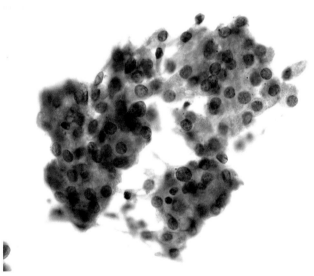

Figure 4.3.4 Hashimoto thyroiditis. These Hurthle cells have abundant cytoplasm. Despite the presence of anisonucleosis, the nuclei remain round and have very regular nuclear contours.

4 THYROID

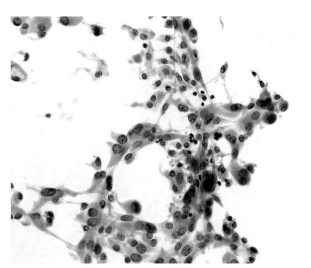

Figure 4.3.5   Hashimoto thyroiditis. Hurthle cells do not have the pale chromatin seen in PTC but may have small or even prominent nucleoli.

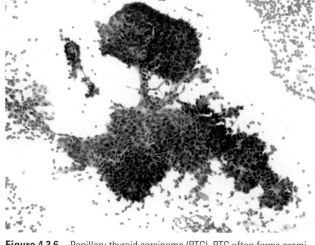

Figure 4.3.6   Papillary thyroid carcinoma (PTC). PTC often forms prominent papillary structures, a feature not seen in Hashimoto thyroiditis.

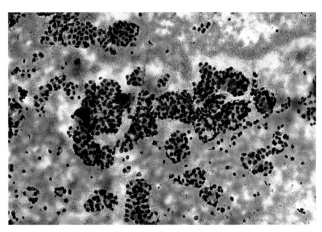

Figure 4.3.7   Papillary thyroid carcinoma (PTC). Numerous monolayer fragments with papillary projections. The specimen is very cellular with neoplastic follicular cells, whereas Hashimoto thyroiditis specimens do not contain a proliferative follicular cell component.

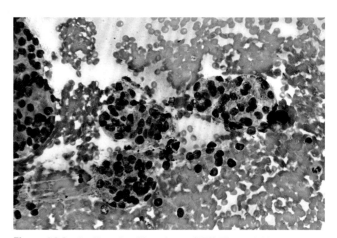

Figure 4.3.8   Papillary thyroid carcinoma (PTC). The nuclei have markedly irregular borders and are enlarged and overlapping. Rare colloid is present as dense, round globules, which should not be considered a reassuring finding.

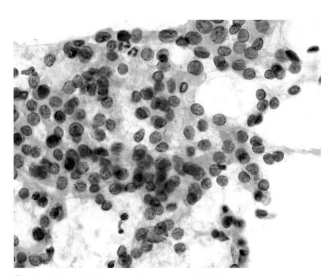

Figure 4.3.9   Papillary thyroid carcinoma (PTC). The nuclei seen here have powdery chromatin with small chromocenters but no distinctive nucleoli.

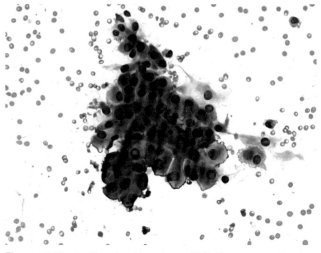

Figure 4.3.10   Papillary thyroid carcinoma (PTC). The presence of nuclear grooves and intranuclear pseudoinclusions are diagnostic of papillary thyroid carcinoma, despite the abundance of cytoplasm seen in these cells.

	Parathyroid Tissue	Adenomatoid Nodule
Age	Middle-aged adults; more commonly women	Mostly young adult and middle-aged women
Location	Anywhere in the neck, including intrathyroidal	Thyroid
Signs and symptoms	Painless nodule(s) in the neck or within the thyroid; symptoms of hyperparathyroidism	Usually a dominant nodule within a multinodular thyroid
Etiology	Parathyroid adenoma or hyperplasia; rarely parathyroid carcinoma	Enlarged thyroid due to iodine deficiency, Hashimoto thyroiditis, or other factors
Cytomorphology	• Tissue fragments with a "packeted" or trabecular configuration *(Figures 4.4.1 and 4.4.2)* • Dispersed single cells and stripped nuclei usually found in the background *(Figures 4.4.1 and 4.4.2)* • Small and monotonous cells with low N/C ratios, granular cytoplasm, and eccentrically placed nuclei *(Figures 4.4.3-4.4.5)* • Small, round nuclei with regular contours and bland often neuroendocrine chromatin *(Figures 4.4.3-4.4.5)* • Colloid is absent	• Tissue fragments, often in three-dimensional sheets, containing monotonous follicular cells that may contain colloid *(Figures 4.4.6-4.4.8)* • Background colloid material • Single cells and stripped nuclei may be absent or present in small numbers in the background *(Figures 4.4.9 and 4.4.10)* • Nuclei are round and have regular nuclear contours *(Figure 4.4.10)*
Special studies	Cells are positive for PTH and GATA-3 and negative for TTF-1, PAX-8, and thyroglobulin by IHC. Needle rinses have elevated PTH levels	Cells are positive for TTF-1, PAX-8, and thyroglobulin and negative for PTH by IHC
Molecular alterations	Loss of heterozygosity in chromosome 1p (parathyroid adenoma)	None
Treatment	Synthetic hormone replacement	Observation or surgery for cosmetic or compressive symptoms
Clinical implications	Generally good with hormone replacement	Excellent

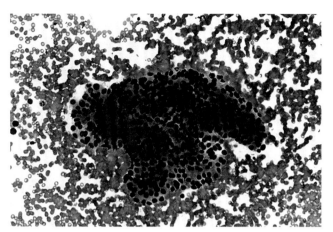

Figure 4.4.1 Parathyroid tissue. A tissue fragment "packet" of parathyroid cells is present with small, round nuclei. A few stripped nuclei can be seen on the left side of the field.

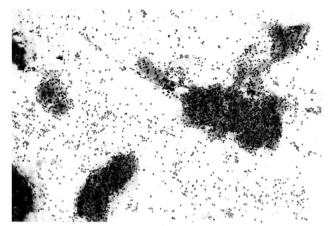

Figure 4.4.2 Parathyroid tissue. Parathyroid cells are seen in fragments as well as dispersed in the background. While adenomatoid nodules can contain dispersed thyroid follicular cells, they are not usually present in such great numbers.

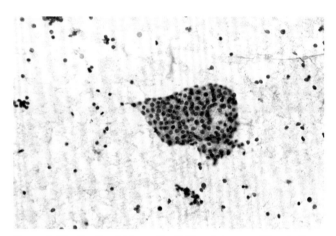

Figure 4.4.3 Parathyroid tissue. The field contains a small "packet" of parathyroid cells and numerous stripped nuclei in the background. The tissue fragment is easily mistaken for benign thyroid follicular cells, and ancillary studies are sometimes needed to prove parathyroid differentiation.

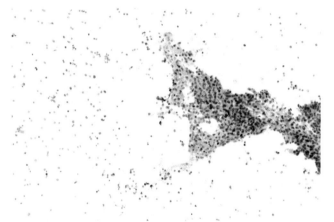

Figure 4.4.4 Parathyroid tissue. A trabecular fragment of parathyroid cells with numerous stripped nuclei in the background.

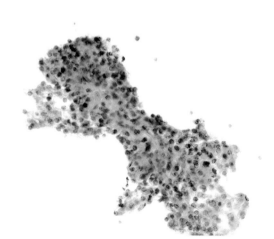

Figure 4.4.5 Parathyroid tissue. The nuclei of parathyroid cells are usually round and have regular borders, and a population of cells often looks monotonous.

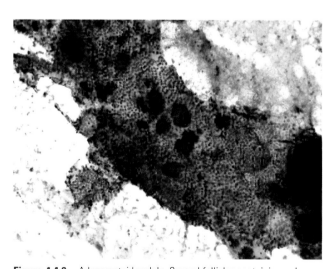

Figure 4.4.6 Adenomatoid nodule. Several follicles containing red-staining colloid can be seen in this fragment.

4 THYROID

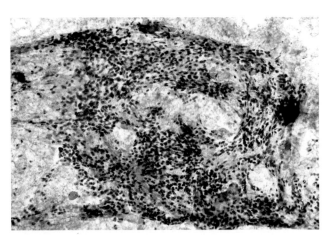

Figure 4.4.7   Adenomatoid nodule. Numerous thyroid follicular cells form swirling structures are associated with pink-staining colloid.

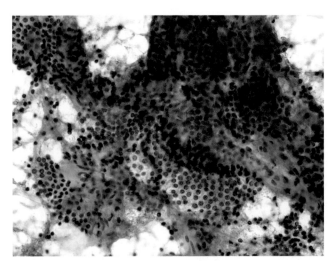

Figure 4.4.8   Adenomatoid nodule. In the absence of colloid, thyroid follicular cells are often bland, with round nuclei and regular nuclear contours. This morphology significantly overlaps with parathyroid tissue, which is much less likely to be sampled during the FNA of a thyroid nodule.

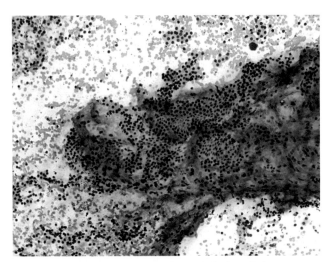

Figure 4.4.9   Adenomatoid nodule. Thyroid follicular cells demonstrate Hurthle cell change, resulting in increased amounts of cytoplasm and slight variations in nuclear size. Hurthle cells are also more likely to appear as single cells in the background, emulating the sampling of parathyroid tissue.

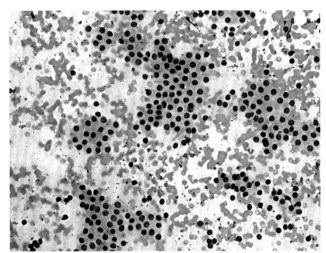

Figure 4.4.10   Adenomatoid nodule. Thyroid follicular cells that appear monotonous with round nuclei and regular nuclear borders. The abundance of cytoplasm indicates Hurthle cell metaplasia; stripped nuclei are present in the background.

	Medullary Thyroid Carcinoma (MTC)	Parathyroid Tissue
Age	Middle-aged adults; younger in familial	Middle-aged adults; more commonly women
Location	Thyroid	Anywhere in the neck, including intrathyroidal
Signs and symptoms	Painless thyroid mass or cervical lymphadenopathy; flushing and diarrhea in metastatic disease	Painless nodule(s) in the neck or within the thyroid; symptoms of hyperparathyroidism
Etiology	Derived from calcitonin-secreting C cells. Associated with familial syndromes MEN 2A, MEN 2B, familial medullary thyroid carcinoma syndrome, von-Hippel-Lindau disease, and neurofibromatosis	Parathyroid adenoma or hyperplasia; rarely parathyroid carcinoma
Cytomorphology	• Loosely cohesive and scattered, monotonous cells (*Figure 4.5.1*) • Background may contain amorphous amyloid material. Colloid is absent • Neoplastic cells are epithelioid or spindled with an eccentrically placed nucleus and abundant cytoplasm (*Figures 4.5.2* and *4.5.3*) • Regular nuclear borders but may demonstrate anisonucleosis (*Figures 4.5.4* and *4.5.5*) • Chromatin has a speckled (neuroendocrine) appearance (*Figure 4.5.5*)	• Tissue fragments with a "packeted" or trabecular configuration (*Figures 4.5.6* and *4.5.7*) • Dispersed single cells and stripped nuclei usually found in the background (*Figures 4.5.8* and *4.5.9*) • Small and monotonous cells with low N/C ratios, granular cytoplasm, and eccentrically placed nuclei (*Figure 4.5.10*) • Small, round nuclei with regular contours and bland chromatin (*Figure 4.5.10*) • Colloid is absent
Special studies	Positive for calcitonin, TTF-1, PAX-8, and neuroendocrine markers and negative for PTH and thyroglobulin by IHC. Amyloid can be identified by a Congo Red special stain. Needle rinses have elevated calcitonin levels	Cells are positive for PTH and GATA-3 and negative for calcitonin, TTF-1, PAX-8, and thyroglobulin by IHC. Needle rinses have elevated PTH levels
Molecular alterations	Mutations in *RET* gene in most familial cases and 50% of sporadic cases. Otherwise, mutations in *HRAS* or *KRAS*	Loss of heterozygosity in chromosome 1p (parathyroid adenoma)
Treatment	Surgical excision	Synthetic hormone replacement
Clinical implications	10-year survival of 75%-85%, worse with distant metastases	Generally good with hormone replacement

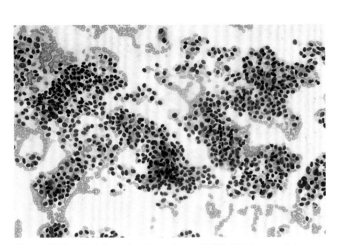

Figure 4.5.1   Medullary thyroid carcinoma (MTC). This hypercellular smear contains a loosely cohesive population of epithelioid cells with faintly colored cytoplasm and predominantly oval-shaped nuclei.

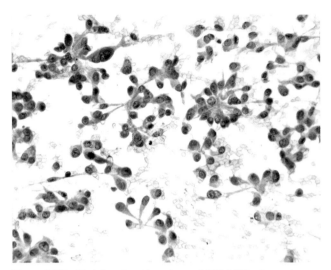

Figure 4.5.2   Medullary thyroid carcinoma (MTC). MTC cells may be spindle shaped or epithelioid. In this field, they are predominantly spindle shaped.

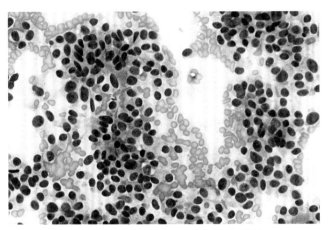

Figure 4.5.3   Medullary thyroid carcinoma (MTC). The field contains a mixture of both epithelioid and spindle-shaped medullary thyroid carcinoma cells.

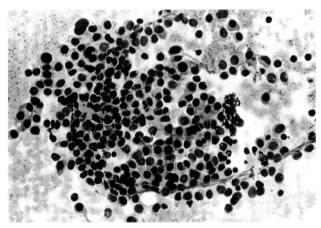

Figure 4.5.4   Medullary thyroid carcinoma (MTC). Medullary thyroid carcinoma cells typically have regular nuclear contours but prominent anisonucleosis may be seen.

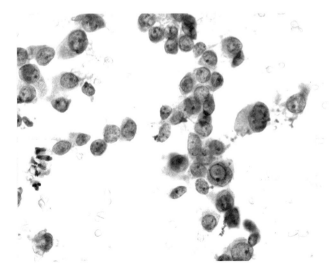

Figure 4.5.5   Medullary thyroid carcinoma (MTC). These cells have a neuroendocrine type chromatin pattern, in which the chromatin is both coarse and finely granular. One nucleus contains an intranuclear pseudo-inclusion, more commonly associated with papillary thyroid carcinoma, but also occasionally seen in MTC.

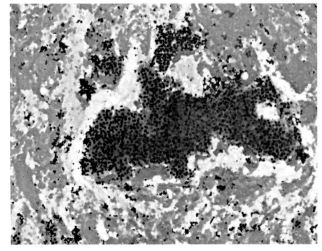

Figure 4.5.6   Parathyroid tissue. In this field, numerous parathyroid cells form a large trabecular fragment.

4 THYROID

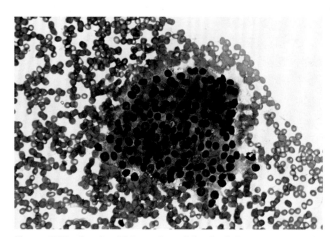

Figure 4.5.7 Parathyroid tissue. A small "packet" of monotonous-appearing parathyroid cells are shown with round nuclei and regular nuclear contours.

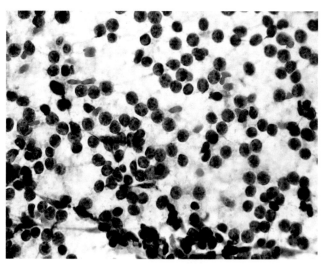

Figure 4.5.8 A Parathyroid tissue. The smears contains a population of dispersed parathyroid cells, mostly with stripped nuclei.

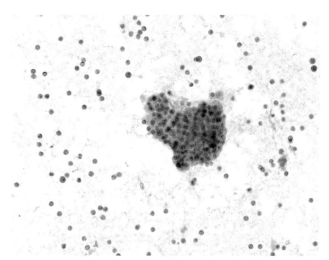

Figure 4.5.9 Parathyroid tissue. Parathyroid cells are present both in a single tissue fragment "packet" as well as singly as stripped nuclei in the background.

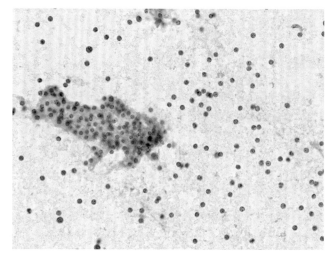

Figure 4.5.10 Parathyroid tissue. The nuclei of these cells are round with regular contours. There is minimal size variation, and the chromatin is bland.

	Cellular Adenomatoid Nodule	Suspicious for a Follicular Neoplasm
Age	Mostly young adult and middle-aged women	Middle-aged adults; more commonly women
Location	Thyroid	Thyroid
Signs and symptoms	Usually a dominant nodule within a multinodular thyroid	Solitary thyroid nodule
Etiology	Enlarged thyroid due to iodine deficiency, Hashimoto thyroiditis, or other factors	Follicular adenoma, follicular variant of PTC, noninvasive follicular thyroid neoplasm with papillary-like nuclear features (NIFTP), or follicular carcinoma
Cytomorphology	• Tissue fragments, often in three-dimensional sheets, containing monotonous follicular cells that may contain colloid (Figures 4.6.1 and 4.6.2) • Background colloid material may be minimal or absent • Single cells and stripped nuclei may be absent or present in small numbers in the background • Hurthle cell metaplasia may cause increased number of stripped nuclei or single dispersed cells (Figure 4.6.3) • Focal or absent microfollicular architecture (Figures 4.6.3-4.6.5) • Nuclei are round and have regular nuclear contours (Figure 4.6.4)	• Cellular specimen with follicular cells present in tissue fragments as well as dispersed microfollicles and single cells in the background (Figures 4.6.5 and 4.6.6) • Absent or rare colloid, which may form dense globules within microfollicles (Figures 4.6.7 and 4.6.8) • Fragments are predominantly constructed from microfollicular structures of less than 12 cells each (Figure 4.6.9) • Minor nuclear changes of papillary carcinoma may be focally present.
Special studies	Cells are positive for TTF-1, PAX-8, and thyroglobulin by IHC	Cells are positive for TTF-1, PAX-8, and thyroglobulin by IHC
Molecular alterations	None	RAS mutations (follicular adenoma, NIFTP, and follicular carcinoma); NRAS, HRAS, PI3CA, and PTEN mutations or PAX8-PPAR gamma rearrangements (follicular carcinoma)
Treatment	Observation or surgery for cosmetic or compressive symptoms	Initially, thyroid lobectomy or total thyroidectomy (if concomitant positive ancillary testing). Subsequent treatment depends on the specific diagnosis
Clinical implications	Excellent	Excellent; for carcinoma, generally good, although distant metastatic disease may persist in PTC and indicate a worse prognosis for FC

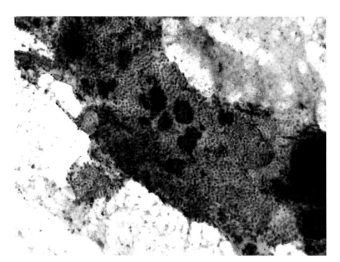

Figure 4.6.1   Cellular adenomatoid nodule. A large, three-dimensional fragment of thyroid follicular cells. Even at this power, the nuclei do not appear to overlap. Follicles of varying size can be seen and contain red-staining colloid.

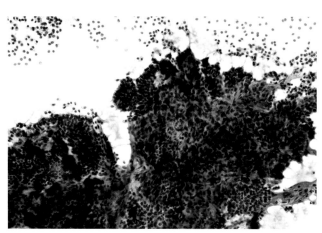

Figure 4.6.2   Cellular adenomatoid nodule. A three-dimensional fragment of thyroid follicular cells, with dispersed single cells in the background. While the papillary architecture may be concerning for papillary thyroid carcinoma, atypical nuclear features are lacking. An underlying microfollicular architecture that would cause concern for a follicular neoplasm is not identified.

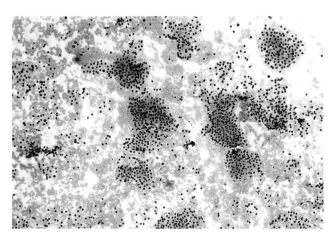

Figure 4.6.3   Cellular adenomatoid nodule. Numerous follicular cells are seen both in monolayer fragments as well as dispersed in the background. The cells have Hurthle cell change, causing nuclear enlargement and an increased amount of cytoplasm. Nuclear atypia is absent, and no microfollicular architecture can be identified. If colloid and lymphocytes are absent and the entire specimen contains Hurthle cells, the specimen would best be diagnosed as "suspicious for a Hurthle cell neoplasm" rather than a benign adenomatoid nodule.

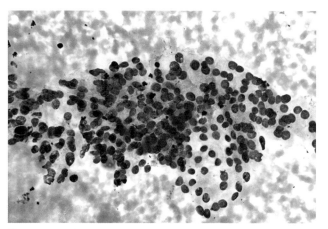

Figure 4.6.4   Cellular adenomatoid nodule. Thyroid follicular cells form a three-dimensional tissue fragment. Some cells are elongated, but the nuclear contours are regular and no other concerning features for PTC can be identified. While some focal microfollicular architecture can be identified, it is not a predominant feature.

4   THYROID

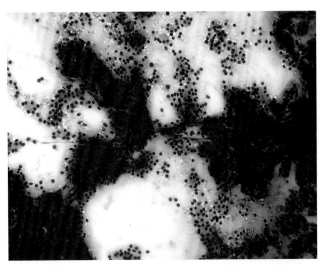

Figure 4.6.5 Suspicious for a follicular neoplasm. Numerous thyroid follicular cells are seen as single cells as well as present in single microfollicles and large tissue fragments. Nuclear features concerning for PTC are absent, as is colloid.

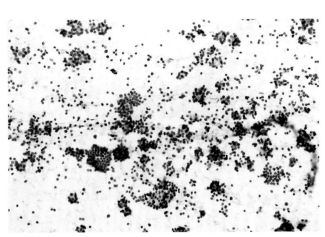

Figure 4.6.6 Suspicious for a follicular neoplasm. The specimen is cellular with thyroid follicular cells which are present singly in the background and also form small microfollicular structures. Nuclear features concerning for PTC are absent, as is colloid.

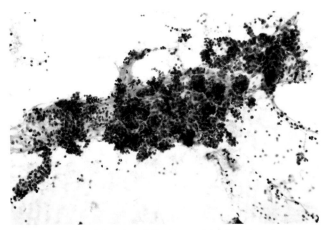

Figure 4.6.7 Suspicious for a follicular neoplasm. This large fragment of follicular cells is constructed from small "rings" of follicular cells (microfollicles), some of which contain dense globules of pink-staining colloid.

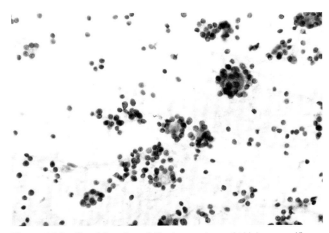

Figure 4.6.8 Suspicious for a follicular neoplasm. At higher magnification, the thyroid follicular cells seen here are small, uniform, and round and form predominantly microfollicles. Colloid is not a reassuring finding if only present in small amounts relative to the large number of follicular cells present.

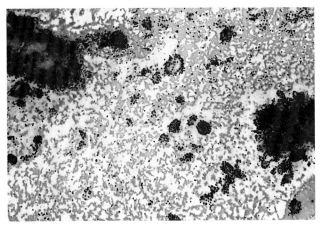

Figure 4.6.9 Suspicious for a follicular neoplasm. Follicular cells are seen in both small and large tissue fragments, but the predominant architecture is microfollicular. The specimen is highly cellular and colloid is absent.

	Cystic Papillary Thyroid Carcinoma	Benign Cystic Degeneration
Age	Mostly young adult and middle-aged women	Mostly young adult and middle-aged women
Location	Thyroid	Thyroid
Signs and symptoms	Usually solitary thyroid nodule; lymphadenopathy	Usually a dominant nodule within a multinodular thyroid
Etiology	Radiation exposure, Hashimoto thyroiditis, familial adenomatous polyposis	Enlarged thyroid due to iodine deficiency, Hashimoto thyroiditis, or other factors
Cytomorphology	• Specimen of varied cellularity containing a mixture of single malignant cells, malignant tissue fragments, and cystic macrophages *(Figures 4.7.1* and *4.7.2)* • The carcinoma cells may be present only in small numbers, or completely absent *(Figure 4.7.1)* • Cystic macrophages contain pigment in cytoplasm *(Figures 4.7.1* and *4.7.2)* • The carcinoma cells often have vacuolated "histiocytic" cytoplasm which causes a lowered N/C ratio *(Figures 4.7.3-4.7.5)* • The carcinoma cells retain the atypical features seen in PTC: enlargement, elongation, irregular nuclear borders, nuclear grooves, and intranuclear pseudoinclusions *(Figures 4.7.2-4.7.5)* • Rare carcinoma cells without vacuolated cytoplasm may be identified *(Figure 4.7.1)*	• Thyroid follicular cells in a background of pigmented cystic macrophages *(Figures 4.7.6-4.7.9)* • If sampled, follicular cells may have spindled cytoplasm, elongated, enlarged nuclei, and mild nuclear border irregularities ("cyst-lining cells"). Nuclear grooves and intranuclear pseudoinclusions are rare *(Figure 4.7.10)*
Special studies	Carcinoma cells are usually positive for TTF-1, PAX-8, and thyroglobulin by IHC, but may be lost in anaplastic areas if present	Cells are positive for TTF-1, PAX-8, and thyroglobulin and negative for PTH by IHC
Molecular alterations	*BRAF* or *RAS* mutations; *RET-PTC* rearrangements	None
Treatment	Surgical excision including cervical lymph node dissection with or without radioactive iodine	Observation or surgery for cosmetic or compressive symptoms
Clinical implications	Generally good but distantly metastatic disease may persist	Excellent

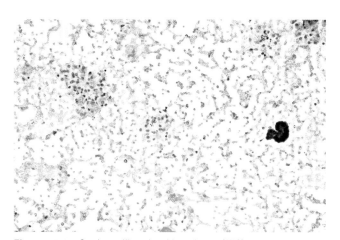

Figure 4.7.1 Cystic papillary thyroid carcinoma (PTC). Predominantly cyst fluid, as evidenced by numerous pigment-laden macrophages. A rare group of papillary thyroid carcinoma cells can be seen on the right-hand side of the field.

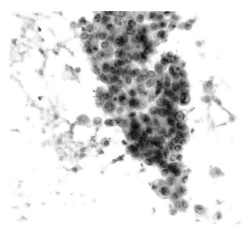

Figure 4.7.2 Cystic papillary thyroid carcinoma (PTC). A fragment of papillary thyroid carcinoma cells with increased amounts of foamy cytoplasm, which creates a deceivingly low N/C ratio. The nuclei are enlarged; the chromatin is powdery; and one cell has a large intranuclear pseudoinclusion.

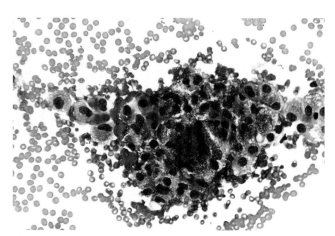

Figure 4.7.3 Cystic papillary thyroid carcinoma (PTC). These papillary thyroid carcinoma cells have a histiocytoid appearance due to their increased amounts of bubbly cytoplasm. The nuclei are enlarged and have irregular borders, creating suspicion for a cystic PTC.

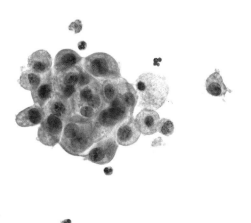

Figure 4.7.4 Cystic papillary thyroid carcinoma (PTC). A small group of papillary thyroid carcinoma cells with abundant foamy cytoplasm. The nuclei are enlarged and demonstrate great variation in size.

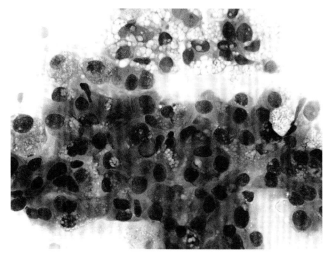

Figure 4.7.5 Cystic papillary thyroid carcinoma (PTC). The carcinoma cells in this fragment have highly irregular nuclear features but low N/C ratios due to their abundant cytoplasm, which is due to cellular uptake of the surrounding cyst fluid.

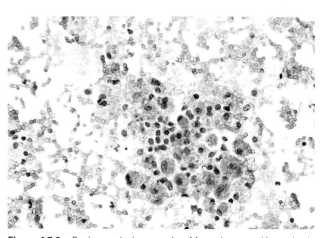

Figure 4.7.6 Benign cystic degeneration. Macrophages and intermixed lymphocytes. The macrophages can be identified by their cytoplasmic pigment and/or their curved nucleus. Their presence ensures that cyst fluid was indeed sampled and present on the preparation.

4 THYROID

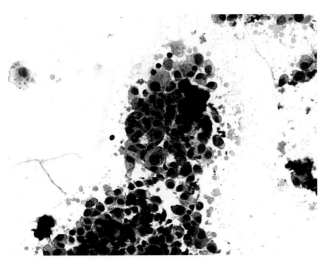

Figure 4.7.7   Benign cystic degeneration. Numerous macrophages cluster together and emulate a tissue fragment. Most of the cells contain cytoplasmic pigment, which helps identify them as macrophages.

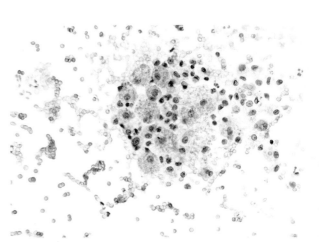

Figure 4.7.8   Benign cystic degeneration. A separate field of pigment-laden cystic macrophages mixed with lymphocytes.

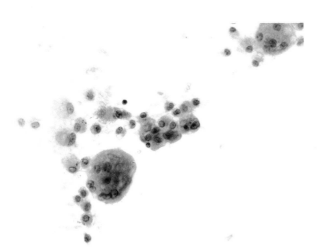

Figure 4.7.9   Benign cystic degeneration. Multinucleated giant cells can sometimes be seen in cyst fluid and are of no particular consequence.

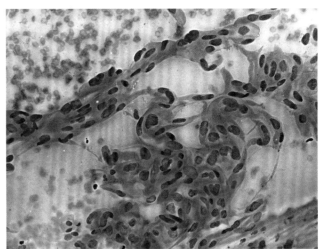

Figure 4.7.10   Benign cystic degeneration. When sampled, the follicular cells lining cyst contents may demonstrate atypia secondary to the forces exerted by the cyst fluid over time. These "cyst-lining cells" may have elongated nuclei and "stretched" cytoplasm but usually only mild nuclear atypia.

4.8 COLLOID NODULE VERSUS CYST FLUID

	Colloid Nodule	Cyst Fluid
Age	Mostly young adult and middle-aged women	Mostly young adult and middle-aged women
Location	Thyroid	Thyroid
Signs and symptoms	Usually a dominant nodule within a multinodular thyroid	Dominant nodule within a multinodular thyroid, or a solitary thyroid nodule if cystic PTC; lymphadenopathy if cystic PTC
Etiology	Enlarged thyroid due to iodine deficiency, Hashimoto thyroiditis, or other factors	Enlarged thyroid due to iodine deficiency, Hashimoto thyroiditis, or other factors, or if cystic PTC, radiation exposure, Hashimoto thyroiditis, familial adenomatous polyposis
Cytomorphology	• Abundant background material that stains purple on Diff-Quik–stained preparations and pink-cyan on Pap stained preparations (Figures 4.8.1 and 4.8.2) • Zones of thick and thin colloid may be present (Figure 4.8.3) • Colloid may form bubbles or crack, which help differentiate colloid from thick serum (Figures 4.8.4 and 4.8.5) • The colloid may contain crystals, macrophages, and rare groups of benign follicular cells (Figures 4.8.1 and 4.8.2)	• Background of granular debris and/or fibrin without features of colloid (Figures 4.8.6 and 4.8.7) • The cyst fluid should contain cystic macrophages to confirm the fluid was properly processed onto the slide (Figures 4.8.8 and 4.8.9) • Crystals may be present (Figure 4.8.10) • Cyst-lining cells are often absent
Special studies	Cells are positive for TTF-1, PAX-8, and thyroglobulin and negative for PTH by IHC	Epithelial cells are usually positive for TTF-1, PAX-8, and thyroglobulin by IHC; cystic macrophages are positive for CD68
Molecular alterations	None	None in benign cyst fluid; for cystic PTC, BRAF or RAS mutations, or RET-PTC rearrangements
Treatment	Observation or surgery for cosmetic or compressive symptoms	FNA is considered non-diagnostic and re-biopsy is indicated. Subsequent treatment depends on re-biopsy result
Clinical implications	Excellent	Excellent. Patients with cystic PTC do well with treatment but distantly metastatic disease may persist

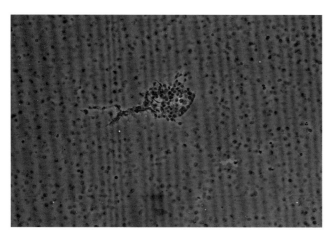

Figure 4.8.1 Colloid nodule. Thick purple-stained colloid covers the entire field and obscures red blood cells. A group of benign-appearing thyroid follicular cells is present in the center, with elongated cytoplasm.

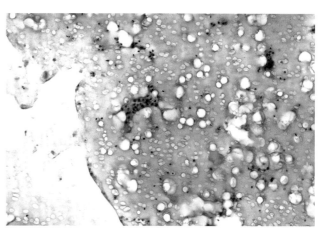

Figure 4.8.2 Colloid nodule. Cystic macrophages and lymphocytes float in pink-staining cyst fluid. Bubbles have formed in the thickened colloid, which would not happen so prominently in thickened serum.

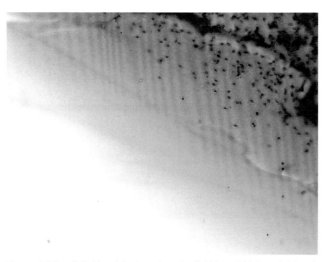

Figure 4.8.3 Colloid nodule. Layering of colloid into thick (top right) and thin (bottom left) layers. The thickened colloid has trapped numerous red blood cells.

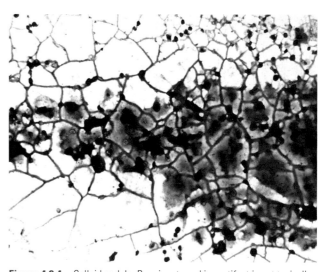

Figure 4.8.4 Colloid nodule. Prominent cracking artifact is not typically seen in thickened serum and provides reassurance that colloid is present in the background.

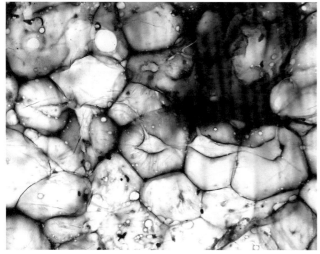

Figure 4.8.5 Colloid nodule. Prominent bubbling of colloid is another feature not typically seen in thickened serum and helps the identification of colloid.

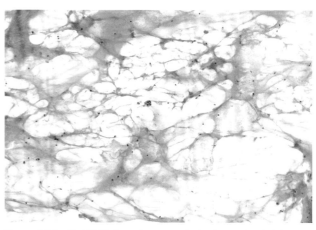

Figure 4.8.6 Cyst fluid. Amorphous granular background material envelopes cystic macrophages and inflammatory cells. This material could represent fibrin and/or cyst contents but is not suggestive of colloid.

4 THYROID

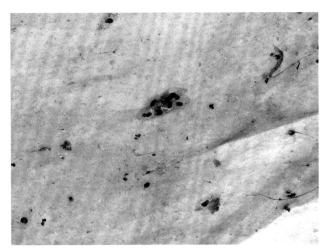

Figure 4.8.7   Cyst fluid. A cluster of macrophages is present in the center of granular debris. Cyst-lining cells are not identified, and thus the nature of the cyst is unknown.

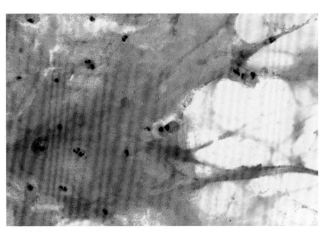

Figure 4.8.8   Cyst fluid. Pigment-laden macrophages are associated with granular debris. Colloid is not identified.

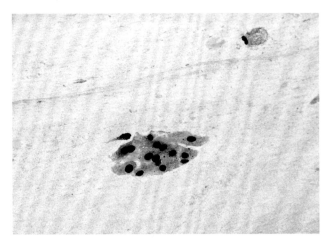

Figure 4.8.9   Cyst fluid. A small cluster of macrophages are present in a background of cyst contents.

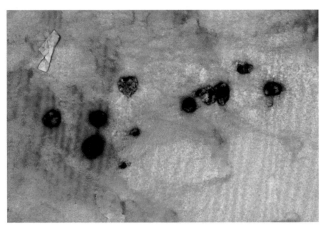

Figure 4.8.10   Cyst fluid. A crystal has formed in this cyst, as seen on the top left of the field. Several macrophages are also present. The background is granular and does not have any features of colloid.

	Papillary Thyroid Carcinoma	Medullary Thyroid Carcinoma (MTC)
Age	Mostly young adult and middle-aged women	Middle-aged adults; younger in familial
Location	Thyroid	Thyroid
Signs and symptoms	Usually solitary thyroid nodule; lymphadenopathy	Painless thyroid mass or cervical lymphadenopathy; flushing and diarrhea in metastatic disease
Etiology	Radiation exposure, Hashimoto thyroiditis, familial adenomatous polyposis	Derived from calcitonin-secreting C cells. Associated with familial syndromes MEN 2A, MEN 2B, familial medullary thyroid carcinoma syndrome, von-Hippel-Lindau disease, and neurofibromatosis
Cytomorphology	• Predominantly cohesive tissue fragments in papillary and/or monolayer sheet configurations (*Figures 4.9.1* and *4.9.2*) • Usually minimal or absent colloid (*Figure 4.9.1*) • Elevated nuclear to cytoplasmic ratios (*Figure 4.9.3*) • Enlarged oval nuclei with powdery chromatin (*Figure 4.9.4*) • Irregular nuclear contours (*Figure 4.9.3*) • Nuclear grooves (*Figure 4.9.4*) • Intranuclear pseudoinclusions may be present (*Figures 4.9.1*, *4.9.4* and *4.9.5*)	• Loosely cohesive and scattered, monotonous cells (*Figures 4.9.6* and *4.9.7*) • Background may contain amorphous amyloid material (*Figure 4.9.8*). Colloid is absent • Neoplastic cells are epithelioid or spindled with an eccentrically placed nucleus and abundant cytoplasm (*Figures 4.9.9* and *4.9.10*) • Regular nuclear borders but may demonstrate anisonucleosis (*Figure 4.9.9*) • Chromatin has a speckled (neuroendocrine) appearance (*Figure 4.9.10*)
Special studies	Carcinoma cells are usually positive for TTF-1, PAX-8, and thyroglobulin by IHC, but may be lost in anaplastic areas if present. Negative for calcitonin	Positive for calcitonin, TTF-1, PAX-8, and neuroendocrine markers and negative for thyroglobulin by IHC. Amyloid can be identified by a Congo Red special stain. Needle rinses have elevated calcitonin levels
Molecular alterations	*BRAF* or *RAS* mutations; *RET-PTC* rearrangements	Mutations in *RET* gene in most familial cases and 50% of sporadic cases. Otherwise, mutations in *HRAS* or *KRAS*
Treatment	Surgical excision including cervical lymph node dissection with or without radioactive iodine	Surgical excision
Clinical implications	Generally good but distantly metastatic disease may persist	10-year survival of 75%-85%, worse with distant metastases

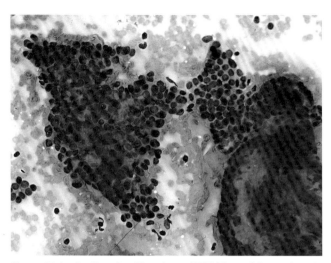

Figure 4.9.1   Papillary thyroid carcinoma (PTC). The nuclei are enlarged and oval shaped. Several intranuclear psuedoinclusions can be seen (top left of fragment), and dense colloid is present (right side of field).

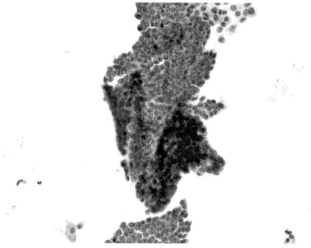

Figure 4.9.2   Papillary thyroid carcinoma (PTC). This folded monolayer of papillary thyroid carcinoma demonstrates nuclear crowding and overlap secondary to nuclear enlargement. The chromatin is powdery, a feature that is always highly suspicious for PTC.

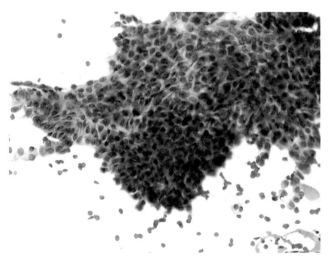

Figure 4.9.3   Papillary thyroid carcinoma (PTC). The nuclei in this fragment are predominantly elongated and crowded, and several have nuclear grooves.

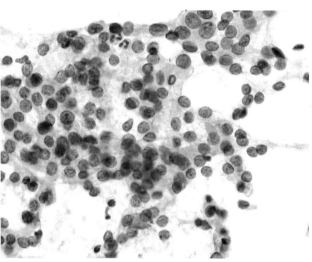

Figure 4.9.4   Papillary thyroid carcinoma (PTC). While the cells in this fragment of PTC have abundant cytoplasm, the nuclei are enlarged and have powdery chromatin. A prominent intranuclear pseudoinclusion can be seen in the top center.

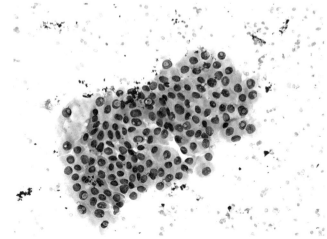

Figure 4.9.5   Papillary thyroid carcinoma (PTC). This fragment of PTC contains numerous intranuclear pseudoinclusions, which have the same color and quality as the cell cytoplasm.

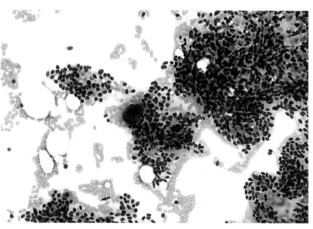

Figure 4.9.6   Medullary thyroid carcinoma (MTC). Cellular and loosely cohesive fragments of MTC are present. The nuclei are predominantly spindled shaped.

4 THYROID

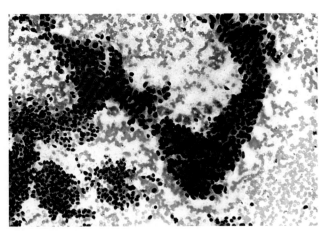

Figure 4.9.7   Medullary thyroid carcinoma (MTC). This fragment of MTC imitates PTC, as it is papillary shaped and the nuclei are oval shaped and crowded. Several cells are dispersed in the background, which should give some consideration to the possibility of MTC; however, dispersed cells can also be seen in PTC.

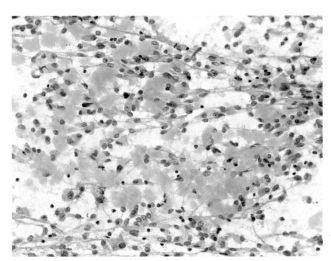

Figure 4.9.8   Medullary thyroid carcinoma (MTC). Numerous spindle-shaped nuclei are associated with cyan-staining amorphous amyloid.

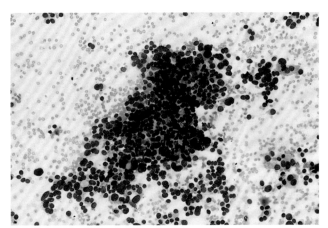

Figure 4.9.9   Medullary thyroid carcinoma (MTC). The field is cellular with numerous individual cells and stripped nuclei. Variation in nuclear size can be seen, similar to what can occur with Hurthle cell metaplasia in follicular cells. For individually dispersed cells with identifiable cytoplasm, the nuclei are eccentrically placed, a feature that suggests MTC.

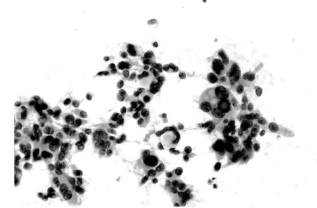

Figure 4.9.10   Medullary thyroid carcinoma (MTC). This medullary thyroid carcinoma is a bit more pleomorphic, with several multinucleated cells and a prominent intranuclear inclusion. There is a hint of "salt-and-pepper" rather than powdery chromatin, which favors MTC rather than PTC.

	Papillary Thyroid Carcinoma	Suspicious for a Follicular Neoplasm
Age	Mostly young adult and middle-aged women	Middle-aged adults; more commonly women
Location	Thyroid	Thyroid
Signs and symptoms	Usually solitary thyroid nodule; lymphadenopathy	Solitary thyroid nodule
Etiology	Radiation exposure, Hashimoto thyroiditis, familial adenomatous polyposis	Follicular adenoma, follicular variant of PTC, noninvasive follicular thyroid neoplasm with papillary-like nuclear features (NIFTP), or follicular carcinoma
Cytomorphology	• Predominantly cohesive tissue fragments in papillary and/or monolayer sheet configurations. May form a predominantly microfollicular architecture (*Figures 4.10.1* and *4.10.2*) • Usually minimal or absent colloid. Colloid may be present as dense globules (*Figures 4.10.1* and *4.10.2*) • Elevated nuclear to cytoplasmic ratios (*Figures 4.10.3* and *4.10.4*) • Enlarged oval nuclei with powdery chromatin (*Figure 4.10.3*) • Irregular nuclear contours (*Figures 4.10.3* and *4.10.5*) • Nuclear grooves (*Figures 4.10.4* and *4.10.5*) • Intranuclear pseudoinclusions may be present	• Highly cellular specimen with follicular cells present in tissue fragments as well as dispersed equisized microfollicles and single cells in the background (*Figures 4.10.6* and *4.10.7*) • Absent or rare colloid, which may form dense globules within microfollicles (*Figure 4.10.8*) • Fragments are predominantly constructed from microfollicular structures of less than 12 cells each (*Figures 4.10.6-4.10.9*)
Special studies	Carcinoma cells are usually positive for TTF-1, PAX-8, and thyroglobulin by IHC, but may be lost in anaplastic areas if present. Negative for calcitonin	Cells are positive for TTF-1, PAX-8, and thyroglobulin by IHC
Molecular alterations	*BRAF* or *RAS* mutations; *RET-PTC* rearrangements	*RAS* mutations (follicular adenoma, NIFTP, and follicular carcinoma); *NRAS*, *HRAS*, *PI3CA*, *PTEN* mutations or *PAX8-PPAR* gamma rearrangements (follicular carcinoma)
Treatment	Surgical excision including cervical lymph node dissection with or without radioactive iodine	Initially, thyroid lobectomy or total thyroidectomy (if concomitant positive ancillary testing). Subsequent treatment depends on the specific diagnosis
Clinical implications	Generally good, but distantly metastatic disease may persist	Excellent; for PTC, generally good, although distant metastatic disease may persist in PTC and indicate a worse prognosis for FC

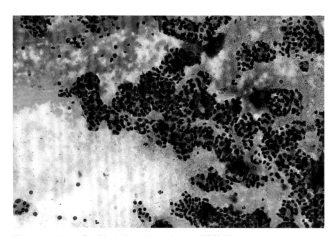

Figure 4.10.1   Papillary thyroid carcinoma (PTC). The nuclei are enlarged and overlapping; colloid is only present as dense globules ("bubble gum colloid").

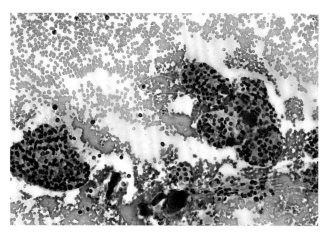

Figure 4.10.2   Papillary thyroid carcinoma (PTC). Separate field.

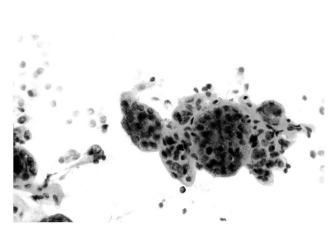

Figure 4.10.3   Papillary thyroid carcinoma (PTC). Some atypical features of papillary thyroid carcinoma include nuclear enlargement, nuclear membrane irregularities, oval nuclear shape, and powdery chromatin.

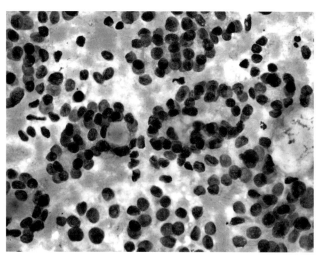

Figure 4.10.4   Papillary thyroid carcinoma (PTC). PTC cells with a microfollicular arrangement, in which some cells encircled blue-staining dense colloid. The nuclei are enlarged and overlapping; several nuclei have prominent grooves.

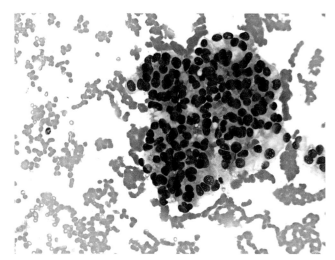

Figure 4.10.5   Papillary thyroid carcinoma (PTC). A fragment of papillary thyroid carcinoma cells built from several small follicles. The nuclei are oval shaped and have prominent nuclear grooves.

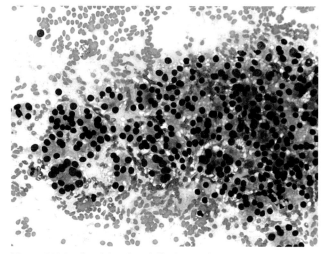

Figure 4.10.6   Suspicious for a follicular neoplasm. Thyroid follicular cells with a predominantly microfollicular arrangement. The cells have enlarged nuclei with anisonucleosis due to Hurthle cell change, but the nuclei are round and lack grooves and contour irregularities.

4   THYROID

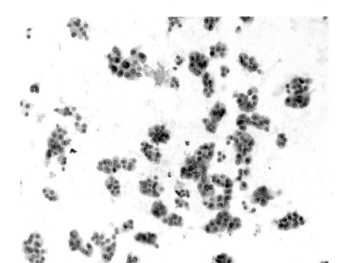

Figure 4.10.7   Suspicious for a follicular neoplasm. Scattered microfol-licles, each containing less than 10 follicular cells. The nuclei are round and have regular borders, and the chromatin seen is not of the "powdery" quality associated with PTC.

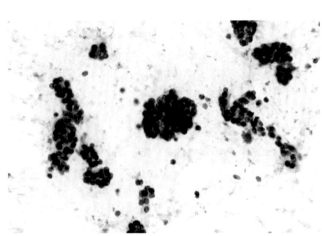

Figure 4.10.8   Suspicious for a follicular neoplasm. Several microfolli-cles are present, either linked together or present singly. Several contain dense, pink-staining colloid. The differential diagnosis includes follicular adenoma, follicular carcinoma, NIFTP, and the follicular variant of PTC, although the latter two are very unlikely due to an absence of atypical nuclear features.

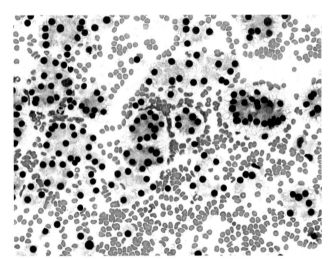

Figure 4.10.9   Suspicious for a follicular neoplasm. Bland-appearing fol-licular cells are present singly in the background and also form microfol-licular structures. The nuclei are round and have regular nuclear contours.

	Papillary Thyroid Carcinoma	Cellular Adenomatoid Nodule
Age	Mostly young adult and middle-aged women	Mostly young adult and middle-aged women
Location	Thyroid	Thyroid
Signs and symptoms	Usually solitary thyroid nodule; lymphadenopathy	Usually a dominant nodule within a multinodular thyroid
Etiology	Radiation exposure, Hashimoto thyroiditis, familial adenomatous polyposis	Enlarged thyroid due to iodine deficiency, Hashimoto thyroiditis, or other factors
Cytomorphology	• Predominantly cohesive tissue fragments in papillary and/or monolayer sheet configurations *(Figures 4.11.1* and *4.11.2)* • Usually minimal or absent colloid *(Figures 4.11.3* and *4.11.4)* • Elevated nuclear to cytoplasmic ratios *(Figure 4.11.5)* • Enlarged oval nuclei with powdery chromatin *(Figure 4.11.5)* • Irregular nuclear contours *(Figures 4.11.3* and *4.11.5)* • Nuclear grooves *(Figure 4.11.3)* • Intranuclear pseudoinclusions may be present *(Figure 4.11.5)*	• Tissue fragments, often in three-dimensional sheets, containing monotonous follicular cells that may contain colloid *(Figures 4.11.6* and *4.11.7)* • Background colloid material *(Figure 4.11.8)* • Single cells and stripped nuclei may be absent or present in small numbers in the background *(Figure 4.11.9)* • Nuclei are round and have regular nuclear contours *(Figure 4.11.10)*
Special studies	Carcinoma cells are usually positive for TTF-1, PAX-8, and thyroglobulin by IHC, but may be lost in anaplastic areas if present	Cells are positive for TTF-1, PAX-8, and thyroglobulin by IHC
Molecular alterations	*BRAF* or *RAS* mutations; *RET-PTC* rearrangements	None
Treatment	Surgical excision including cervical lymph node dissection with or without radioactive iodine	Observation or surgery for cosmetic or compressive symptoms
Clinical implications	Generally good but distantly metastatic disease may persist	Excellent

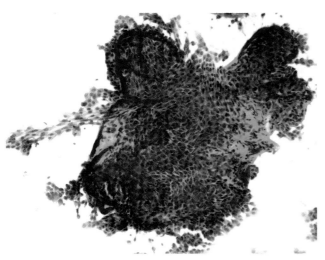

Figure 4.11.1 Papillary thyroid carcinoma (PTC). A fragment of papillary thyroid carcinoma with an associated fibrovascular core. The nuclei are elongated and overlapping due to high N/C ratios.

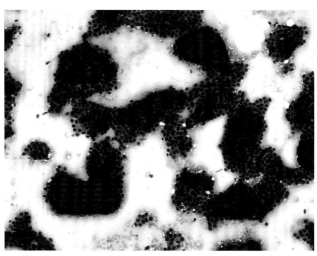

Figure 4.11.2 Papillary thyroid carcinoma (PTC). Papillary fragments containing monotonous populations of thyroid carcinoma cells. The cells have nuclei which are round to oval and have irregular shapes. The N/C ratios are elevated, and colloid is absent in the background.

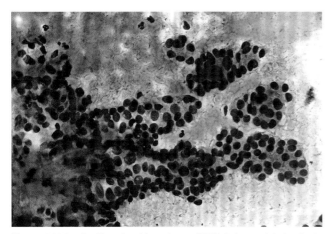

Figure 4.11.3 Papillary thyroid carcinoma (PTC). A dense globule of colloid is found associated with one group of cells. The cells have enlarged nuclei with irregular shapes; some have nuclear grooves.

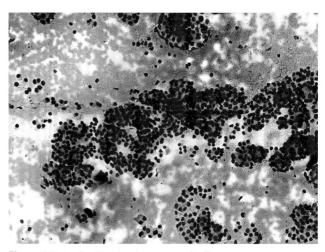

Figure 4.11.4 Papillary thyroid carcinoma (PTC). A small amount of dense colloid can be seen in this field. The cells form monolayer tissue fragments with papillary architecture. The nuclei are mostly elongated and enlarged.

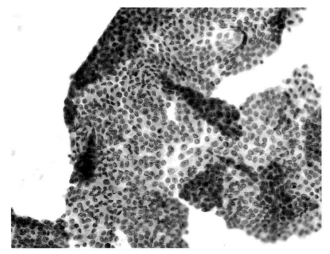

Figure 4.11.5 Papillary thyroid carcinoma (PTC). This monolayer fragment contains nuclei with powdery chromatin, elongation, irregular nuclear borders, nuclear grooves, and occasional intranuclear pseudoinclusions. A psammoma body can be seen at the top right-hand side of the field.

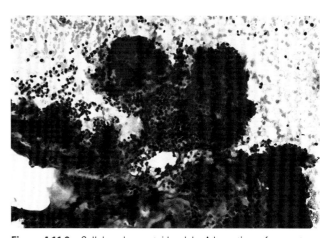

Figure 4.11.6 Cellular adenomatoid nodule. A large tissue fragment from an adenomatoid nodule is associated with vessels and appears to form papillary architecture. However, the cells have round and monotonous nuclei that do not overlap.

4   THYROID

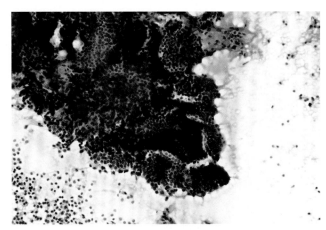

Figure 4.11.7   Cellular adenomatoid nodule. A folded sheet of benign follicular cells is seen adjacent to numerous dispersed individual cells in the background. The nuclei are round and monotonous and do not overlap. Pink-staining colloid is seen both within the tissue fragment as well as in the background.

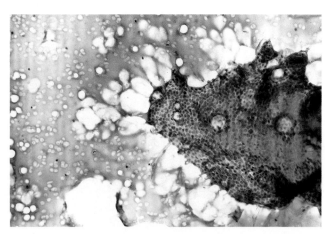

Figure 4.11.8   Cellular adenomatoid nodule. A large tissue fragment contains numerous benign follicular cells. The cells have round nuclei, each respecting their own space within the fragment. Pink-staining colloid is seen in the background, with negative images of red blood cells creating a "swiss cheese" appearance.

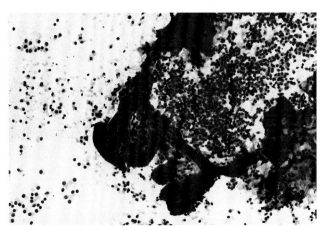

Figure 4.11.9   Cellular adenomatoid nodule. FNA of an adenomatoid nodule has yielded a cellular specimen, with individually dispersed cells as well as a papillary tissue fragment associated with fibrovascular cores. While colloid is not identified in this field, the small round nuclei of these cells provide reassurance that they are benign.

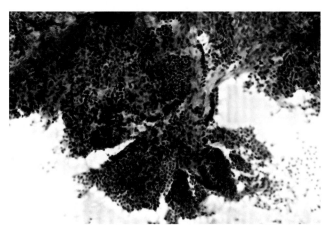

Figure 4.11.10   Cellular adenomatoid nodule. This benign fragment is cellular and papillary-like and contains a fibrovascular core. Although cellular, the spaces can be seen between the round, small nuclei even at this low magnification, indicating a benign process.

	Cyst-Lining Cells	Cystic Papillary Thyroid Carcinoma
Age	Mostly young adult and middle-aged women	Mostly young adult and middle-aged women
Location	Thyroid	Thyroid
Signs and symptoms	Usually a dominant nodule within a multinodular thyroid	Usually solitary thyroid nodule; lymphadenopathy
Etiology	Enlarged thyroid due to iodine deficiency, Hashimoto thyroiditis, or other factors	Radiation exposure, Hashimoto thyroiditis, familial adenomatous polyposis
Cytomorphology	• Small to medium fragments of cyst-lining cells have elongated cytoplasm and may contain bipolar processes (Figures 4.12.1 and 4.12.2) • Nuclei may be enlarged and/or elongated but only rarely contain nuclear grooves or intranuclear pseudoinclusions (Figures 4.12.3 and 4.12.4) • Chromatin does not have a powdery appearance (Figure 4.12.4) • Background of cyst fluid, cystic macrophages, and/or colloid (Figure 4.12.5)	• Specimen of varied cellularity containing a mixture of single malignant cells, malignant tissue fragments, and cystic macrophages (Figures 4.12.6 and 4.12.7) • The carcinoma cells may be present only in small numbers or completely absent (Figure 4.12.8) • Cystic macrophages contain pigment in cytoplasm (Figures 4.12.7 and 4.12.8) • The carcinoma cells may have bubbly cytoplasm which causes a lowered N/C ratio (Figure 4.12.1) • The carcinoma cells retain the atypical features seen in PTC: enlargement, elongation, irregular nuclear borders, nuclear grooves, and intranuclear pseudoinclusions (Figures 4.12.9 and 4.12.10)
Special studies	Cells are positive for TTF-1, PAX-8, and thyroglobulin and negative for PTH by IHC	Carcinoma cells are usually positive for TTF-1, PAX-8, and thyroglobulin by IHC, but may be lost in anaplastic areas if present
Molecular alterations	None	*BRAF* or *RAS* mutations; *RET-PTC* rearrangements
Treatment	Observation or surgery for cosmetic or compressive symptoms	Surgical excision including cervical lymph node dissection with or without radioactive iodine
Clinical implications	Excellent	Generally good but distantly metastatic disease may persist

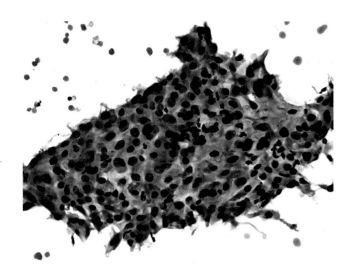

Figure 4.12.1   Cyst-lining cells. A fragment of benign cyst-lining cells with abundant cytoplasm, nuclear enlargement, and nuclear elongation.

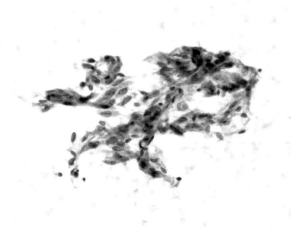

Figure 4.12.2   Cyst-lining cells. A small group of benign cyst-lining cells with bipolar, tapered cytoplasm and anisonucleosis. The chromatin does not have the powdery quality seen in PTC.

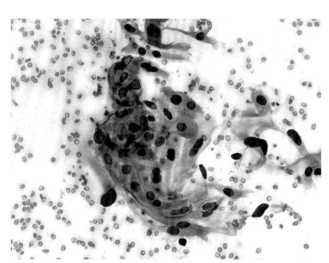

Figure 4.12.3   Cyst-lining cells. Cyst-lining cells can sometimes have irregular nuclear borders and nuclear elongation, which may cause concern for PTC. In some instances, it may be necessary to diagnose such a specimen as *Atypia of Undetermined Significance* rather than dismiss the changes as benign.

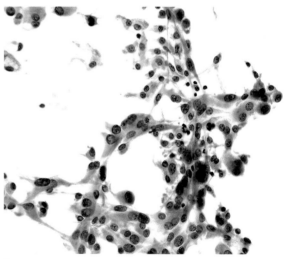

Figure 4.12.4   Cyst-lining cells. The cells seen here have elongated and enlarged nuclei. Missing are other features of PTC, such as powdery chromatin, nuclear grooves, and intranuclear pseudoinclusions.

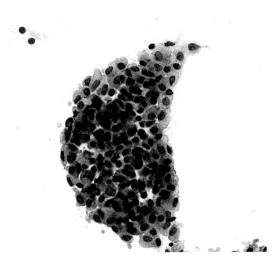

Figure 4.12.5   Cyst-lining cells. The field contains a cluster of cystic macrophages, many containing blue-staining cytoplasmic pigment. In cystic lesions, clusters of macrophages may aggregate to form pseudofragments and emulate a neoplasm.

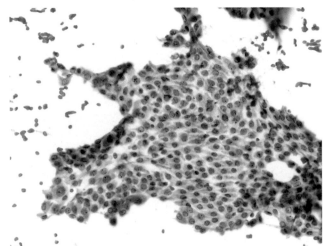

Figure 4.12.6   Cystic papillary thyroid carcinoma (PTC). The cells have an increased amount of cytoplasm, which appears "stretched" from the forces exerted by the cyst fluid. Despite having low N/C ratios, the nuclear features of PTC remain enlarged nuclei with powdery chromatin, some with nuclear grooves.

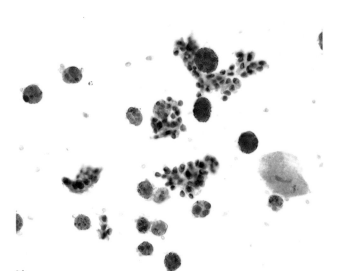

Figure 4.12.7   Cystic papillary thyroid carcinoma (PTC). The field shows groups of papillary thyroid carcinoma admixed with pigment-laden cystic macrophages. Cystic lesions may contain only small numbers of cyst-lining cells, limiting a definitive diagnosis.

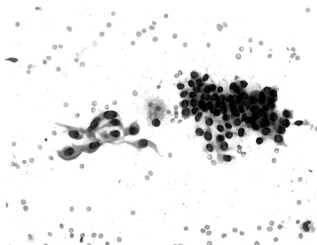

Figure 4.12.8   Cystic papillary thyroid carcinoma (PTC). Some of the cells have seen prominent cyst-lining change (left side of field) and others have less cytoplasm and higher N/C ratios (right side of field).

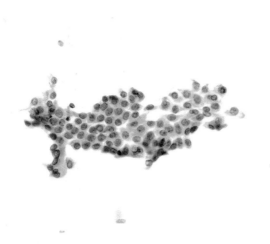

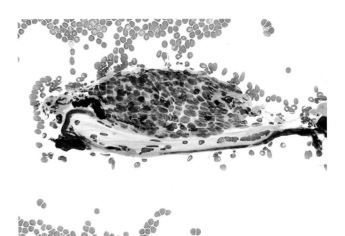

Figure 4.12.9   Cystic papillary thyroid carcinoma (PTC). This fragment contains cells with nuclear enlargement, powdery chromatin, and a prominent intranuclear pseudoinclusion.

Figure 4.12.10   Cystic papillary thyroid carcinoma (PTC). This small fragment of cells contains cells with elongated nuclei that overlap due to decreased N/C ratios. The elongated nuclei appear to "stream" in one direction, a feature seen in papillary thyroid carcinoma.

4 THYROID

	Noninvasive Follicular Thyroid Neoplasm with Papillary-like Nuclear Features (NIFTP)	Papillary Thyroid Carcinoma, Follicular Variant
Age	Mostly young adult and middle-aged women	Mostly young adult and middle-aged women
Location	Thyroid	Thyroid
Signs and symptoms	Solitary thyroid nodule	Usually solitary thyroid nodule; lymphadenopathy
Etiology	Under investigation	Radiation exposure, Hashimoto thyroiditis, familial adenomatous polyposis
Cytomorphology	• Cohesive tissue fragments that predominantly have an underlying microfollicular architecture *(Figures 4.13.1 and 4.13.2)* • Usually minimal or absent colloid. Colloid may be present as dense globules • Elevated nuclear to cytoplasmic ratios *(Figure 4.13.3)* • Enlarged oval nuclei with powdery chromatin *(Figures 4.13.4 and 4.13.5)* • Irregular nuclear contours *(Figure 4.13.3)* • Nuclear grooves may or may not be present *(Figures 4.13.4 and 4.13.5)* • Intranuclear pseudoinclusions may be present but are rare	• Cohesive tissue fragments that have an underlying microfollicular architecture but may also form monolayer fragments with papillary architecture *(Figures 4.13.6 and 4.13.7)* • Usually minimal or absent colloid. Colloid may be present as dense globules *(Figure 4.13.8)* • Elevated nuclear to cytoplasmic ratios *(Figure 4.13.9)* • Enlarged oval nuclei with powdery chromatin *(Figure 4.13.10)* • Irregular nuclear contours *(Figure 4.13.9)* • Nuclear grooves more common *(Figures 4.13.9 and 4.13.10)* • Intranuclear pseudoinclusions more common but may be absent
Special studies	Cells are positive for TTF-1, PAX-8, and thyroglobulin by IHC	Carcinoma cells are usually positive for TTF-1, PAX-8, and thyroglobulin by IHC, but may be lost in anaplastic areas if present
Molecular alterations	*RAS* mutations	*RAS* mutations; *BRAF* mutations less common. *RET-PTC* and *PAX8-PPAR gamma* rearrangements
Treatment	Thyroid lobectomy	Surgical excision including cervical lymph node dissection with or without radioactive iodine
Clinical implications	Excellent	Generally good but distantly metastatic disease may persist

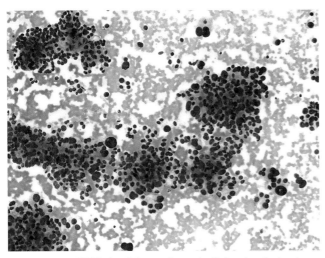

Figure 4.13.1   NIFTP. A cellular specimen of cells forming single microfollicles as well as larger tissue fragments with an underlying microfollicular architecture. The nuclei are enlarged, and some are elongated. Colloid is absent, and no intranuclear pseudoincusions can be identified.

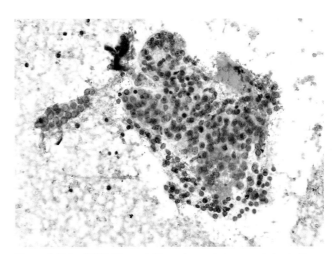

Figure 4.13.2   NIFTP. The nuclei here demonstrate some, but not all, features of papillary thyroid carcinoma: enlargement, oval shapes, and powdery chromatin.

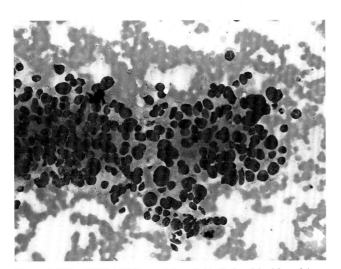

Figure 4.13.3   NIFTP. NIFTP cannot be reliably distinguished from follicular carcinoma, follicular adenoma, or the follicular variant of papillary thyroid carcinoma on cytology alone. Specimens usually contain incompletely features of PTC. A predominance of microfollicular architecture should be interpreted with caution.

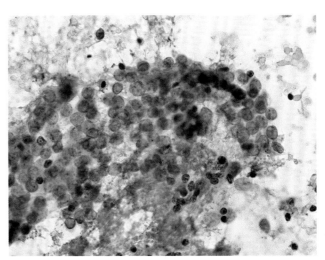

Figure 4.13.4   NIFTP. The nuclei are enlarged and overlapping, and some have nuclear grooves. The chromatin has a powdery appearance, usually only seen in PTC.

4   THYROID

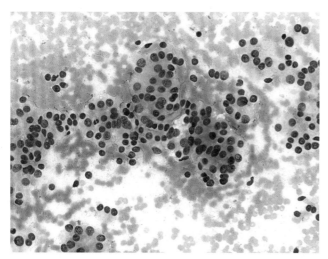

Figure 4.13.5 NIFTP. A predominance of microfollicular formations should raise suspicion for a possible NIFTP, even in the presence of intranuclear pseudoinclusions (seen here).

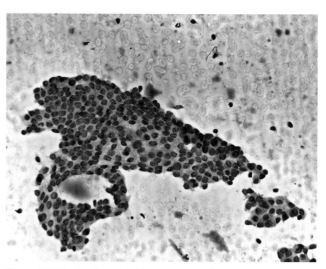

Figure 4.13.6 Papillary thyroid carcinoma (PTC). This field shows a small monolayer fragment without microfollicular architecture. Some areas of the follicular variant of PTC may not form microfollicular architecture.

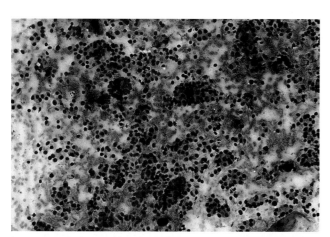

Figure 4.13.7 Papillary thyroid carcinoma (PTC). A cellular field containing dispersed cells, small microfollicles, and small fragments of cohesive microfollicles. While this could be seen in NIFTP, the subsequent specimen was diagnosed as a follicular variant of PTC.

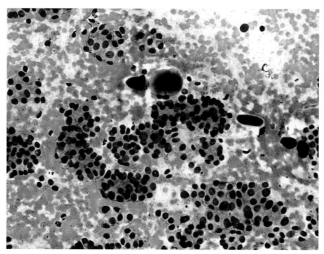

Figure 4.13.8 Papillary thyroid carcinoma (PTC). Thyroid carcinomas can sometimes contain dense globules of colloid ("bubble gum colloid") that should not be misinterpreted as a benign finding. Note the enlarged, overlapping, oval nuclei.

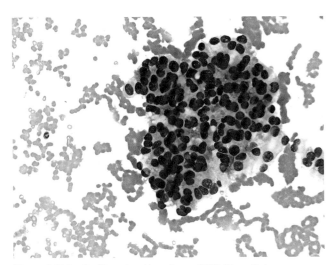

Figure 4.13.9 *Papillary thyroid carcinoma (PTC). The cells have sufficient nuclear atypia to cause concern for PTC—nuclear enlargement, irregular nuclear borders, oval-shaped nuclei, and nuclear grooves. The predominant microfollicular architecture may justify an indeterminate diagnosis, with a note suggesting the possibility of either NIFTP or the follicular variant of PTC.*

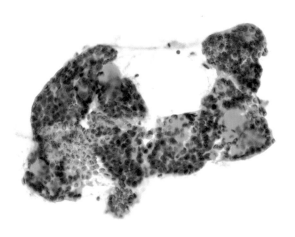

Figure 4.13.10 *Papillary thyroid carcinoma (PTC). This monolayer fragment has papillary architecture and does not have a microfollicular architecture. It likely represents a more conventional component within the follicular variant of PTC. Dense globules of colloid can be seen within the fragment.*

	Anaplastic Thyroid Carcinoma	Metastatic Cancers
Age	Older adults	Middle aged and older adults
Location	Thyroid	Thyroid
Signs and symptoms	Rapidly enlarging thyroid mass causing dysphagia and/or dyspnea	One or multiple thyroid nodules
Etiology	Unknown; may arise in a long-standing well-differentiated thyroid carcinoma	Invasion by adjacent squamous cell carcinoma of head and neck or metastasis of a kidney, lung, or breast carcinoma, or melanoma
Cytomorphology	• Highly pleomorphic cells present singly and/or in tissue fragments *(Figures 4.14.1 and 4.14.2)* • Background necrosis *(Figure 4.14.3)* • Giant cells, spindle cells, and/or squamous differentiation may be seen *(Figures 4.14.4 and 4.14.5)* • Areas of more conventional thyroid carcinoma may be seen	• Singly dispersed cells and/or cells seen in tissue fragments • Morphology varies based on primary site • Renal cell carcinoma cells have abundant, vacuolated cytoplasm with eccentrically placed nuclei and nucleolar prominence and are rarely pleomorphic *(Figure 4.14.6)* • Conventional adenocarcinoma have enlarged nuclei, irregular nuclear borders, may form glands, and are pleomorphic when poorly differentiated *(Figures 4.14.7 and 4.14.8)* • Squamous cell carcinoma have dense, waxy cytoplasm and may have keratinaceous debris *(Figures 4.14.9 and 4.14.10)* • Melanoma can look epithelioid or spindled with binucleation, cytoplasmic pigment, and/or cytopasmic tails
Special studies	Cells may lack most thyroid markers by IHC; PAX-8 is the most sensitive marker	Varies based on site of origin; the lung may be TTF-1 positive, and the kidney may be PAX-8 positive by IHC. Melanoma markers.
Molecular alterations	*RAS* mutations	Varies based on site of origin and neoplasm type
Treatment	Surgery and/or chemoradiation; some targeted therapies available	Chemoradiation and/or targeted therapies/immunotherapy depending on carcinoma type and marker status
Clinical implications	Poor prognosis; <20% survive one year	Varies based on neoplasm type and status

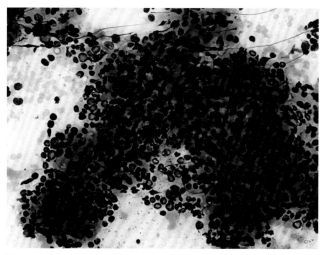

Figure 4.14.1   Anaplastic thyroid carcinoma. A fragment of cells with loosely cohesive and single cells at the fragment edges. Even at this low magnification, the nuclei are enlarged and pleomorphic, giving no clue as to a site of origin.

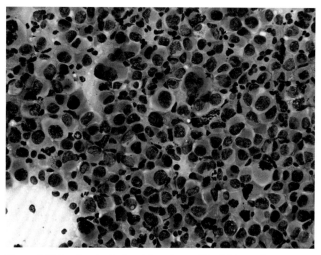

Figure 4.14.2   Anaplastic thyroid carcinoma. The field contains a sea of large, pleomorphic cells with abundant cytoplasm and enlarged nuclei with irregular shapes.

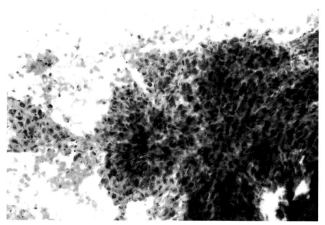

Figure 4.14.3   Anaplastic thyroid carcinoma. The cells form a cellular fragment, with abundant necrotic debris in the background.

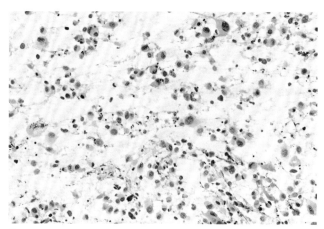

Figure 4.14.4   Anaplastic thyroid carcinoma. Singly dispersed pleomorphic cells can be seen in a background of necrotic debris. There is great variation in nuclear size.

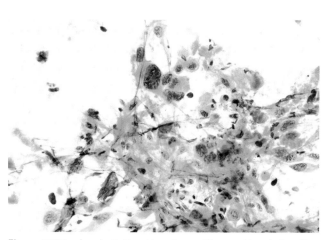

Figure 4.14.5   Anaplastic thyroid carcinoma. Pleomorphic spindle cells have enlarged, oval nuclei and hyperchromasia. A fragment of pink-staining keratinaceous debris suggests the tumor may have squamous differentiation.

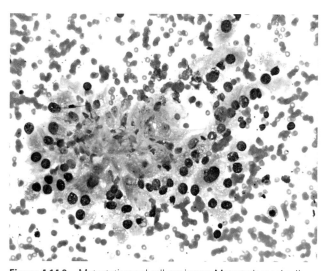

Figure 4.14.6   Metastatic renal cell carcinoma. Metastatic renal cell carcinoma is the most common metastasis to the thyroid. The cells usually have round nuclei with regular borders, in contrast to anaplastic thyroid carcinoma.

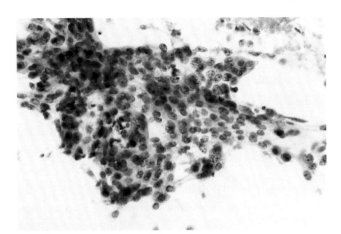

Figure 4.14.7   Metastatic breast ductal adenocarcinoma. The malignant cells have formed a three-dimensional tissue fragment of cells with high N/C ratios, dark chromatin, and irregular nuclear borders. The pleomorphism is less than what is seen in anaplastic thyroid carcinoma.

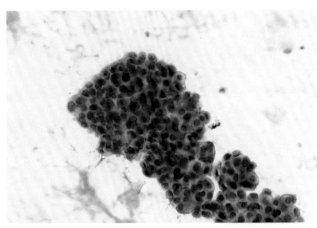

Figure 4.14.8   Metastatic breast ductal adenocarcinoma. A three-dimensional papillary fragment contains cells with enlarged, dark nuclei. Anaplastic features are absent and are uncommonly seen in most metastatic adenocarcinomas.

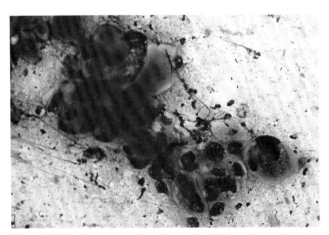

Figure 4.14.9   Squamous cell carcinoma. The field contains malignant cells with dense, waxy cytoplasm and large, dark nuclei with irregular borders and variation in size. Squamous cell carcinoma may metastasize to the thyroid or extend from adjacent structures in the head and neck.

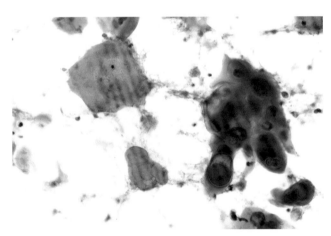

Figure 4.14.10   Squamous cell carcinoma. One fragment of malignant cells can be seen adjacent to irregularly shaped anucleate fragments of keratin. Most always, patients with squamous cell carcinoma in the thyroid will have a history or clinical suspicion of head and neck squamous cell carcinoma, helping to exclude an anaplastic thyroid carcinoma with squamous differentiation.

	Insular Thyroid Carcinoma	Papillary Thyroid Carcinoma
Age	Older adults	Mostly young adult and middle-aged women
Location	Thyroid	Thyroid
Signs and symptoms	Thyoid mass; lymphadenopathy	Usually solitary thyroid nodule; lymphadenopathy
Etiology	Unknown; may arise from the dedifferentiated of a well-differentiated thyroid carcinoma	Radiation exposure, Hashimoto thyroiditis, familial adenomatous polyposis
Cytomorphology	• Cellular specimen with neoplastic cells present predominantly in tight tissue fragment "packets" *(Figures 4.15.1* and *4.15.2)* • Nuclei are round to oval, enlarged, and overlap in tissue fragments *(Figures 4.15.3* and *4.15.4)* • Nuclear palisading around tissue fragment edges *(Figure 4.15.1)* • Nuclear contours are regular *(Figure 4.15.5)* • The cells do not demonstrate nuclear grooves, powdery chromatin, or intranuclear pseudoinclusions; the chromatin may have a neuroendocrine appearance	• Predominantly cohesive tissue fragments in papillary and/or monolayer sheet configurations *(Figures 4.15.6* and *4.15.7)* • Usually minimal or absent colloid *(Figure 4.15.8)* • Elevated nuclear to cytoplasmic ratios *(Figure 4.15.9)* • Enlarged oval nuclei with powdery chromatin *(Figure 4.15.9)* • Irregular nuclear contours *(Figure 4.15.10)* • Nuclear grooves *(Figure 4.15.10)* • Intranuclear pseudoinclusions may be present
Special studies	Cells are positive for TTF-1, PAX-8, and thyroglobulin by IHC	Carcinoma cells are usually positive for TTF-1, PAX-8, and thyroglobulin by IHC, but may be lost in anaplastic areas if present. Negative for calcitonin
Molecular alterations	*BRAF* or *RAS* mutations	*BRAF* or *RAS* mutations; *RET-PTC* rearrangements
Treatment	Thyroidectomy with cervical lymph node dissection with or without radioactive iodine	Surgical excision including cervical lymph node dissection with or without radioactive iodine
Clinical implications	More aggressive; often recurs and higher rate of aggressive distant metastases	Generally good but distantly metastatic disease may persist

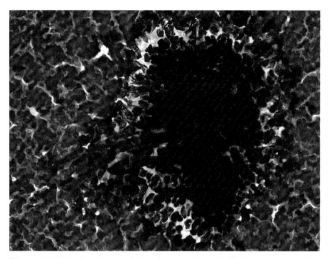

Figure 4.15.1   Insular thryoid carcinoma. A "packet" of carcinoma cells is shown. The cells are mostly oval, crowded, and palisade along the edges of the fragment.

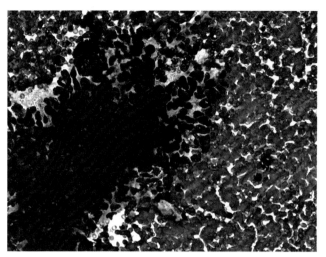

Figure 4.15.2   Insular thryoid carcinoma. Elongated cells palisade along the fragment edges. The nuclei are enlarged but lack nuclear grooves and intranuclear pseudoinclusions.

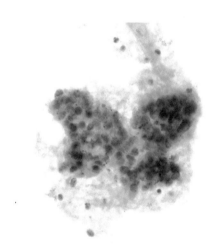

Figure 4.15.3   Insular thryoid carcinoma. A "packet" of more epithelioid insular carcinoma cells. The cells lack most distinctive features of well-differentiated thyroid carcinomas, such as microfollicular formation in follicular carcinoma and nuclear grooves of PTC.

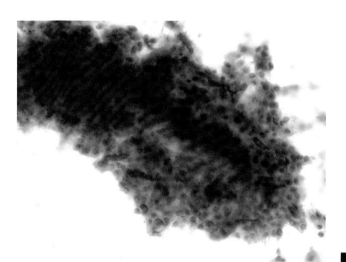

Figure 4.15.4   Insular thryoid carcinoma. A papillary fragment emulates PTC. Insular carcinoma on FNA is usually cellular and unusual enough to cause suspicion for a neoplasm but is difficult to definitively diagnose on cytomorphology alone.

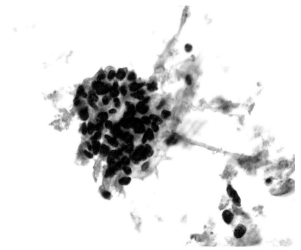

Figure 4.15.5   Insular thryoid carcinoma. A "packet" of cells with enlargement and elongation can be seen. The cells have uniform, dark chromatin, and rare intranuclear pseudoinclusions.

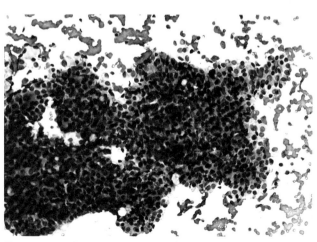

Figure 4.15.6   Papillary thyroid carcinoma (PTC). This papillary fragment contains cells with enlarged, oval nuclei.

4   THYROID

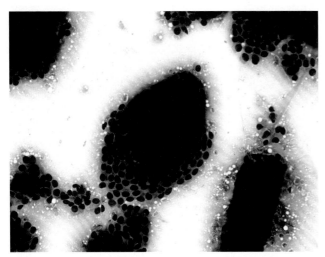

Figure 4.15.7 Papillary thyroid carcinoma (PTC). These fragments contain oval-shaped nuclei, some with grooves. An intranuclear pseudoinclusion is present at the bottom right.

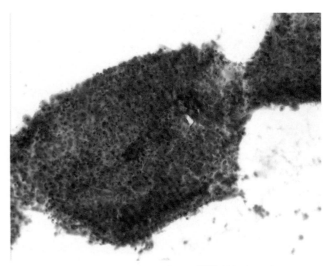

Figure 4.15.8 Papillary thyroid carcinoma (PTC). This tissue fragment is cellular and contains disorganized cells with oval-shaped nuclei. Small globules of red-staining colloid can be seen within the fragment.

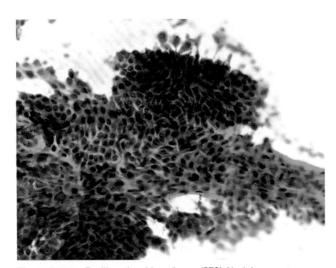

Figure 4.15.9 Papillary thyroid carcinoma (PTC). Nuclei appear to "stream" within this fragment. The nuclei are oval shaped, and several have nuclear grooves.

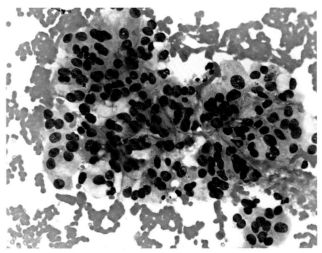

Figure 4.15.10 Papillary thyroid carcinoma (PTC). Many of the cells in this fragment have abundant cytoplasm, but they also have enlarged nuclei, many with oval shapes.

	Hyalinizing Trabecular Adenoma (Tumor)	Papillary Thyroid Carcinoma
Age	Middle-aged and older women	Mostly young adult and middle-aged women
Location	Thyroid	Thyroid
Signs and symptoms	Solitary thyroid nodule	Usually solitary thyroid nodule; lymphadenopathy
Etiology	Unknown; can be associated with lymphocytic thyroiditis	Radiation exposure, Hashimoto thyroiditis, familial adenomatous polyposis
Cytomorphology	• Cellular specimen containing neoplastic cells in loosely cohesive fragments and present singly (Figures 4.16.1 and 4.16.2) • Neoplastic cells are associated with hyaline material (Figures 4.16.3 and 4.16.4) • Neoplastic cells contain features of PTC, such as nuclear elongation, nuclear grooves, and numerous intranuclear pseudoinclusions (Figures 4.16.4 and 4.16.5) • Often vacuolated cytoplasm • Nuclei may be oval-to-spindle shaped	• Predominantly cohesive tissue fragments in papillary and/or monolayer sheet configurations (Figures 4.16.6 and 4.16.7) • Usually minimal or absent colloid (Figure 4.16.8) • Elevated nuclear to cytoplasmic ratios (Figure 4.15.6) • Enlarged oval nuclei with powdery chromatin (Figure 4.16.9) • Irregular nuclear contours (Figure 4.16.6) • Nuclear grooves (Figure 4.15.9) • Intranuclear pseudoinclusions may be present (Figure 4.16.10)
Special studies	Cells are positive for TTF-1, PAX-8, and thyroglobulin by IHC	Carcinoma cells are usually positive for TTF-1, PAX-8, and thyroglobulin by IHC, but may be lost in anaplastic areas if present
Molecular alterations	*RET-PTC* rearrangements	*BRAF* or *RAS* mutations; *RET-PTC* rearrangements
Treatment	Thyroid lobectomy	Surgical excision including cervical lymph node dissection with or without radioactive iodine
Clinical implications	Excellent	Generally good but distantly metastatic disease may persist

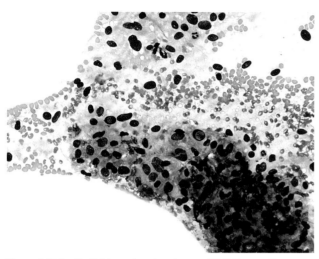

Figure 4.16.1 Hyalinizing trabecular adenoma (HTA). These cells are present singly as well as in a loosely cohesive tissue fragment. The cells have nuclear enlargement and elongation. A prominent intranuclear pseudoinclusion is present in the center of the field.

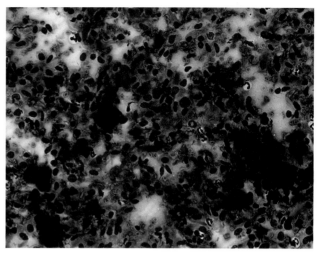

Figure 4.16.2 Hyalinizing trabecular adenoma (HTA). The cells have elongated and enlarged nuclei. Hyaline material is associated with some of the cells and has stained a dark purple color.

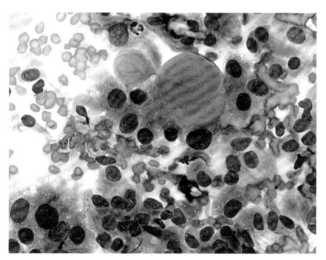

Figure 4.16.3 Hyalinizing trabecular adenoma (HTA). Two large pink hyaline globules are associated with several cells. These globules may be mistaken for colloid.

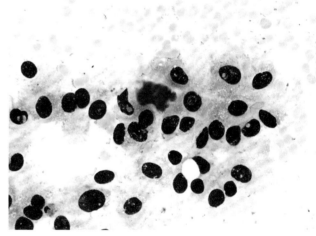

Figure 4.16.4 Hyalinizing trabecular adenoma (HTA). Several cells have prominent intranuclear pseudoinclusions in this field. A small fragment of magenta hyaline material is associated with a few of the cells.

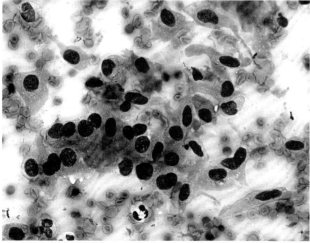

Figure 4.16.5 Hyalinizing trabecular adenoma (HTA). The cells here have enlarged and elongated nuclei. Some cells are associated with thin, wispy, magenta hyaline material.

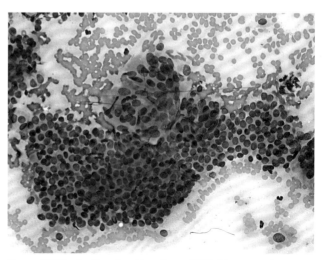

Figure 4.16.6 Papillary thyroid carcinoma (PTC). A large monolayer fragment is associated with a multinucleated giant cell. The nuclei are enlarged, elongated, and overlapping. Several nuclei have grooves.

4 THYROID

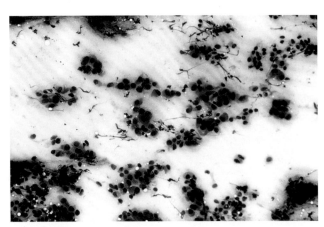

Figure 4.16.7 Papillary thyroid carcinoma (PTC). Background lymphocytes can be seen as chromatin streaks, and likely explain the oncocytic nature of the neoplastic cells.

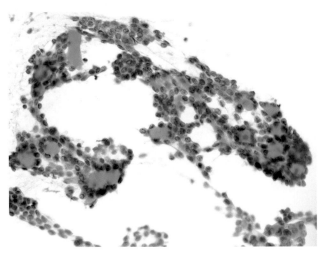

Figure 4.16.8 Papillary thyroid carcinoma (PTC). These cells have powdery chromatin, elongated nuclei, and nuclear grooves. Several dense cyan globules of colloid are present.

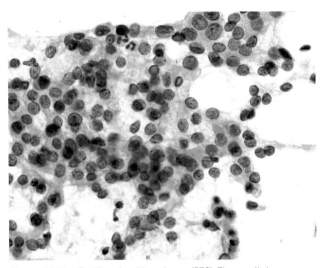

Figure 4.16.9 Papillary thyroid carcinoma (PTC). These cells have enlarged nuclei with powdery chromatin and nuclear grooves. A prominent intranuclear pseudoinclusion can be seen at the top center of the field.

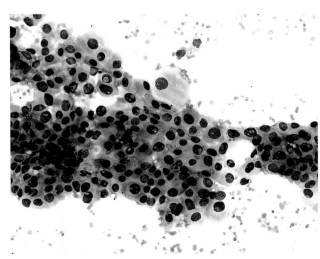

Figure 4.16.10 Papillary thyroid carcinoma (PTC). This fragment has several cells with abundant cytoplasm, but the nuclei are enlarged and have irregular shapes. Numerous intranuclear pseudoinclusions can be seen.

	Graves' Disease	Papillary Thyroid Carcinoma
Age	Middle-aged women	Mostly young adult and middle-aged women
Location	Thyroid	Thyroid
Signs and symptoms	Diffuse thyromegaly, swelling of extremeties, clubbing, and pretibial myxedema	Usually solitary thyroid nodule; lymphadenopathy
Etiology	Autoimmune disease in which anti-TSH receptor antibodies activate the receptor	Radiation exposure, Hashimoto thyroiditis, familial adenomatous polyposis
Cytomorphology	• Cellular specimen containing follicular cells in sheets and loosely cohesive fragments (*Figures 4.17.1* and *4.17.2*) • Background lymphocytes • Columnar cells with abundant cytoplasm containing granules and/or vacuoles (*Figures 4.17.3* and *4.17.4*) • "Flame cells" may be seen, with pink frayed edges to the cytoplasm (*Figure 4.17.3*) • Enlarged nuclei with nucleoli (*Figure 4.17.5*) • Vascular proliferations may impart papillary-like architectural patterns	• Cohesive tissue fragments that have an underlying microfollicular architecture but may also form monolayer fragments with papillary architecture (*Figures 4.17.6* and *4.17.7*) • Usually minimal or absent colloid. Colloid may be present as dense globules • Elevated nuclear to cytoplasmic ratios (*Figure 4.17.8*) • Enlarged oval nuclei with powdery chromatin (*Figure 4.17.9*) • Irregular nuclear contours (*Figure 4.17.8*) • Elongated nuclei and nuclear grooves (*Figure 4.17.10*) • Intranuclear pseudoinclusions more common but may be absent (*Figure 4.17.8*)
Special studies	Lesional cells are positive for TTF-1, PAX-8, and thyroglobulin by IHC	Carcinoma cells are usually positive for TTF-1, PAX-8, and thyroglobulin by IHC but may be lost in anaplastic areas if present. Negative for calcitonin
Molecular alterations	None	*BRAF* or *RAS* mutations; *RET-PTC* rearrangements
Treatment	Beta blockers; PTU; radioactive iodine; surgery	Surgical excision including cervical lymph node dissection with or without radioactive iodine
Clinical implications	Excellent	Generally good, but distantly metastatic disease may persist

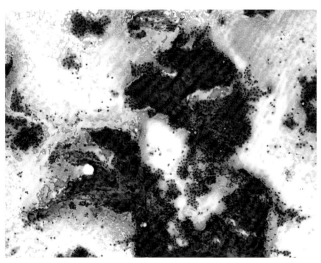

Figure 4.17.1 Graves' disease. Numerous follicular cells are present both in large papillary fragments as well as dispersed in the background.

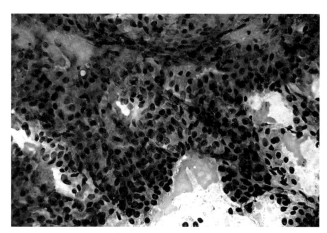

Figure 4.17.2 Graves' disease. Follicular cells are associated with a fibrovascular core and have enlarged, oval nuclei with granular cytoplasm.

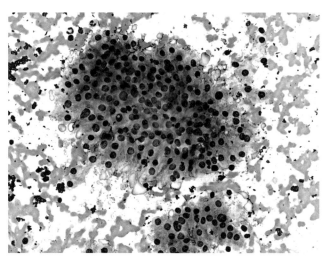

Figure 4.17.3 Graves' disease. The cells at the edges of this fragment are columnar. The edges of the fragment also appear frayed and associated with red-magenta material, giving rise to the name "flame cells."

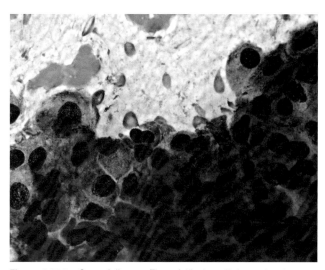

Figure 4.17.4 Graves' disease. These follicular cells have abundant, granular cytoplasm and enlarged round to oval nuclei. Magenta-colored material can be seen at the tissue fragment's edge.

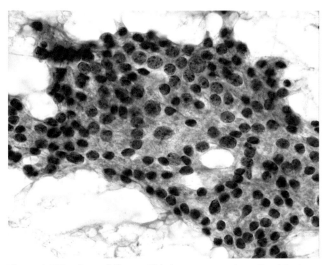

Figure 4.17.5 Graves' disease. This fragment contains cells with abundant, granular cytoplasm and enlarged round to oval nuclei. Some cells have small yet distinct nucleoli. The powdery chromatin pattern seen in PTC is absent.

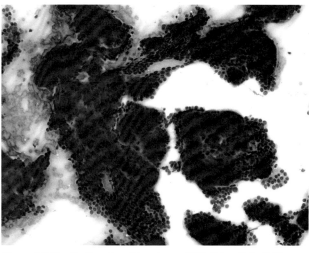

Figure 4.17.6 Papillary thyroid carcinoma (PTC). This cellular field contains numerous tissue fragments with papillary architecture. Even at this low magnification, cells with large and crowded nuclei can be identified.

4 THYROID

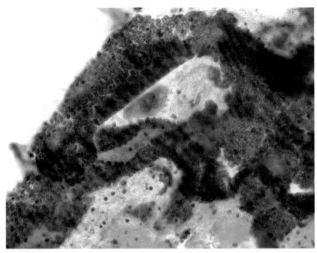

Figure 4.17.7 Papillary thyroid carcinoma (PTC). This papillary fragment is packed with nuclei, and very little cytoplasm is visible. The nuclei are oval shaped and enlarged and have powdery chromatin.

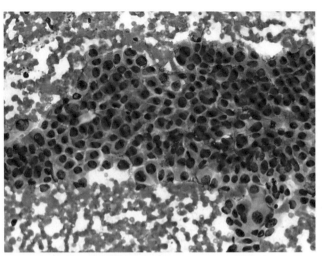

Figure 4.17.8 Papillary thyroid carcinoma (PTC). This carcinoma contains cells with abundant cytoplasm, but the nuclei are enlarged with irregular borders, and several prominent intranuclear pseudoinclusions can be seen.

Figure 4.17.9 Papillary thyroid carcinoma (PTC). The cells here form papillary structures with bulbous projections. Nuclei palisade along the edges of the fragment.

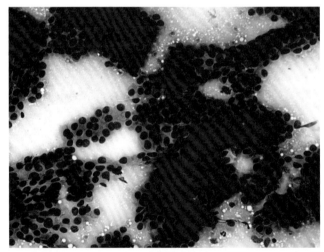

Figure 4.17.10 Papillary thyroid carcinoma (PTC). The nuclei in these papillary tissue fragments are enlarged and oval shaped, and some have grooves.

	Hyalinizing Trabecular Adenoma (Tumor)	Medullary Thyroid Carcinoma (MTC)
Age	Middle-aged and older women	Middle-aged adults; younger in familial
Location	Thyroid	Thyroid
Signs and symptoms	Solitary thyroid nodule	Painless thyroid mass or cervical lymphadenopathy; flushing and diarrhea in metastatic disease
Etiology	Unknown; can be associated with lymphocytic thyroiditis	Derived from calcitonin-secreting C cells. Associated with familial syndromes MEN 2A, MEN 2B, familial medullary thyroid carcinoma syndrome, von-Hippel-Lindau disease, and neurofibromatosis
Cytomorphology	• Cellular specimen containing neoplastic cells in loosely cohesive fragments and present singly (Figures 4.18.1 and 4.18.2) • Neoplastic cells are associated with hyaline material (Figures 4.18.1 and 4.18.3) • Neoplastic cells contain features of PTC, such as nuclear elongation, nuclear grooves, and numerous intranuclear pseudoinclusions (Figures 4.18.4 and 4.18.5) • Vascular proliferations may impart papillary-like architectural patterns	• Loosely cohesive and scattered, monotonous cells (Figures 4.18.6 and 4.18.7) • Background may contain amorphous amyloid material. Colloid is absent • Neoplastic cells are epithelioid or spindled with an eccentrically placed nucleus and abundant cytoplasm (Figure 4.18.8) • Regular nuclear borders but may demonstrate anisonucleosis (Figure 4.18.9) • Chromatin has a speckled (neuroendocrine) appearance (Figure 4.18.10)
Special studies	Cells are positive for TTF-1, PAX-8, and thyroglobulin by IHC. Negative for calcitonin	Positive for calcitonin, TTF-1, PAX-8, and neuroendocrine markers and negative for thyroglobulin by IHC. Amyloid can be identified by a Congo Red special stain. Needle rinses have elevated calcitonin levels
Molecular alterations	RET-PTC rearrangements	Mutations in RET gene in most familial cases and 50% of sporadic cases. Otherwise, mutations in HRAS or KRAS
Treatment	Thyroid lobectomy	Surgical excision
Clinical implications	Excellent	10 y survival of 75%-85%, worse with distant metastases

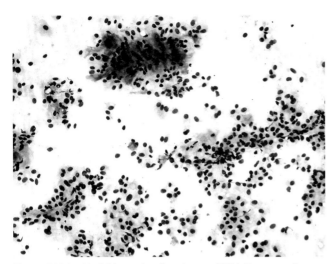

Figure 4.18.1 Hyalnizing trabecular adenoma (HTA). Numerous dispersed as well as loosely cohesive fragments of cells are seen. The cells have delicate cytoplasm and oval to spindled nuclei. Several cells are associated with magenta hyaline material (top center).

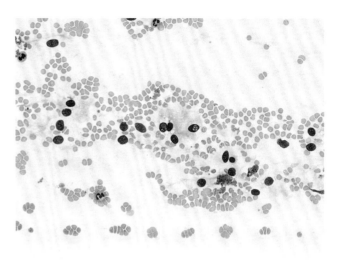

Figure 4.18.2 Hyalnizing trabecular adenoma (HTA). These cells are singly dispersed, and a few stripped nuclei can be seen in the background. Several cells have finely vacuolated cytoplasm and prominent intranuclear pseudoinclusions.

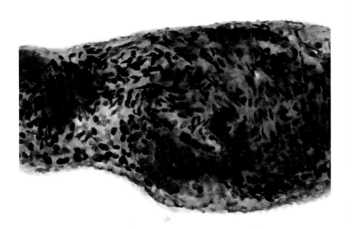

Figure 4.18.3 Hyalnizing trabecular adenoma (HTA). These cells with spindled nuclei emulate a mesenchymal tumor, as they are embedded in hyaline matrix material, causing them to appear more cohesive.

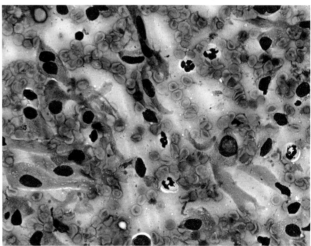

Figure 4.18.4 Hyalnizing trabecular adenoma (HTA). These cells have elongated cytoplasm, some with bipolar processes. The nuclei are enlarged and oval to spindle shaped. One cell has a large intranuclear pseudoinclusion.

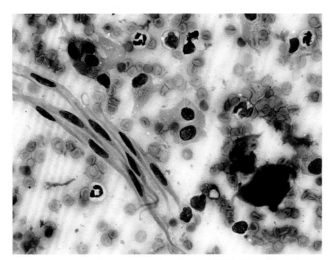

Figure 4.18.5   Hyalnizing trabecular adenoma (HTA). The cells on the left have a stretched appearance, similar to what may be seen in cyst-lining cells. Other cells in the field are more epithelioid and have abundant granular cytoplasm. One cell has a large intranuclear pseudoinclusion.

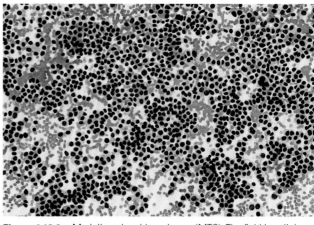

Figure 4.18.6   Medullary thyroid carcinoma (MTC). The field is cellular with dispersed cells. The nuclei are monotonous and round to oval with regular borders and minimal size variation, providing a monotonous look to the cellular population.

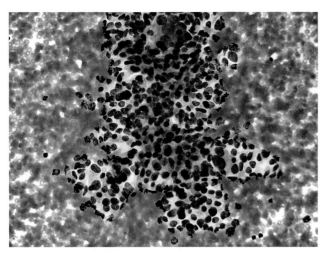

Figure 4.18.7   Medullary thyroid carcinoma (MTC). Many of the cells in this fragment have abundant cytoplasm, and the nuclei are oval shaped. Despite the prominent anisonucleosis, the nuclear contours are regular. Intranuclear pseudoinclusions and nuclear grooves are absent.

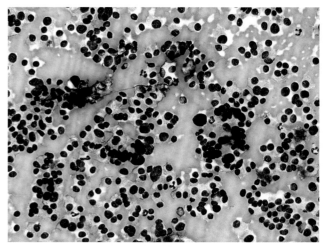

Figure 4.18.8   Medullary thyroid carcinoma (MTC). These dispersed cells have abundant cytoplasm and eccentrically placed nuclei.

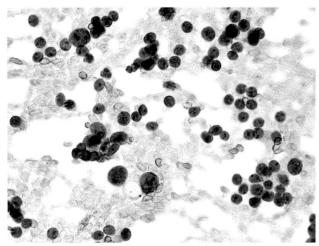

Figure 4.18.9   Medullary thyroid carcinoma (MTC). The nuclei of these cells are round to oval and have regular nuclear borders. Many of the nuclei have been stripped of their cytoplasm, while others have delicate, granular cytoplasm.

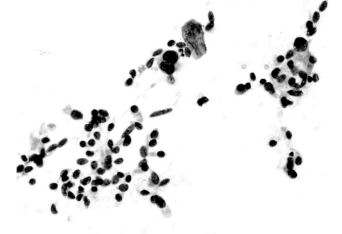

Figure 4.18.10   Medullary thyroid carcinoma (MTC). The nuclei of these cells are predominantly spindle shaped, although a few are oval. The chromatin has a "salt-and-pepper" appearance.

5

Pancreas

	Benign Pancreatic Acinar Tissue	Acinar Cell Carcinoma
Age	Any age	Older age; usually men
Location	Anywhere in pancreas	Anywhere in pancreas
Signs and symptoms	Usually sampled during FNA of a mass lesion seen on imaging; symptoms may be associated with mass lesion	Weight loss; may cause lipase hypersecretion syndrome
Etiology	May be sampled if a mass lesion is missed, or as part of a mass lesion (eg, chronic pancreatitis)	Malignancy with acinar cell differentiation
Cytomorphology	• Monotonous cells in acinar formations, which may form fragments of different sizes ("bunch of grapes") *(Figures 5.1.1 and 5.1.2)* • In large fragments, acinar groups are associated with ducts *(Figures 5.1.3 and 5.1.4)* • Single cells may be seen adjacent to fragments in the plane of smear preparation • Acinar cells have abundant granular cytoplasm and uniform nuclei with regular nuclear contours *(Figure 5.1.5)* • Bland chromatin pattern *(Figure 5.1.5)* • Specimen is often hypocellular *(Figure 5.1.5)*	• Cells in discohesive groups and present singly *(Figures 5.1.6 and 5.1.7)* • Cellular specimen • Microglandular formations may be seen *(Figure 5.1.8)* • Prominent nucleoli *(Figure 5.1.9)* • Eccentrically placed nucleus *(Figure 5.1.10)* • Numerous naked nuclei • Granular cytoplasm • Vascular proliferations can be seen
Special studies	BCL-10, PAS and PAS/D, trypsin, chymotrypsin, lipase, and amylase (same as acinar cell carcinoma)	BCL-10, PAS and PAS/D, trypsin, chymotrypsin, lipase, and amylase
Molecular alterations	None	Amplifications in 20q and 19p
Treatment	None	Not standardized; usually surgery and/or chemotherapy
Clinical implications	Reassessment of the lesion seen on imaging studies and possible re-biopsy	Better than pancreatic ductal adenocarcinoma, but still prognosis (mean survival 18 months after diagnosis); often metastatic at time of diagnosis

Figure 5.1.1   Benign pancreatic acinar tissue. The group looks like a cluster of grapes due to the formation of cells into acini. Small single cells and acini can be seen immediately adjacent to the fragment.

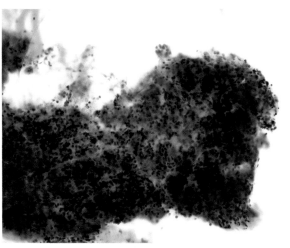

Figure 5.1.2   Benign pancreatic acinar tissue. These cells forming a grapelike architecture. Such architecture is not seen in acinar cell carcinoma.

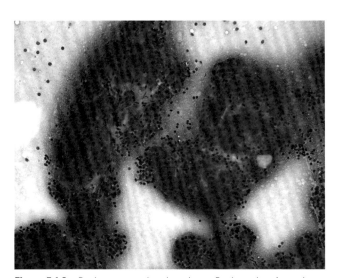

Figure 5.1.3   Benign pancreatic acinar tissue. Benign acinar formations can be seen, some connected by less cellular ductal structures. This normal architecture reassures against acinar cell carcinoma, although acinar cell carcinoma often has vessels that may appear similar.

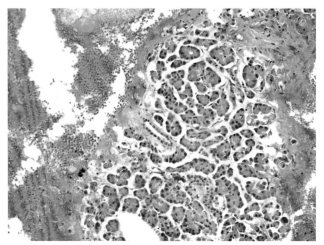

Figure 5.1.4   Benign pancreatic acinar tissue. This cell block section shows the normal grapelike arrangement of acinar cells in association with a duct.

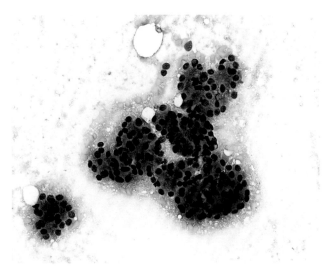

Figure 5.1.5   Benign pancreatic acinar tissue. At high magnification, benign acinar cells have abundant granular cytoplasm and small, uniform nuclei with regular borders. Importantly, the chromatin pattern is bland and nucleoli are absent.

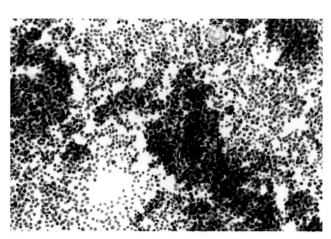

Figure 5.1.6   Acinar cell carcinoma. The field is cellular with monotonous cells both forming loosely cohesive fragments as well as singly dispersed in the background.

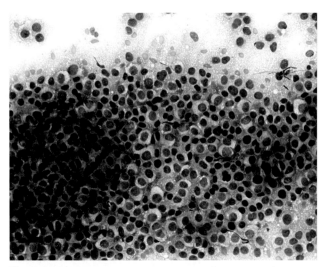

Figure 5.1.7   Acinar cell carcinoma. This acinar cell carcinoma has lost all architecture and appears predominantly as single cells. Given their monotonous and discohesive nature and eccentrically placed nuclei, a pancreatic neuroendocrine tumor is high on the differential diagnosis.

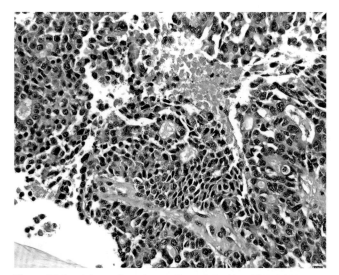

Figure 5.1.8   Acinar cell carcinoma. The cells in this cell block have the morphology of acinar cells (abundant granular cytoplasm) but form a disorganized architecture, including some microglandular formations.

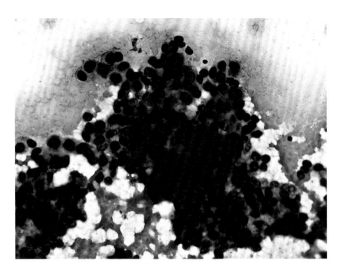

Figure 5.1.9 Acinar cell carcinoma. This carcinoma has atypical architecture but also atypical cytomorphology. Note the prominent nucleoli seen in many of the cells.

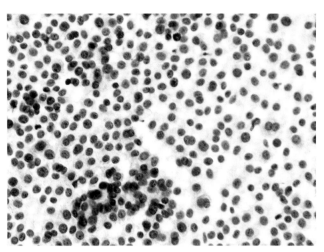

Figure 5.1.10 Acinar cell carcinoma. This field contains a monotonous population of acinar cells which are individually dispersed and have a plasmacytoid configuration. The differential diagnosis primarily includes a pancreatic neuroendocrine tumor.

	Pancreatic Neuroendocrine Tumor (PanNET)	Well-Differentiated Adenocarcinoma
Age	Usually middle-aged adults but can occur at any age	Usually older adults
Location	Anywhere in pancreas	Anywhere in pancreas
Signs and symptoms	Asymptomatic and incidentally discovered, or obstructive symptoms; functional tumors are associated with clinical syndromes	Weight loss; painless jaundice; back pain; migratory thrombophlebitis
Etiology	Neoplasms with neuroendocrine differentiation; can be associated with various syndromes (MEN1, neurofibromatosis type 1, von Hippel-Lindau, tuberous sclerosis)	Smoking, alcohol abuse, obesity, diabetes, chronic pancreatitis. Associated familial syndromes (Peutz-Jeghers, hereditary pancreatitis, Lynch syndrome, familial adenomatous polyposis, and others)
Cytomorphology	• Cellular specimen with monotonous cells in small fragments and individually dispersed (*Figures 5.2.1* and *5.2.2*) • Eccentrically placed round nucleus with regular nuclear contours (*Figure 5.2.3*) • Abundant granular cytoplasm (*Figures 5.2.3* and *5.2.4*) • "Salt and pepper" (neuroendocrine type) chromatin pattern (*Figure 5.2.4*) • Poorly differentiated tumors may have different features and more closely resemble adenocarcinoma (*Figure 5.2.5*)	• Predominantly cohesive cells in tissue fragments (*Figures 5.2.6* and *5.2.7*) • Nuclei are disorganized within tissue fragment ("drunken honeycomb") (*Figure 5.2.8*) • Nuclear size variation and nuclear border irregularities (*Figures 5.2.9* and *5.2.10*) • Nucleoli may be seen (*Figure 5.2.10*)
Special studies	Positive for INSM1, chromogranin, synaptophysin, and CD56 by immunohistochemistry	Usually negative or only weakly/focally positive for neuroendocrine markers
Molecular alterations	For sporadic tumors, mutations in MEN1, DAXX, ATRX, TSC2, and/or PTEN, among others	Commonly mutations in KRAS, CDKN2A, TP53, and SMAD4
Treatment	Surgical removal; sometimes chemotherapy. Targeted therapies available	Surgical removal; chemoradiation
Clinical implications	5 y survival of 55% for localized, resected tumors	Poor survival; often not resectable at time of diagnosis

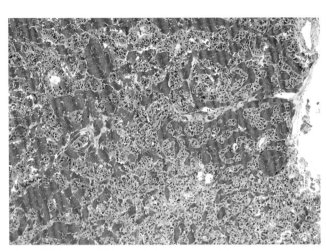

Figure 5.2.1 PanNET. A cell block section containing numerous, monotonous cells forming predominantly small cellular strips ("ribbons").

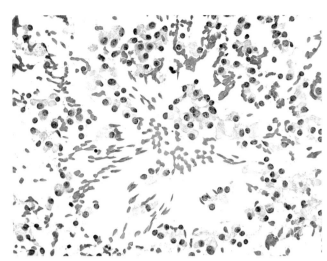

Figure 5.2.2 PanNET. The neoplasm is seen predominantly as a dispersed population of single cells with eccentric nuclei and abundant cytoplasm.

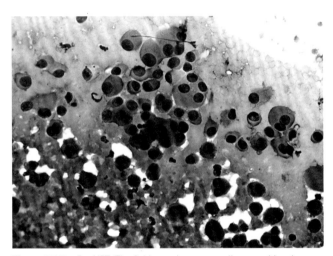

Figure 5.2.3 PanNET. The field contains tumor cells, some binucleated, with eccentrically placed round nuclei and granular cytoplasm. The nuclear borders are regular.

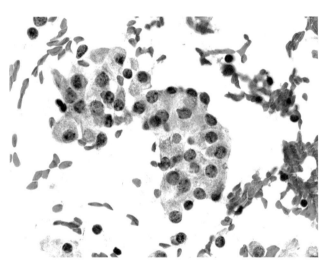

Figure 5.2.4 PanNET. This small fragment contains neoplastic cells with abundant, granular cytoplasm and eccentrically placed nuclei. The chromatin is both powdery and coarse, compatible with neuroendocrine differentiation.

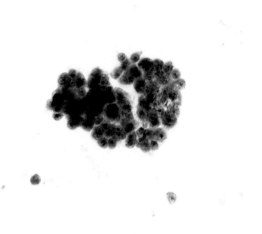

Figure 5.2.5   PanNET. The cells have high N/C ratios and prominent nucleoli, features not seen in a well-differentiated neuroendocrine tumor. The differential diagnosis includes acinar cell carcinoma and ductal adenocarcinoma.

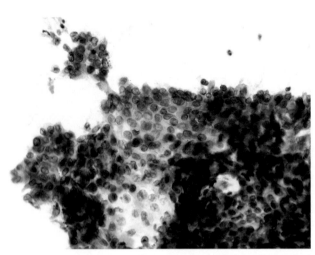

Figure 5.2.6   Adenocarcinoma. The nuclei are crowded and disorganized within the fragment. Some pancreatic adenocarcinomas contain powdery, bland chromatin such as is seen in this case.

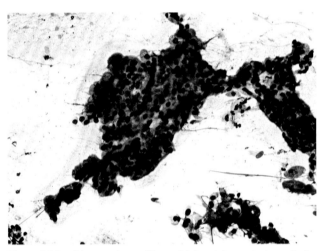

Figure 5.2.7   Adenocarcinoma. The nuclei do not demonstrate much size variation but are disorganized within the fragment. Closer examination may reveal nuclear border irregularities.

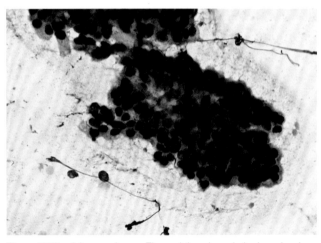

Figure 5.2.8   Adenocarcinoma. The nuclei are irregularly shaped and disorganized within the fragment.

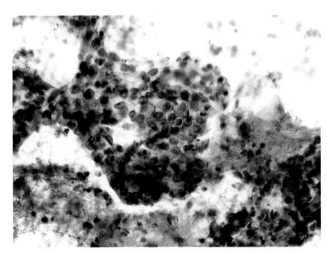

Figure 5.2.9   Adenocarcinoma. The field contains cells with nuclear size variation and irregular nuclear contours. The nuclei are disorganized within the fragment.

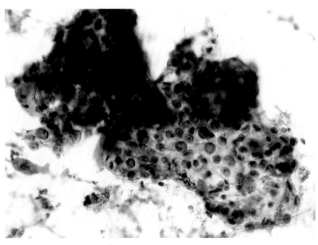

Figure 5.2.10   Adenocarcinoma. These cells have enlarged nuclei, anisonucleosis, nuclear border irregularities, and some nucleolar prominence.

	Well-Differentiated Adenocarcinoma	Benign Ductal Cells
Age	Usually older adults	Any age
Location	Anywhere in pancreas	Anywhere in pancreas
Signs and symptoms	Weight loss; painless jaundice; back pain; migratory thrombophlebitis	Usually sampled during FNA of a mass lesion seen on imaging; symptoms may be associated with mass lesion
Etiology	Smoking, alcohol abuse, obesity, diabetes, chronic pancreatitis. Associated familial syndromes (Peutz-Jeghers, hereditary pancreatitis, Lynch syndrome, familial adenomatous polyposis, and others)	May be sampled if a mass lesion is missed, or as part of a mass lesion (eg, chronic pancreatitis)
Cytomorphology	• Predominantly cohesive cells in tissue fragments *(Figures 5.3.1 and 5.3.2)* • Nuclei are disorganized within tissue fragment ("drunken honeycomb") *(Figure 5.3.3)* • Nuclear size variation and nuclear border irregularities *(Figure 5.3.4)* • Nucleoli may be seen	• Fragments and small strips of cells; occasionally individual cells in background sheared during smearing *(Figures 5.3.5 and 5.3.6)* • Organized, honeycomb arrangement of nuclei *(Figure 5.3.7)* • Uniform, round nuclei with regular borders and pale chromatin *(Figure 5.3.8)* • May have small nucleoli and be slightly enlarged • Brushing specimens may demonstrate significant reactive and artifactual atypia
Special studies	DPC4 nuclear expression lost in ~50% and indicates malignancy	Usually same markers as pancreatic ductal carcinoma; DPC4 retained.
Molecular alterations	Commonly mutations in KRAS, CDKN2A, TP53, and SMAD4.	N/A
Treatment	Surgical removal; chemoradiation	N/A
Clinical implications	Poor survival; often not resectable at time of diagnosis	May indicate poor sampling of a lesion and require re-biopsy

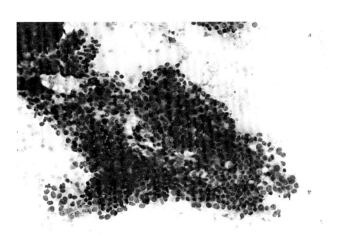

Figure 5.3.1 Adenocarcinoma. The nuclei are enlarged, crowded, and disorganized within the fragment.

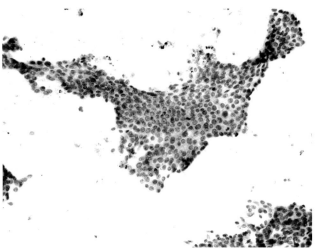

Figure 5.3.2 Adenocarcinoma. The nuclei in this fragment of adenocarcinoma are deceivingly bland and well-organized. Well-differentiated adenocarcinomas may be difficult to distinguish from benign ductal epithelium or gastrointestinal contamination. Benign ductal epithelium typically does not form large, papillary structures.

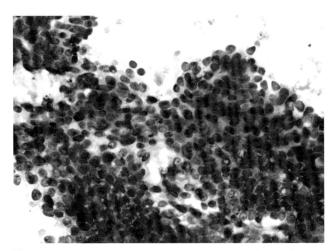

Figure 5.3.3 Adenocarcinoma. At higher magnification, it is easier to see that the nuclei have size variation and nuclear border irregularities.

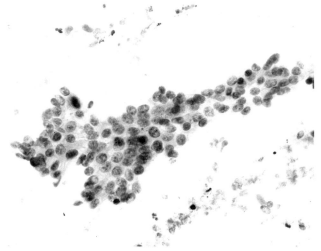

Figure 5.3.4 Adenocarcinoma. These cells demonstrate only mild anisonucleosis but are not arranged in a honeycomb, as would be expected if they were benign ductal cells.

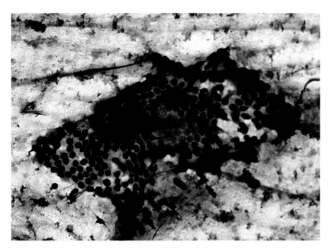

Figure 5.3.5   Benign ductal tissue. The nuclei are uniform and have regular borders. The nuclei are arranged in a honeycomb, although the irregular shape to the fragment causes some disruption to this appearance.

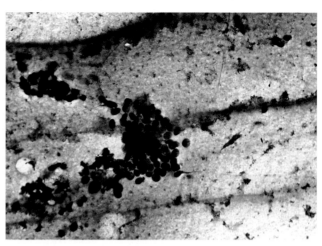

Figure 5.3.6   Benign ductal tissue. A few cells are present singly adjacent to the fragment. During aspiration and smearing, benign ductal cells may become singly dispersed in the background, but usually only in small numbers.

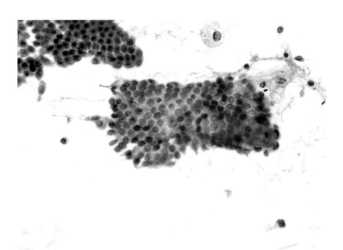

Figure 5.3.7   Benign ductal tissue. This fragment contains well-organized benign ductal cells that form a honeycomb architecture. The nuclei are round and have regular contours. The chromatin is bland.

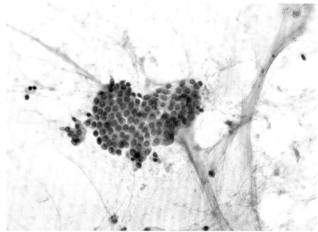

Figure 5.3.8   Benign ductal tissue. The cells are organized within the fragment and have round nuclei with regular borders.

	Pancreatic Neuroendocrine Tumor (PanNET)	Solid Pseudopapillary Neoplasm
Age	Usually middle-aged adults but can occur at any age	Young women
Location	Anywhere in pancreas	Pancreatic body or tail
Signs and symptoms	Asymptomatic and incidentally discovered, or obstructive symptoms; functional tumors are associated with clinical syndromes	Abdominal pain/discomfort; abdominal mass; nausea; vomiting
Etiology	Neoplasms with neuroendocrine differentiation; can be associated with various syndromes (MEN1, neurofibromatosis type 1, von Hippel-Lindau, tuberous sclerosis)	Unknown; usually caused by point mutation in CTNNB1 (beta catenin gene)
Cytomorphology	• Cellular specimen with monotonous cells in small fragments and individually dispersed (Figures 5.4.1 and 5.4.2) • Eccentrically placed round nucleus with regular nuclear contours (Figure 5.4.3) • Abundant granular cytoplasm (Figures 5.4.3 and 5.4.4) • "Salt and pepper" (neuroendocrine type) chromatin pattern (Figure 5.4.4) • Poorly differentiated tumors may have different features and more closely resemble adenocarcinoma (Figure 5.4.5)	• Cellular smears with tumor cells loosely attached to vessels and present singly in the background (Figure 5.4.6) • Fragments have characteristic complex branching architecture (Figures 5.4.6-5.4.8) • Monotonous cells with eccentric nuclei (Figure 5.4.9) • Oval nuclei with fine chromatin and occasional grooves (Figure 5.4.10) • Cytoplasmic vacuoles and/or globules
Special studies	Positive for INSM1, chromogranin, synaptophysin, and CD56 by immunohistochemistry. Negative for B-catenin	Positive for B-catenin, CD56, and synaptophysin by IHC; negative for chromogranin.
Molecular alterations	For sporadic tumors, mutations in MEN1, DAXX, ATRX, TSC2, and/or PTEN, among others	Point mutation in CTNNB1 (beta catenin gene)
Treatment	Surgical removal; sometimes chemotherapy. Targeted therapies available	Surgical removal
Clinical implications	5 y survival of 55% for localized, resected tumors	Excellent following surgical removal; males have more aggressive tumors

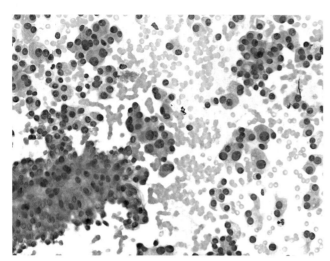

Figure 5.4.1 PanNET. The cells are loosely cohesive and singly dispersed. The cells are monotonous and have abundant cytoplasm, eccentric round nuclei, and regular nuclear contours

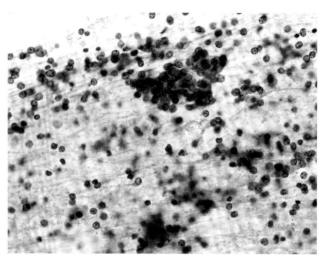

Figure 5.4.2 PanNET. A predominantly dispersed population of cells should raise PanNET as the likely diagnosis, although less common entities such as solid pseudopapillary neoplasm and acinar cell carcinoma can present as a predominantly single cell population.

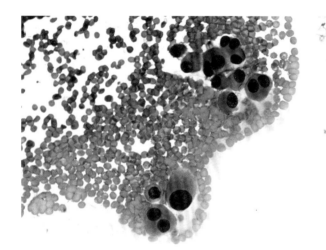

Figure 5.4.3 PanNET. Pancreatic neuroendocrine tumors may occasionally demonstrate anisonucleosis and binucleation. However, the cells here have round nuclei with regular nuclear borders. Poorly differentiated neoplasms are less uniform and may resemble adenocarcinoma.

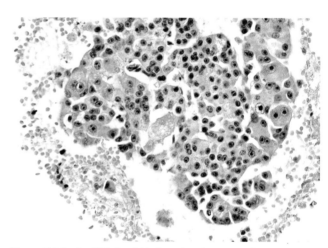

Figure 5.4.4 PanNET. A cell block section of a pancreatic neuroendocrine tumor is shown. The cells have abundant, granular cytoplasm. Some cells here have prominent nucleoli, not commonly seen in well-differentiated PanNETs.

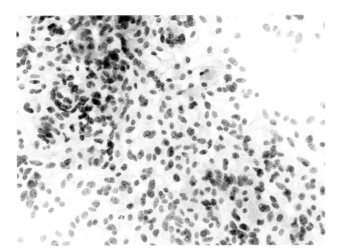

Figure 5.4.5   PanNET. These dispersed cells have abundant, delicate cytoplasm which blends in with the background. While most PanNETs have epithelioid nuclei, some may have elongated nuclei such as seen here.

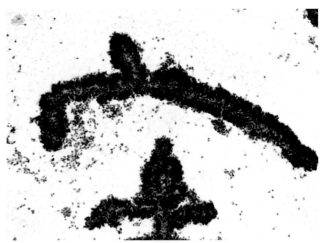

Figure 5.4.6   Solid pseudopapillary neoplasm. Solid pseudopapillary neoplasm is characterized by the presence of thin papillary fragments with irregular branches. Neoplastic cells form thin layers on these fragments and are also present in the background as individually dispersed cells.

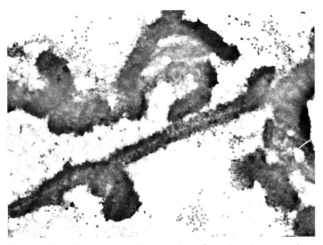

Figure 5.4.7   Solid pseudopapillary neoplasm. Several poorly preserved fragments can be seen with irregularly branching architecture. Numerous monotonous neoplastic cells are singly dispersed throughout the background.

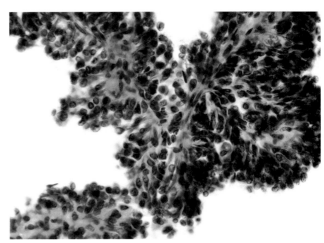

Figure 5.4.8   Solid pseudopapillary neoplasm. The cells are monotonous and line a vessel that is thin and branching.

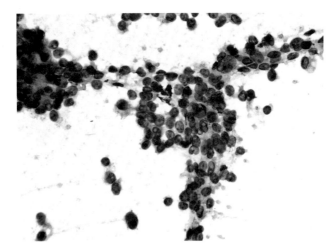

Figure 5.4.9   Solid pseudopapillary neoplasm. The cells are loosely cohesive and their cytoplasm is delicate and difficult to visualize, but the cells are predominantly in a plasmacytoid configuration.

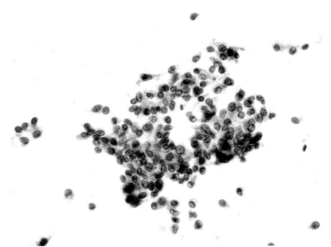

Figure 5.4.10   Solid pseudopapillary neoplasm. The neoplastic cells have uniform, oval-shaped nuclei with powdery chromatin and occasional nuclear grooves.

	Pancreatic Neuroendocrine Tumor (PanNET)	Acinar Cell Carcinoma
Age	Usually middle-aged adults, but can occur at any age	Older age; usually men
Location	Anywhere in pancreas	Anywhere in pancreas
Signs and symptoms	Asymptomatic and incidentally discovered, or obstructive symptoms; functional tumors are associated with clinical syndromes	Weight loss; may cause lipase hypersecretion syndrome
Etiology	Neoplasms with neuroendocrine differentiation; can be associated with various syndromes (MEN1, neurofibromatosis type 1, von Hippel-Lindau, tuberous sclerosis)	Malignancy with acinar cell differentiation
Cytomorphology	• Cellular specimen with monotonous cells in small fragments and individually dispersed (Figures 5.5.1 and 5.5.2) • Eccentrically placed round nucleus with regular nuclear contours (Figure 5.5.3) • Abundant granular cytoplasm (Figures 5.5.3 and 5.5.4) • "Salt and pepper" (neuroendocrine type) chromatin pattern (Figures 5.5.3 and 5.5.4) • Stripped nuclei may be numerous (Figure 5.5.5) • Poorly differentiated tumors may have different features and more closely resemble adenocarcinoma (Figure 5.2.5)	• Cells in discohesive groups and present singly (Figures 5.5.6 and 5.5.7) • Cellular specimen (Figure 5.5.8) • Microglandular formations may be seen • Prominent nucleoli may be seen • Eccentrically placed nucleus and maintained cytoplasm (Figure 5.5.9) • Numerous naked nuclei • Granular cytoplasm • Vascular proliferations can be seen
Special studies	Positive for INSM1, chromogranin, synaptophysin, and CD56 by immunohistochemistry	Positive for BCL-10, PAS and PAS/D, trypsin, chymotrypsin, lipase, and amylase
Molecular alterations	For sporadic tumors, mutations in MEN1, DAXX, ATRX, TSC2, and/or PTEN, among others	Amplifications in 20q and 19p
Treatment	Surgical removal; sometimes chemotherapy. Targeted therapies available	Not standardized; usually surgery and/or chemotherapy
Clinical implications	5 y survival of 55% for localized, resected tumors	Better than pancreatic ductal adenocarcinoma, but still prognosis (mean survival 18 months after diagnosis); often metastatic at time of diagnosis

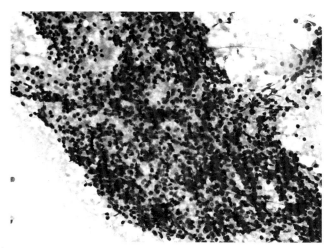

Figure 5.5.1 PanNET. The field is hypercellular and contains a dispersed, monotonous of neuroendocrine cells. At this magnification, the cells may look lymphoid, and closer examination is needed to exclude an intrapancreatic lymph node or splenule.

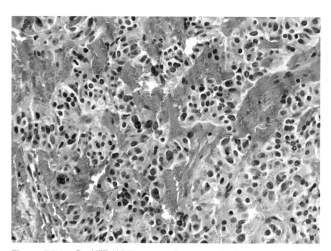

Figure 5.5.2 PanNET. While pancreatic neuroendocrine tumors usually show a dispersed population of single cells, they can sometimes present with tissue fragments. This cell block material shows PanNET cells in ribbon formations, a common architecture seen in neuroendocrine neoplasms.

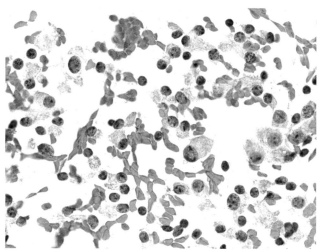

Figure 5.5.3 PanNET. The field contains singly dispersed pancreatic neuroendocrine tumor cells with abundant granular cytoplasm and eccentrically placed nuclei. The nuclei are round and have regular borders.

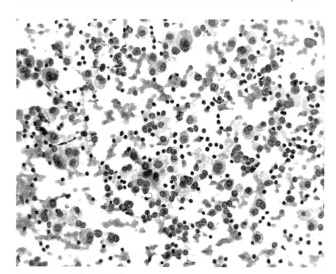

Figure 5.5.4 PanNET. Singly dispersed pancreatic neuroendocrine tumor cells admixed with lymphocytes. The tumor cells have abundant cytoplasm.

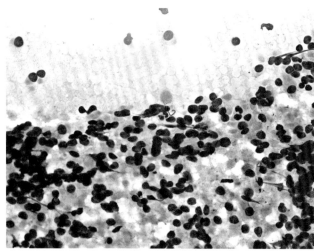

Figure 5.5.5 PanNET. Several pancreatic neoplasms can present with stripped nuclei, making assessment of the cytoplasm difficult. In this case, the pancreatic neuroendocrine tumor cells closely resemble lymphocytes.

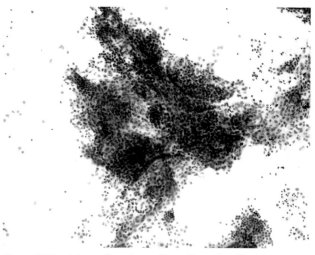

Figure 5.5.6 Acinar cell carcinoma. The cells are in a tissue fragment as well as present as singly dispersed cells. At this magnification, the cells look monotonous and the differential includes a pancreatic neuroendocrine tumor as well as solid pseudopapillary neoplasm.

5 PANCREAS

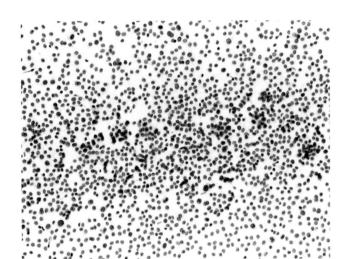

Figure 5.5.7   Acinar cell carcinoma. Acinar differentiation is not obvious given the scant, delicate cytoplasm seen in these cells. This field alone would be most suspicious for a pancreatic neuroendocrine tumor, and so ancillary studies as well as clinicoradiologic correlation become important.

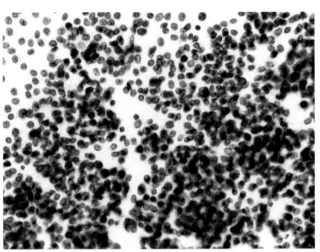

Figure 5.5.8   Acinar cell carcinoma. This acinar cell carcinoma closely resembles a pancreatic neuroendocrine tumor as the cells are singly dispersed and have little cytoplasm. The chromatin also has a neuroendocrine appearance, causing additional diagnostic difficulty.

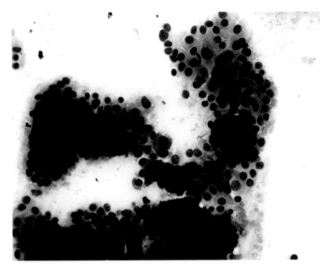

Figure 5.5.9   Acinar cell carcinoma. This three-dimensional fragment contains cells with abundant, granular cytoplasm. The nuclei are round, uniform, and eccentrically placed. While these cells have some acinar differentiation, a pancreatic neuroendocrine neoplasm cannot be completely excluded.

	Solid Pseudopapillary Neoplasm	Acinar Cell Carcinoma
Age	Young women	Older age; usually men
Location	Pancreatic body or tail	Anywhere in pancreas
Signs and symptoms	Abdominal pain/discomfort; abdominal mass; nausea; vomiting	Weight loss; may cause lipase hypersecretion syndrome
Etiology	Unknown; usually caused by point mutation in CTNNB1 (beta catenin gene)	Malignancy with acinar cell differentiation
Cytomorphology	• Cellular smears with tumor cells loosely attached to vessels and present singly in the background *(Figures 5.6.1* and *5.6.2)* • Fragments have characteristic complex branching architecture *(Figure 5.6.1)* • Monotonous cells with eccentric nuclei *(Figure 5.6.3)* • Oval nuclei with fine chromatin and occasional grooves *(Figures 5.6.4* and *5.6.5)* • Cytoplasmic vacuoles and/or globules	• Cells in discohesive groups and present singly *(Figures 5.6.6* and *5.6.7)* • Cellular specimen *(Figure 5.6.7)* • Microglandular formations may be seen • Granular cytoplasm *(Figure 5.6.8)* • Prominent nucleoli may be seen • Eccentrically placed round nucleus with regular borders *(Figures 5.6.9* and *5.6.10)* • Numerous naked nuclei • Granular cytoplasm • Vascular proliferations can be seen
Special studies	Positive for B-catenin, CD56, and synaptophysin by IHC; negative for chromogranin.	Positive for BCL-10, PAS and PAS/D, trypsin, chymotrypsin, lipase, and amylase by immunohistochemistry
Molecular alterations	Point mutation in CTNNB1 (beta catenin gene)	Amplifications in 20q and 19p
Treatment	Surgical removal	Not standardized; usually surgery and/or chemotherapy
Clinical implications	Excellent following surgical removal; males have more aggressive tumors	Better than pancreatic ductal adenocarcinoma, but still prognosis (mean survival 18 months after diagnosis) often metastatic at time of diagnosis

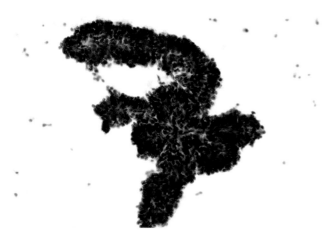

Figure 5.6.1   Solid pseudopapillary neoplasm. This tissue fragment with thin papillary fronds is covered by monotonous neoplastic cells. The irregular branching is characteristic of solid pseudopapillary neoplasm.

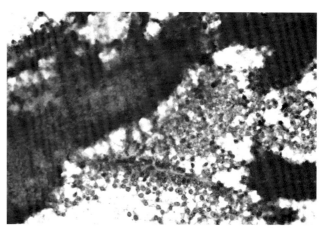

Figure 5.6.2   Solid pseudopapillary neoplasm. The background contains poorly preserved large branching structures. Numerous small, monotonous neoplastic cells are scattered throughout the background.

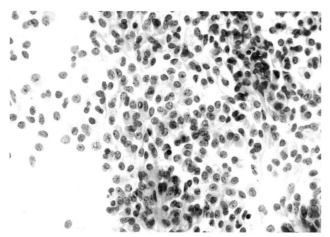

Figure 5.6.3   Solid pseudopapillary neoplasm. The nuclei are eccentrically placed and the cells have mostly tapered cytoplasm. The differential diagnosis includes pancreatic neuroendocrine tumor and, less likely, acinar cell carcinoma.

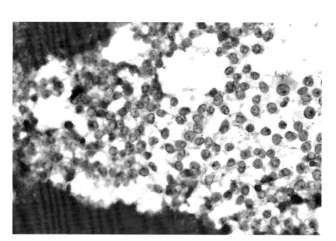

Figure 5.6.4   Solid pseudopapillary neoplasm. The neoplastic cells are small and monotonous and in this case have been stripped of their cytoplasm. The chromatin pattern is bland.

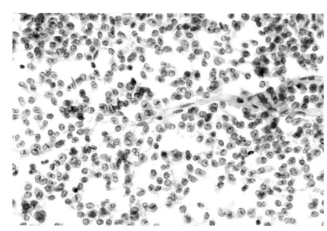

Figure 5.6.5   Solid pseudopapillary neoplasm. Here, numerous discohesive cells are seen adjacent to a thin vessel. The cells have delicate cytoplasm and round, regular nuclei. These findings are consistent with a solid pseudopapillary neoplasm but do not exclude a neuroendocrine neoplasm. Ancillary studies can help confirm the diagnosis.

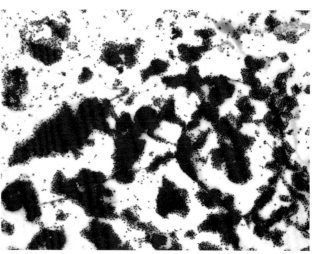

Figure 5.6.6   Acinar cell carcinoma. Large irregularly shaped fragments of acinar cell carcinoma. At this magnification, the structures seem similar to the irregularly branching fragments seen in solid pseudopapillary neoplasm (SPN). However, some of these branches seem thick, whereas SPN usually has thin structures.

5 PANCREAS

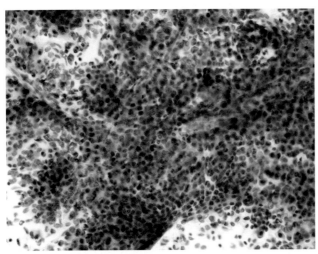

Figure 5.6.7 Acinar cell carcinoma. This densely packed field contains numerous monotonous cells, which form a fragment and are also seen loosely in the background. The cells are associated with vessels, but this is a nonspecific finding.

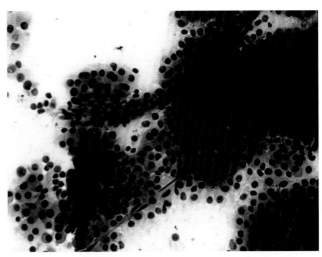

Figure 5.6.8 Acinar cell carcinoma. These neoplastic cells have abundant, granular cytoplasm, which is consistent with their acinar differentiation. The nuclei are round and eccentrically placed. A pancreatic neuroendocrine tumor should be ruled out before a diagnosis of acinar cell carcinoma is made.

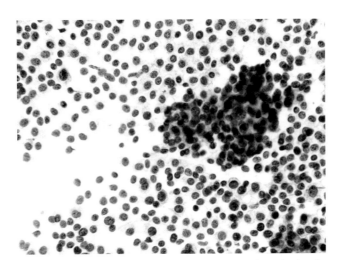

Figure 5.6.9 Acinar cell carcinoma. A small fragment of neoplastic cells is seen amid numerous dispersed single tumor cells. The fragment has an underlying acinar architecture that may help suggest acinar cell carcinoma. However, this architecture can appear similar to rosette structures formed in neuroendocrine neoplasms.

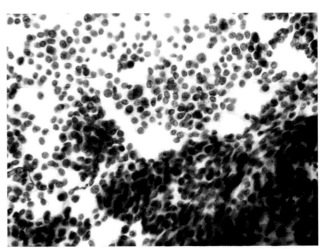

Figure 5.6.10 Acinar cell carcinoma. The field contains monotonous neoplastic cells with small, round nuclei with regular borders. Cytoplasm is scant. The tumor cells form fragments and are present singly, and ancillary studies would be required to prove an acinar cell carcinoma.

	Chronic Pancreatitis	Well-Differentiated Adenocarcinoma
Age	Usually middle-aged to older men	Usually older adults
Location	"Groove pancreatitis" is associated with alcoholism and forms between the pancreas and duodenum	Anywhere in pancreas
Signs and symptoms	Elevated amylase, weight loss, abdominal pain, diabetes, steatorrhea	Weight loss; painless jaundice; back pain; migratory thrombophlebitis
Etiology	Alcohol abuse, smoking, cystic fibrosis, familial hereditary pancreatitis, pancreatic divisum, hyperlipidemia, among others. Sometimes unknown etiology	Smoking, alcohol abuse, obesity, diabetes, chronic pancreatitis. Associated familial syndromes (Peutz-Jeghers, hereditary pancreatitis, Lynch syndrome, familial adenomatous polyposis, and others)
Cytomorphology	• Few fragments of ductal and/or acinar epithelium in an inflammatory background (Figures 5.7.1 and 5.7.2) • Ductal cells may demonstrate reactive atypia with enlarged nuclei and nucleoli (Figures 5.7.1 and 5.7.2) • Inflammatory cells may be closely associated with benign tissue fragments (Figures 5.7.3 and 5.7.4)	• Predominantly cohesive cells in tissue fragments (Figure 5.7.5) • Nuclei are disorganized within tissue fragment ("drunken honeycomb") (Figures 5.7.6 and 5.7.7) • Nuclear size variation and nuclear border irregularities (Figures 5.7.2 and 5.7.8) • Nucleoli may be seen • Necrosis with associated acute inflammatory cells may be present (Figures 5.7.5 and 5.7.9)
Special studies	N/A	Loss of nuclear DPC4 expression in ~50%
Molecular alterations	PRSS1 (trypsinogen gene) mutation (familial hereditary pancreatitis)	Commonly mutations in KRAS, CDKN2A, TP53, and SMAD4.
Treatment	Pain management and lifestyle changes; pancreatic duct drainage; surgery	Surgical removal; chemoradiation
Clinical implications	Damage is irreversible; increases risk for pancreatic adenocarcinoma	Poor survival; often not resectable at time of diagnosis

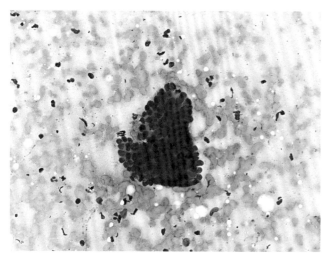

Figure 5.7.1   Chronic pancreatitis. The field contains a single fragment of benign ductal epithelial cells. The nuclei are enlarged and oval-shaped, and some mild nuclear contour irregularities can be seen. However, the nuclei are uniform and regularly arranged in a honeycomb pattern. Inflammatory cells are seen in the background.

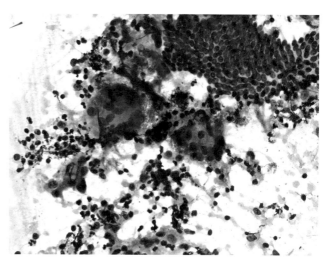

Figure 5.7.2   Chronic pancreatitis. The field is cellular and filled with inflammatory cells, multinucleated giant cells, and histiocytes. While inflammation can be associated with the necrosis of an adenocarcinoma, the ductal epithelium seen here have nuclei arranged in a honeycomb pattern and atypia is not seen.

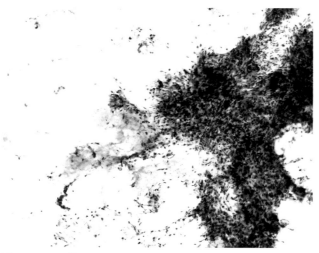

Figure 5.7.3   Chronic pancreatitis. Adenocarcinoma may be associated with desmoplasia and may morphologically overlap with pancreatitis. However, in this field, granulomatous inflammation forms a large fragment that may mimic an atypical epithelial fragment.

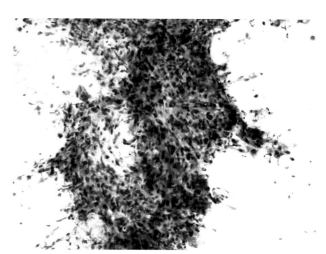

Figure 5.7.4   Chronic pancreatitis. Examination at higher magnification reveals a mixture of lymphocytes, lymphocyte tangles, and epithelioid histiocytes. Granulomatous inflammation is a benign finding that inexperienced pathologists sometimes mistake for a neoplasm.

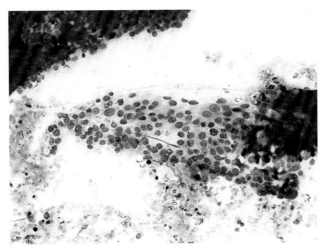

Figure 5.7.5 Adenocarcinoma. A fragment of atypical ductal cells is seen in a background of granular debris (necrosis). The cells have enlarged nuclei with size variation. The cells have a "drunken honeycomb" arrangement within the fragment.

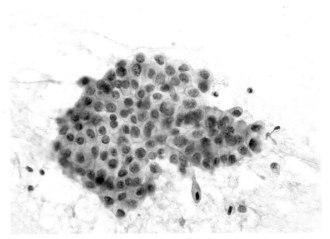

Figure 5.7.6 Adenocarcinoma. The nuclei in this fragment are of different sizes and have nuclear border irregularities. Well-differentiated adenocarcinomas usually do not demonstrate 4:1 variations in nuclear size that is diagnostic of adenocarcinoma, and thus other features are required for a diagnosis. In this case, the normal honeycomb architecture is disrupted.

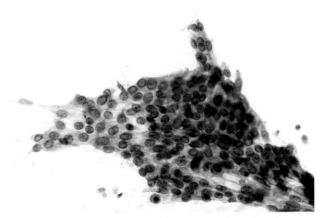

Figure 5.7.7 Adenocarcinoma. This fragment contains enlarged, overlapping nuclei with small nucleoli. The chromatin pattern is otherwise bland. This disrupted honeycomb architecture raises suspicion for an adenocarcinoma.

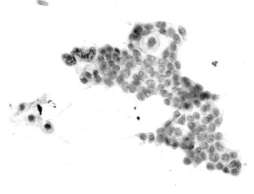

Figure 5.7.8 Adenocarcinoma. This small fragment contains cells with enlarged nuclei with irregular borders. There is a moderate amount of anisonucleosis. The larger nuclei at the top left-hand side of the fragment are quite atypical, and adenocarcinoma is suspected.

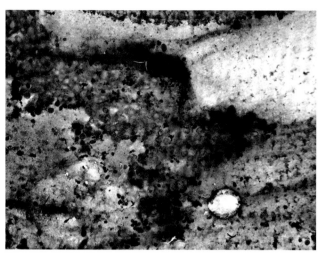

Figure 5.7.9   Adenocarcinoma. A poorly preserved fragment of adenocarcinoma is present in a background of necrosis. The visible nuclei are enlarged and have irregular borders. The diagnosis of adenocarcinoma should rely on the atypia seen in epithelial cells and not be based on the presence of necrosis.

	Adenocarcinoma	Metastatic Renal Cell Carcinoma
Age	Usually older adults	Middle-aged and older adults
Location	Anywhere in pancreas	Anywhere in pancreas; most commonly head followed by the tail
Signs and symptoms	Weight loss; painless jaundice; back pain; migratory thrombophlebitis	Asymptomatic and incidentally discovered, or obstructive symptoms. May recur years to decades after treatment of primary tumor
Etiology	Smoking, alcohol abuse, obesity, diabetes, chronic pancreatitis. Associated familial syndromes (Peutz-Jeghers, hereditary pancreatitis, Lynch syndrome, familial adenomatous polyposis, and others)	Metastatic disease
Cytomorphology	• Predominantly cohesive cells in tissue fragments *(Figure 5.8.1)* • Nuclei are disorganized within tissue fragment ("drunken honeycomb") *(Figure 5.8.2)* • Cell cytoplasm may be foamy with mucin *(Figures 5.8.2 and 5.8.3)* • Nuclear size variation and nuclear border irregularities *(Figures 5.8.4 and 5.8.5)* • Nucleoli may be seen	• Neoplastic cells in fragments and may also be present singly *(Figure 5.8.6)* • Fragments may be associated with vessels and form papillary architecture *(Figures 5.8.6 and 5.8.7)* • Neoplastic cells have abundant, vacuolated cytoplasm *(Figure 5.8.8)* • Enlarged round, eccentric nuclei with regular borders *(Figure 5.8.9)* • Prominent nucleoli *(Figure 5.8.10)* • Higher-grade neoplasms may have more nuclear atypia and pleomorphism
Special studies	Negative for PAX-8, RCC, CAIX, CD10, and RCC	Positive for PAX-8; typically is clear cell RCC and positive for CAIX, CD10, and RCC.
Molecular alterations	Commonly mutations in KRAS, CDKN2A, TP53, and SMAD4	VHL gene alterations
Treatment	Surgical removal; chemoradiation	Surgical removal and systemic therapy
Clinical implications	Poor survival; often not resectable at time of diagnosis	May do well if solitary metastasis and complete resection is possible

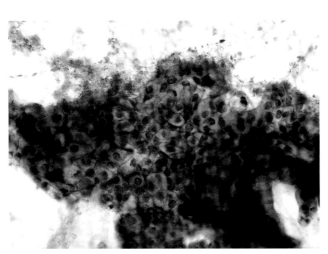

Figure 5.8.1   Adenocarcinoma. This fragment contains cells with nuclei of similar size but with marked nuclear border irregularities. The foamy cytoplasm and well-defined cytoplasmic borders may mimic clear cell renal cell carcinoma.

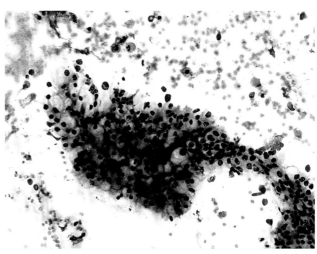

Figure 5.8.2   Adenocarcinoma. This papillary fragment contains cells with foamy cytoplasm that may mimic the "clear" cytoplasm of renal cell carcinoma. However, clear cell renal cell carcinoma typically has vacuolated cytoplasm on cytologic preparations, which is not seen here.

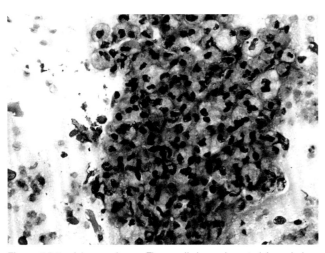

Figure 5.8.3   Adenocarcinoma. These cells have elongated, irregularly shaped nuclei and foamy cytoplasm. The appearance of cytoplasmic vacuoles should cause at least some consideration for a metastatic renal cell carcinoma, as it is the most common metastatic tumor to the pancreas.

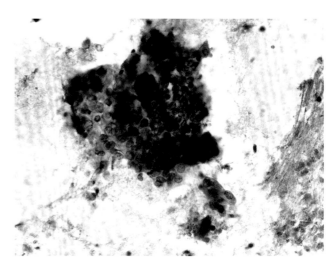

Figure 5.8.4   Adenocarcinoma. This pancreatic adenocarcinoma has a classic appearance, containing cells with enlarged nuclei with irregular borders (note the nuclear grooves). The nuclei are disorganized within the fragment ("drunken honeycomb").

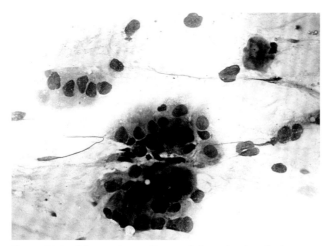

Figure 5.8.5 Adenocarcinoma. These cells have abundant, finely vacuolated, foamy cytoplasm. The nuclei are enlarged and have irregular borders.

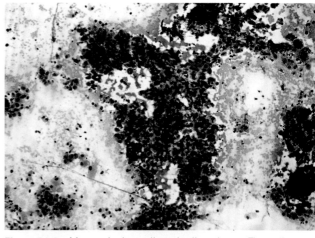

Figure 5.8.6 Metastatic clear cell renal cell carcinoma. The malignant cells are present in papillary fragments; dispersed single cells can also be seen in the background. The cells contain abundant granular cytoplasm; cytoplasmic vacuoles are difficult to assess at this low magnification.

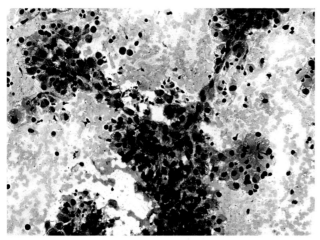

Figure 5.8.7 Metastatic clear cell renal cell carcinoma. The neoplastic cells are loosely associated with vessels. The cells have abundant cytoplasm containing small vacuoles. The differential diagnosis includes adenocarcinoma, and clear cell RCC may be missed if the patient's history is not known.

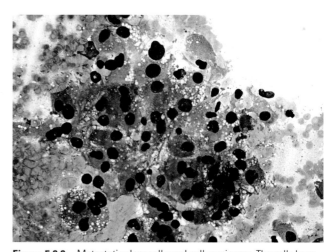

Figure 5.8.8 Metastatic clear cell renal cell carcinoma. The cells have enlarged nuclei and significant nuclear size variation. The presence of prominent nucleoli is also a characteristic of renal cell carcinoma, although they can be seen in some pancreatic adenocarcinomas.

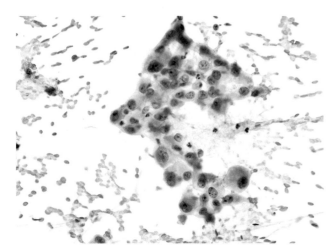

Figure 5.8.9 Metastatic clear cell renal cell carcinoma. The cells have abundant, granular cytoplasm and enlarged nuclei with small nucleoli. The nuclei are deceiving round and regular for a malignant neoplasm.

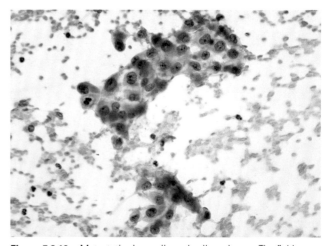

Figure 5.8.10 Metastatic clear cell renal cell carcinoma. The field shows cells with enlarged nuclei containing nucleoli. Renal cell carcinoma may be found in the pancreas many years (even decades) after the patient's first diagnosis of RCC.

	Mucin-Producing Neoplastic Cyst	Gastrointestinal Contamination
Age	Middle-aged women (mucinous cystic neoplasm); any age (IPMN)	Any
Location	Tail (mucinous cystic neoplasm); anywhere but more often head (IPMN)	Anywhere in pancreas
Signs and symptoms	Detected incidentally, or with symptoms of obstruction, especially if there is an invasive component	Found during sampling of a pancreatic lesion; signs and symptoms specific for that lesion may be present
Etiology	Mucinous cystic neoplasm: may be due to ectopic ovarian stroma and associated hormonal growth factors IPMN: Noninvasive mucinous neoplasm associated with main duct or branch ducts; can be associated with familial adenomatous polyposis and Peutz-Jeghers syndrome	Sampling of duodenal or gastric epithelium during endoscopic biopsy of the pancreas
Cytomorphology	• Specimen cellularity is low to moderate • Papillary fragments of neoplastic cells (Figures 5.9.1 and 5.9.2) • Mucinous columnar epithelium (Figure 5.9.3) • Mild nuclear atypia (mild enlargement, size variation, and nuclear contour irregularities) (Figure 5.9.1) • High-grade dysplasia can resemble adenocarcinoma and is characterized by cells with high N/C ratios • Background of "clean mucin," which may contain macrophages and lacks debris, inflammation, and bacteria (Figures 5.9.4 and 5.9.5)	• Bland columnar cells with uniform, oval nuclei with regular borders (Figure 5.9.6) • Duodenal epithelium contains goblet cells, which should be seen in medium-sized and large fragments (Figures 5.9.6-5.9.8) • Gastric foveolar epithelium is mucinous and lacks goblet cells (Figure 5.9.9) • Large fragments may have three-dimensional architecture of the GI tract (such as gastric pits) • Background of "dirty mucin," which contains debris, inflammatory cells, and/or bacteria (Figures 5.9.9 and 5.9.10)
Special studies	MCN: Ovarian stroma is positive for CD10, ER, PR, inhibin, SMA, though not usually found in FNA specimens IPMN: IHC is not usually useful in FNA specimens Elevated CEA in cyst fluid in both MCN and IPMN	None
Molecular alterations	MCN: KRAS in invasive areas IPMN: GNAS and KRAS mutations	N/A
Treatment	Surgical removal	N/A

	Mucin-Producing Neoplastic Cyst	**Gastrointestinal Contamination**
Clinical implications	MCN: Most are not aggressive; may be precursors to invasive adenocarcinoma IPMN: Precursor to invasive adenocarcinoma; a large minority are associated with invasive adenocarcinoma on resection	If lesional cells are not sampled, the patient may have to undergo re-biopsy

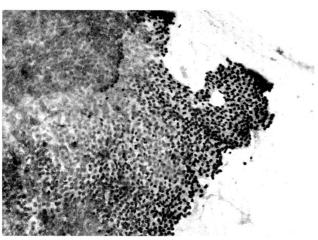

Figure 5.9.1 Mucin-producing neoplastic cyst. The field shows a large fragment of mucinous epithelial cells with small, uniform nuclei. This is not duodenal contamination because it does not contain goblet cells; if the lesion were sampled through the stomach, the architecture would be three-dimensional.

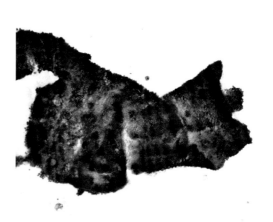

Figure 5.9.2 Mucin-producing neoplastic cyst. A folded, papillary fragment of epithelial cells is shown. Goblet cells are missing. Examination at higher magnification will likely show some mild nuclear atypia, as all mucin-producing neoplastic cysts by definition have at least low-grade dysplasia. The differential diagnosis would include contamination with background foveolar epithelium if the procedure sampled the lesion through the stomach.

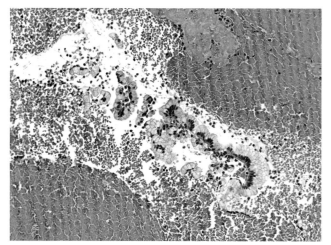

Figure 5.9.3 Mucin-producing neoplastic cyst. The field shows small strips of mucinous epithelium that could represent gastrointestinal contamination or the lining of a mucin-producing neoplastic cyst. The epithelium does not contain goblet cells and would not be compatible with duodenal epithelium.

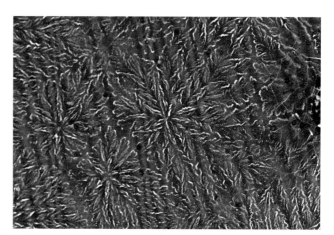

Figure 5.9.4 Mucin-producing neoplastic cyst. Thick mucin containing macrophages and is otherwise clean of bacteria, debris, and inflammatory cells. Such "clean" mucin is found in sterile environments such as neoplastic cyst contents and not in the gastrointestinal tract.

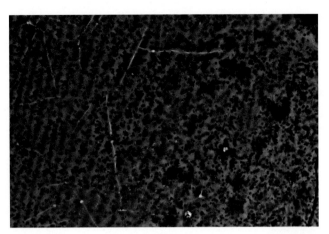

Figure 5.9.5 Mucin-producing neoplastic cyst. This field contains thick mucin, which has begun to crack, similar to what is seen in smears made from thyroid colloid nodules. This thick mucin is found in mucin-producing neoplastic cysts and not in the gastrointestinal tract.

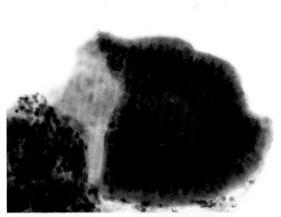

Figure 5.9.6 Gastrointestinal contamination. Duodenal epithelium containing bland columnar cells with uniform, oval nuclei. The presence of goblet cells (with pink staining intracytoplasmic mucin vacuoles) confirms this fragment as gastrointestinal contamination.

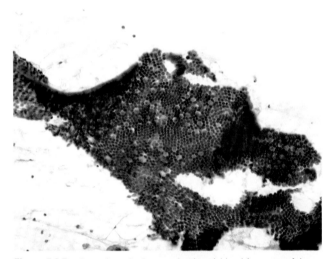

Figure 5.9.7 Gastrointestinal contamination. A bland fragment of duodenal epithelium containing uniform nuclei in a honeycomb arrangement. Numerous goblet cells are easily identified.

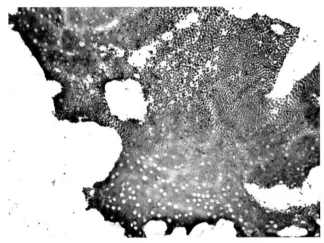

Figure 5.9.8 Gastrointestinal contamination. On Diff-Quik stained preparations, goblet cells are identified by empty "punched out" spaces in a tissue fragment (as seen here).

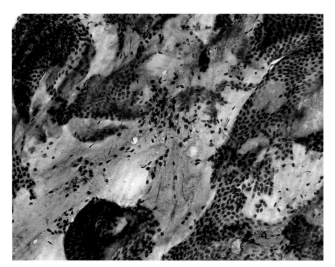

Figure 5.9.9 Gastrointestinal contamination. Foveolar epithelium from the stomach can be seen when pancreatic body and tail lesions are sampled. Goblet cells are not seen, making it challenging to determine whether the epithelium is from the gastrointestinal tract or cyst lining. In this case, "dirty mucin" is seen in the background and indicates the associated epithelial cells are from the gastrointestinal tract.

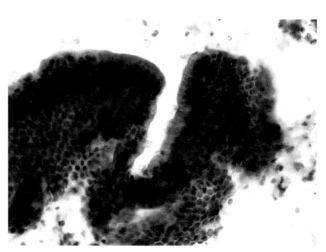

Figure 5.9.10 Gastrointestinal contamination. A fragment of duodenal epithelium containing duodenal cells in a background of "dirty mucin." The mucin contains inflammatory cells and granular debris; at higher magnification, bacteria may be identified.

	Pseudocyst	Lymphoepithelial Cyst
Age	Adults	Middle-aged to older adults
Location	Anywhere in pancreas	Anywhere in pancreas
Signs and symptoms	Pain radiating to back; nausea; vomiting; mass on imaging studies	Incidental finding; pain or nausea
Etiology	Collection of pancreatic secretions following pancreatitis or obstruction of pancreatic duct; does not contain an epithelial lining	Congenital cyst of uncertain etiology
Cytomorphology	• Granular debris *(Figures 5.10.1 and 5.10.2)* • Pigmented macrophages *(Figures 5.10.3 and 5.10.4)* • Hematoidin pigment *(Figure 5.10.5)* • Crystalloids and crystals but not cholesterol crystals *(Figure 5.10.5)* • Only rare lymphocytes • No squamous epithelium	• Keratinaceous debris *(Figures 5.10.6 and 5.10.7)* • Benign, mature squamous cells and anucleate squames *(Figures 5.10.8 and 5.10.9)* • Rare lymphocytes *(Figures 5.10.7-5.10.9)* • Crystalloids • Cholesterol crystals are a specific feature but may be absent *(Figure 5.10.9)* • Cystic macrophages
Special studies	Elevated fluid amylase and low fluid CEA	None usually performed; elevated CEA but not amylase in cyst fluid
Molecular alterations	N/A	N/A
Treatment	Surgical removal or drainage	Does not need to be removed if asymptomatic but often is due to nondiagnostic preceding FNA
Clinical implications	If not treated can rupture and become fatal	Benign

Figure 5.10.1   Pseudocyst. The field shows pseudocyst contents, with a mixture of granular debris and pigment-laden macrophages.

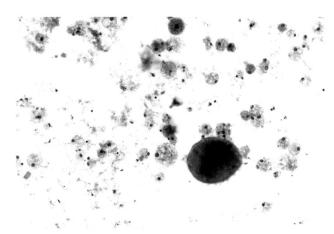

Figure 5.10.2   Pseudocyst. Pigment-laden macrophages are seen in a background of granular debris. Rare golden-staining hematoidin pigment can be seen, which is strongly suggestive of a pseudocyst.

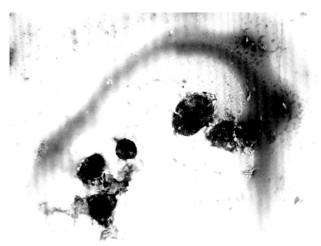

Figure 5.10.3   Pseudocyst. Cystic macrophages and granular debris can be seen in a background of thick, purple-staining proteinaceous fluid.

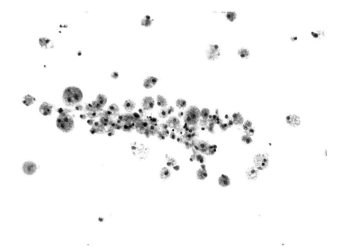

Figure 5.10.4   Pseudocyst. The presence of pigment-laden macrophages is a nonspecific finding and can be found in any cystic lesion. Pseudocysts do not contain an epithelial lining, making a definitive diagnosis challenging in some cases. Measurement of cyst fluid amylase levels is helpful, as pseudocysts often have highly elevated levels of amylase.

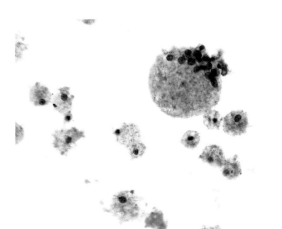

Figure 5.10.5   Pseudocyst. The field contains small pigment-laden cystic macrophages and a multinucleated giant cell. The cells contain golden hematoidin pigment, which is suggestive of a pseudocyst.

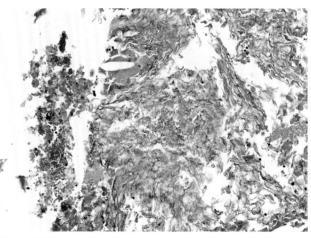

Figure 5.10.6   Lymphoepithelial cyst. A cell block section of a lymphoepithelial cyst demonstrating predominantly keratinaceous debris with rare lymphocytes.

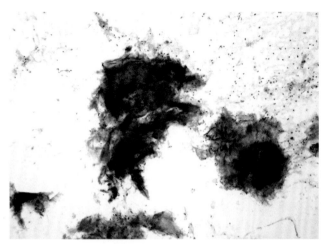

Figure 5.10.7   Lymphoepithelial cyst. A Pap-stained smear shows keratinaceous debris and scattered lymphocytes. Mature squamous cells are not identified at this low magnification.

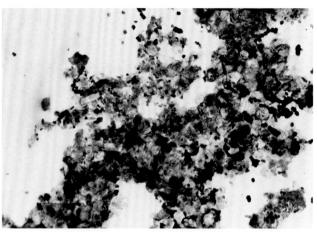

Figure 5.10.8   Lymphoepithelial cyst. The field contains intermixed lymphocytes, mature squamous cells, macrophages, and keratinaceous debris.

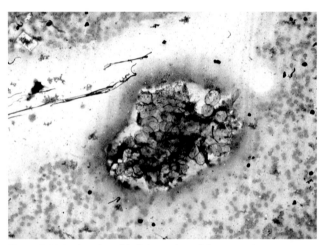

Figure 5.10.9   Lymphoepithelial cyst. A small fragment of mature squamous cells with platelike cytoplasm and rare small nuclei is seen. The background contains rare mature lymphocytes. The top left-hand corner contains a rectangular cholesterol crystal.

	Pancreatic Neuroendocrine Tumor (PanNET)	Accessory Spleen (Splenule)
Age	Usually middle-aged adults but can occur at any age	Any age
Location	Anywhere in pancreas	Pancreatic tail
Signs and symptoms	Asymptomatic and incidentally discovered, or obstructive symptoms; functional tumors are associated with clinical syndromes	Incidentally found on imaging studies; may be multiple
Etiology	Neoplasms with neuroendocrine differentiation; can be associated with various syndromes (MEN1, neurofibromatosis type 1, von Hippel-Lindau, tuberous sclerosis)	Ectopic rest of splenic tissue
Cytomorphology	• Cellular specimen with monotonous cells in fragments and individually dispersed *(Figures 5.11.1* and *5.11.2)* • Eccentrically placed round nucleus with regular nuclear contours *(Figure 5.11.3)* • Abundant granular cytoplasm *(Figures 5.11.3* and *5.11.4)* • "Salt and pepper" (neuroendocrine type) chromatin pattern *(Figure 5.11.3)* • Stripped nuclei may be numerous *(Figure 5.11.5)* • Poorly differentiated tumors may have different features and more closely resemble adenocarcinoma	• Lymphocytes in cohesive fragments intermixed with larger endothelial (sinusoid) cells or predominantly dispersed lymphocytes *(Figures 5.11.6* and *5.11.7)* • Lymphocytes are polymorphous, have angulated nuclei, and a thin rim of cytoplasm *(Figures 5.11.8* and *5.11.9)* • Lymphoid tangles from crushed lymphocyte nuclei may be seen *(Figures 5.11.9* and *5.11.10)* • Cell block preparations better illustrate the spenic architecture
Special studies	Positive for INSM1, chromogranin, synaptophysin, and CD56 by immunohistochemistry	CD8 immunostain will highlight sinusoids on cell block material
Molecular alterations	For sporadic tumors, mutations in MEN1, DAXX, ATRX, TSC2, and/or PTEN, among others.	N/A
Treatment	Surgical removal; sometimes chemotherapy. Targeted therapies available.	N/A
Clinical implications	5 y survival of 55% for localized, resected tumors	N/A

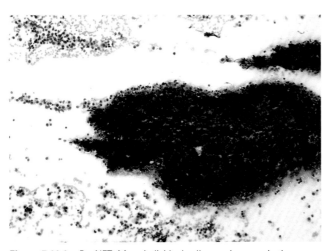

Figure 5.11.1   PanNET. Many individual cells are also seen in the background and have abundant cytoplasm and round, uniform, eccentric nuclei. By contrast, the lymphocytes found in a splenule typically do not contain this much cytoplasm.

Figure 5.11.2   Pancreatic neuroendocrine cells PanNet. These cells are forming small rosettes as well as are singly dispersed in the background. Lymphocytes do not form rosette structures, and the dispersed population of cells makes PanNET high on the differential diagnosis.

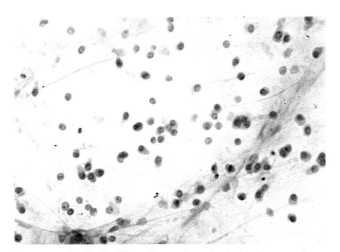

Figure 5.11.3   PanNet. These dispersed neoplastic cells have round, regular nuclei and a plasmacytoid configuration. The chromatin pattern is compatible with a neuroendocrine differentiation.

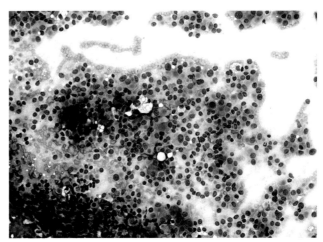

Figure 5.11.4   Numerous loosely cohesive PanNET cells with abundant cytoplasm PanNET. Some cells contain a pink intracytoplasmic inclusion, giving them a rhabdoid appearance.

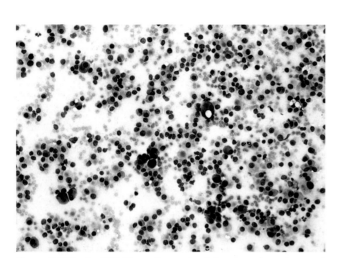

Figure 5.11.5   PanNET. These dispersed cells have round, regular nuclei and little nuclear size variation. Some cells have cytoplasm and stripped (bare) nuclei can also be seen in the background.

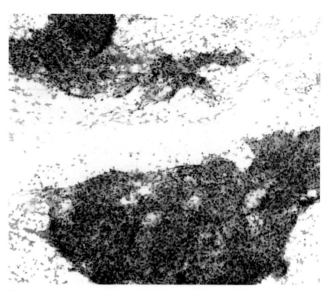

Figure 5.11.6   Accessory spleen. Even at this power, lymphoid tangles (streaked chromatin) can be seen within the fragment. Several punched-out spaces can be seen, likely sinusoids, which would stain positively for CD8 on cell block material.

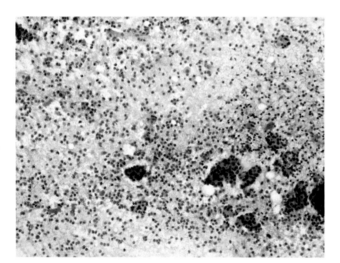

Figure 5.11.7   Accessory spleen. A dispersed population of lymphocytes can be seen among benign pancreatic acinar cells. The acinar cells may be mistaken for rosette structures of a PanNET, causing a diagnostic pitfall. Close examination of dispersed small cells will usually help distinguish them as either lymphocytes or neuroendocrine cells.

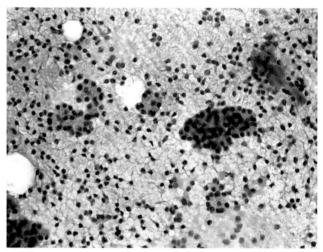

Figure 5.11.8   Accessory spleen. As opposed to neuroendocrine cells, lymphocytes have angulated nuclei and a thin rim of cytoplasm. Neuroendocrine cells usually have round nuclei and more cytoplasm than lymphocytes.

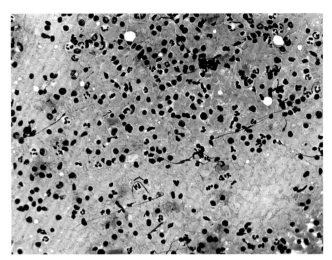

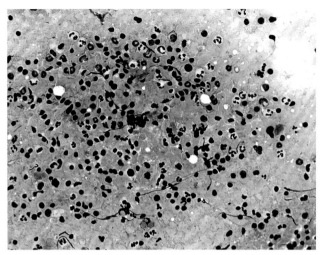

Figure 5.11.9 Accessory spleen. The field contains a polymorphous population of lymphocytes and a few lymphoid tangles. The differential diagnosis includes an intrapancreatic lymph node as well as a splenule.

Figure 5.11.10 Accessory spleen. The field contains numerous polymorphous lymphocytes and rare benign pancreatic acinar cells. Lymphoid tangles are present. The preparation of cell block material can help identify small fragments of a splenule and also allow for the performance of ancillary studies.

	Gastrointestinal Contamination	Well-Differentiated Adenocarcinoma
Age	Any	Usually older adults
Location	Anywhere in pancreas	Anywhere in pancreas
Signs and symptoms	Found during sampling of a pancreatic lesion; signs and symptoms specific for that lesion may be present	Weight loss; painless jaundice; back pain; migratory thrombophlebitis
Etiology	Sampling of duodenal or gastric epithelium during endoscopic biopsy of the pancreas	Smoking, alcohol abuse, obesity, diabetes, chronic pancreatitis. Associated familial syndromes (Peutz-Jeghers, hereditary pancreatitis, Lynch syndrome, familial adenomatous polyposis, and others)
Cytomorphology	• Bland columnar cells with uniform, oval nuclei with regular borders *(Figure 5.12.1)* • Duodenal epithelium contains goblet cells, which should be seen in medium-sized and large fragments *(Figures 5.12.2 and 5.12.3)* • Gastric foveolar epithelium is mucinous and lacks goblet cells *(Figures 5.12.1 and 5.12.4)* • Large fragments may have three-dimensional architecture of the GI tract (such as gastric pits) *(Figures 5.12.4 and 5.12.5)*	• Predominantly cohesive cells in tissue fragments *(Figure 5.12.6)* • Nuclei are disorganized within tissue fragment ("drunken honeycomb") *(Figures 5.12.7 and 5.12.8)* • Nuclear size variation and nuclear border irregularities *(Figures 5.12.9 and 5.12.10)* • Nucleoli may be seen
Special studies	None	Usually negative or only weakly/focally positive for neuroendocrine markers
Molecular alterations	N/A	Commonly mutations in KRAS, CDKN2A, TP53, and SMAD4.
Treatment	N/A	Surgical removal; chemoradiation
Clinical implications	If lesional cells are not sampled, the patient may have to undergo re-biopsy	Poor survival; often not resectable at time of diagnosis

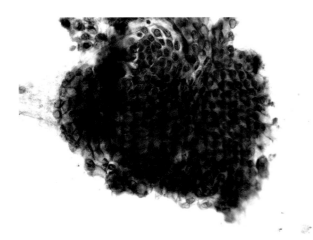

Figure 5.12.1   Gastrointestinal contamination. The field contains a bland fragment of glandular epithelium, representing foveolar epithelium contaminated as the needle passed through the stomach. GI contamination may have reactive changes but is often very bland, containing uniform, oval-shaped nuclei with regular borders. The cells are organized within the fragment.

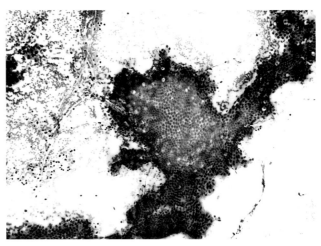

Figure 5.12.2   Gastrointestinal contamination. Contaminating duodenal epithelium is evidenced by the "punched-out" spaces containing goblet cells at regular intervals. The presence of goblet cells automatically dismisses a fragment as GI contamination.

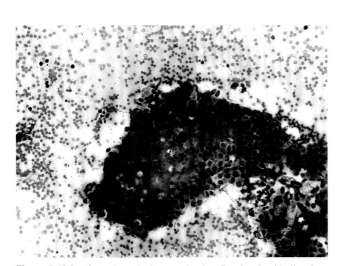

Figure 5.12.3   Gastrointestinal contamination. Duodenal epithelium is seen during the sampling of pancreatic head lesions.

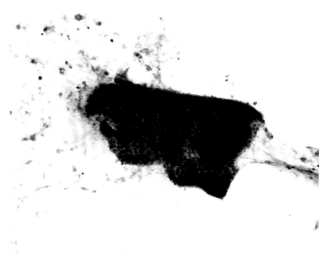

Figure 5.12.4   Gastrointestinal contamination. This specimen contains foveolar epithelium contaminating the specimen from the stomach. These procedures typically sample pancreatic head or tail lesions. The absence of goblet cells makes it difficult to exclude this fragment as lesional. However, the fragment is associated with "dirty" mucin from the gastrointestinal tract, suggesting the fragment is also from the GI tract.

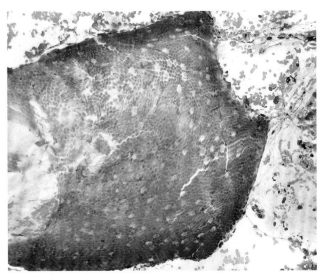

Figure 5.12.5   Gastrointestinal contamination. The field shows a large, wrinkled sheet of contaminating duodenal epithelium. Goblet cells can be seen, and the cells within the fragment are well-organized.

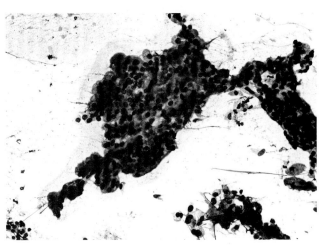

Figure 5.12.6   Adenocarcinoma. A fragment of ductal adenocarcinoma forms a papillary structure; this architecture not seen in GI contamination. The nuclei are enlarged and disorganized within the fragment.

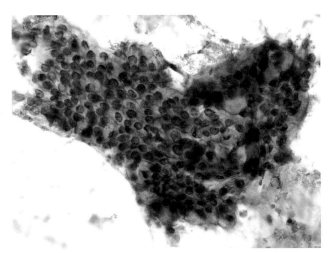

Figure 5.12.7   Adenocarcinoma. The cells have enlarged nuclei and irregular nuclear borders and nuclear grooves. The cells form microglandular structures (top right), a finding seen in adenocarcinoma and not in gastrointestinal contamination.

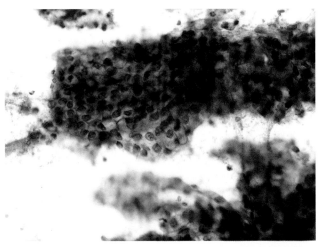

Figure 5.12.8   Adenocarcinoma. These cells have enlarged nuclei with irregular borders. The nuclei are disorganized within the fragment. Owing to the mucin contained within these cells, the N/C ratios are lower than what is seen in other adenocarcinomas.

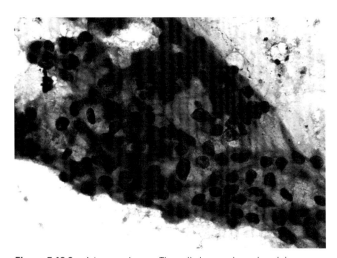

Figure 5.12.9   Adenocarcinoma. The cells have enlarged nuclei, some with markedly irregular borders. This level of atypia suggests an adenocarcinoma.

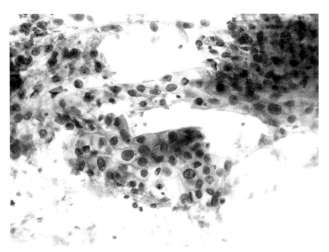

Figure 5.12.10   Adenocarcinoma. The cells are disorganized within the fragment and have enlarged nuclei, anisonucleosis, and irregular nuclear borders. Some nuclei vary in size by more than 4:1 compared with adjacent nuclei, a feature diagnostic of adenocarcinoma.

6

Serous Effusions

	Mesothelial Hyperplasia	Metastatic Adenocarcinoma
Age	Usually adults	Usually older adults
Location	Pericardial, pleural, and peritoneal cavities	Pericardial, pleural, and peritoneal cavities
Signs and symptoms	Often an incidental finding	Pleural effusion; ascites; pericardial effusion
Etiology	Reactive/reparative process in which hyperplasia of the mesothelial lining	Metastasis, commonly from lung or breast (pleural and pericardial effusions) or gynecologic, gastrointestinal, or pancreatobiliary tract (ascites)
Cytomorphology	• Small clusters and/or dispersed mesothelial cells; large clusters or fragments not usually seen *(Figures 6.1.1* and *6.1.2)* • Abundant cytoplasm and round nuclei with regular borders *(Figure 6.1.3)* • "Lacy skirt" appearance due to two-toned cytoplasm • Empty spaces ("windows") between adjoining mesothelial cells • Occasional cytoplasmic vacuolization *(Figure 6.1.3)* • May be multinucleated • May have nucleoli *(Figure 6.1.2)* • Occasional mitotic figures • Sometimes associated psammomatous calcification *(Figure 6.1.4)*	• Single cells, small fragments, and/or three-dimensional glandular structures *(Figures 6.1.5* and *6.1.6)* • Spherical or papillary structures with empty or mucin-containing glandular centers *(Figure 6.1.7)* • Single cells with mucinous vacuoles *(Figure 6.1.8)* • Cytomorphology varies with tumor type but classic features of adenocarcinoma: enlarged cells, enlarged nuclei, high N/C ratios, irregular nuclear borders, coarse chromatin, hyperchromasia, and anisonucleosis *(Figure 6.1.9.)*
Special studies	Negative for BerEP4/MOC-31. Positive for calretinin and often also nuclear WT1. Usually negative for EMA. BAP1 nuclear expression retained	Usually positive for BerEP4/MOC-31 and negative for calretinin
Molecular alterations	N/A	Depends on primary tumor site and type
Treatment	None, or tissue biopsy if mesothelioma cannot be excluded	Depends on primary tumor site and type
Clinical implications	N/A	Involvement of serous cavity usually indicates high stage disease and a poor prognosis

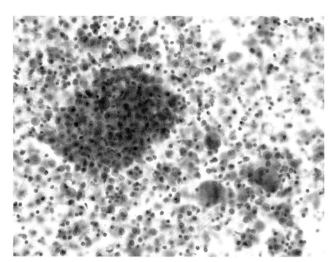

Figure 6.1.1   Reactive mesothelial cells. A small fragment of mesothelial cells is seen in a background of reactive mesothelial cells, lymphocytes, and histiocytes. A few enlarged multinucleated giant cells can be seen, but their nuclei are small and round, with regular borders and bland chromatin.

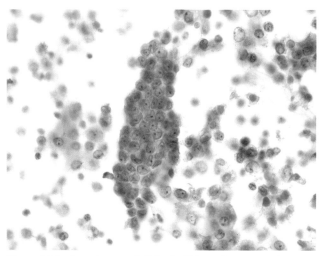

Figure 6.1.2   Reactive mesothelial cells. This small monolayer fragment contains mesothelial cells with slight nuclear contour irregularities and small nucleoli. The cells also have small amounts of cytoplasm and an adenocarcinoma should be considered.

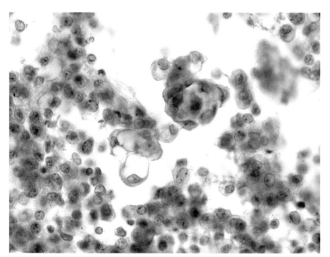

Figure 6.1.3   Reactive mesothelial cells. This specimen contains an increased number of mesothelial cells. The cells have enlarged nuclei, coarse chromatin or nucleoli, and relatively regular nuclear contours. Most cells have low N/C ratios and some cells have large cytoplasmic vacuoles, which may mimic the mucinous vacuoles of some adenocarcinomas.

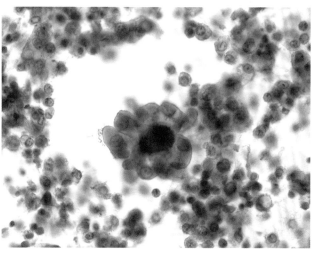

Figure 6.1.4   Reactive mesothelial cells. The central field contains a psammoma body surrounded by bland mesothelial cells. Psammomatous calcification can be seen in both benign and malignant conditions.

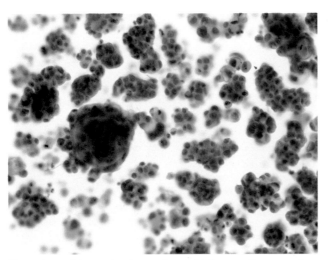

Figure 6.1.5   Metastatic adenocarcinoma. Malignant cells are seen in small three-dimensional fragments. The cells have high N/C ratios and moderate variation in nuclear size. Some nuclei have markedly irregular contours.

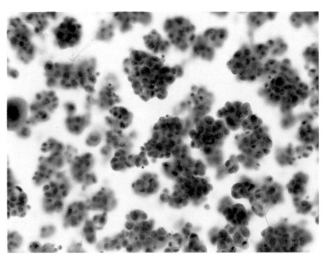

Figure 6.1.6   Metastatic adenocarcinoma. These fragments form three-dimensional, papillary fragments. This architecture is not typically seen in mesotheliomas. The cells are overtly malignant, given their high N/C ratios, irregular nuclear borders, anisonucleosis, and hyperchromasia.

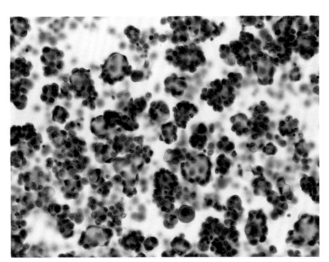

Figure 6.1.7   Metastatic adenocarcinoma. This metastatic adenocarcinoma has prominent gland formation. The glands appear as empty spaces, whereas mesothelioma cells do not form true glands but may surround a central core of "ground substance."

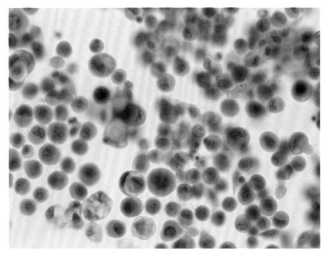

Figure 6.1.8   Metastatic adenocarcinoma. Adenocarcinoma cells are seen as a predominantly dispersed, single cell population. The cells are large and have enlarged nuclei with irregular borders and coarse chromatin. Mesothelioma can occasionally present as a single cell population, a potential pitfall.

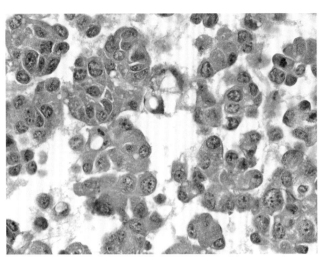

Figure 6.1.9 Metastatic adenocarcinoma. These cells demonstrate all the features of malignancy: high N/C ratios, anisonucleosis, coarse chromatin, irregular nuclear borders, and large cell size. Some cells contain intracytoplasmic vacuoles that may stain for mucin; however, mesotheliomas can also contain vacuoles.

	Metastatic Adenocarcinoma	Endosalpingiosis
Age	Usually older adults	Usually middle-aged and older women
Location	Peritoneal cavity.	Peritoneal cavity.
Signs and symptoms	Pleural effusion; ascites; pericardial effusion	Usually detected asymptomatically in fluid specimens; may cause pelvic pain
Etiology	Metastasis, commonly from lung or breast (pleural and pericardial effusions) or gynecologic, gastrointestinal, or pancreatobiliary tract (ascites)	Ectopic fallopian tube epithelium
Cytomorphology	• Single cells, small fragments, and/or three-dimensional glandular structures *(Figures 6.2.1 and 6.2.2)* • Three-dimensional glandular structures which may contain mucinous vacuoles *(Figure 6.2.3)* • Single cells with mucinous vacuoles *(Figure 6.2.4)* • Cytomorphology varies with tumor type but classic features of adenocarcinoma: enlarged cells, enlarged nuclei, high N/C ratios, irregular nuclear borders, hyperchromasia, and anisonucleosis *(Figures 6.2.1-6.2.5)*	• Fragments of various sizes containing columnar cells with regular, oval-shaped nuclei *(Figures 6.2.6 and 6.2.7)* • Nuclei are well organized within tissue fragments *(Figures 6.2.6-6.2.10)* • Tissue fragment edges contain terminal bars and/or cilia *(Figures 6.2.6-6.2.8)* • Cilia may not be well identified, causing a diagnostic dilemma *(Figures 6.2.9 and 6.2.10)*
Special studies	Usually positive for BerEP4/MOC-31 and negative for calretinin	Positive for BerEP4/MOC-31, ER, PAX-8, and WT-1. Wild-type p53. Negative for calretinin
Molecular alterations	Depends on primary tumor site and type	N/A
Treatment	Depends on primary tumor site and type	N/A
Clinical implications	Involvement of serous cavity usually indicates high-stage disease and a poor prognosis	N/A

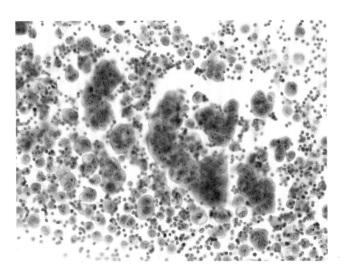

Figure 6.2.1   Metastatic adenocarcinoma. These cells are forming papillary tissue fragments as well as single cells in the background. The cells are enlarged and have large nuclei with prominent nucleoli. Cytoplasmic vacuoles can be seen, likely containing mucin.

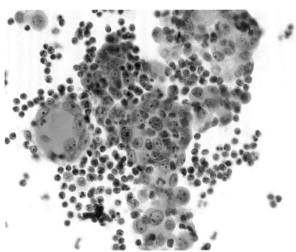

Figure 6.2.2   Metastatic adenocarcinoma. These malignant cells are seen in a background of lymphocytes and histiocytes. The malignant cells are large and have large nuclei with irregular borders, anisonucleosis, and prominent nucleoli.

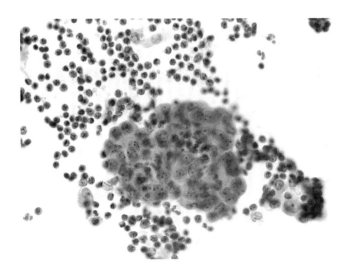

Figure 6.2.3   Metastatic adenocarcinoma. A three-dimensional group contains cells with high N/C ratios and coarse chromatin. This atypia is too marked to be a benign process, and the cells lack cilia and terminal bars.

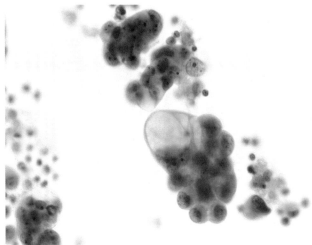

Figure 6.2.4   Metastatic adenocarcinoma. The field shows overtly malignant cells, some containing mucinous vacuoles. The cells are very large compared with the background benign cells and have nuclei of varied size and coarse chromatin.

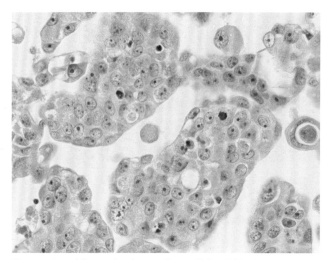

Figure 6.2.5 Metastatic adenocarcinoma. This cell block preparation shows cells with microglandular formations, large irregular nuclei, and coarse chromatin. Cilia are not identified.

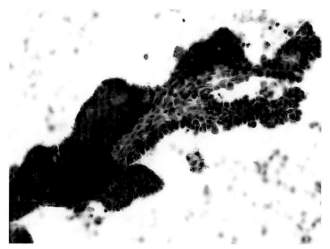

Figure 6.2.6 Endosalpingiosis. This papillary structure is lined by columnar cells with oval, uniform nuclei. The cells are organized within the tissue fragment. It is difficult to confirm the presence of cilia at this low magnification, but they may be seen at a higher magnification, which would help confirm this process as endosalpingiosis.

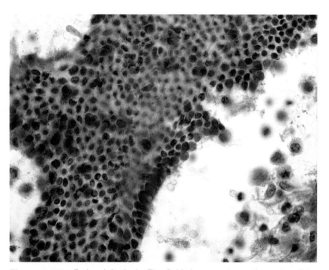

Figure 6.2.7 Endosalpingiosis. The field shows a sheet of round nuclei that form a slightly disorganized honeycomb. The edge of the tissue fragment is flat due to the presence of cellular terminal bars, at which red-staining cilia are attached.

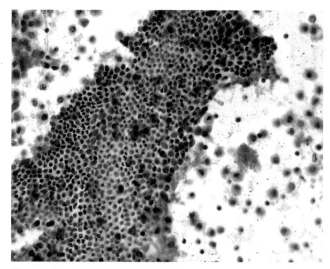

Figure 6.2.8 Endosalpingiosis. This large monolayer fragment contains cells with bland-appearing nuclei that are well organized within the fragment. The edges of the fragment contain red-staining cilia, which are difficult to see at this low magnification.

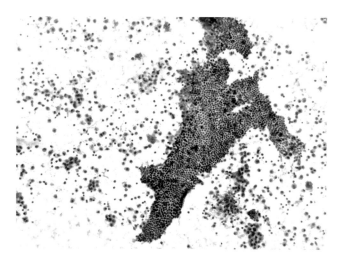

Figure 6.2.9 Endosalpingiosis. Even at this low magnification, the nuclei are small and spaces can be seen between nuclei, indicating that their architecture is not disrupted. Cilia are not identified at this low magnification.

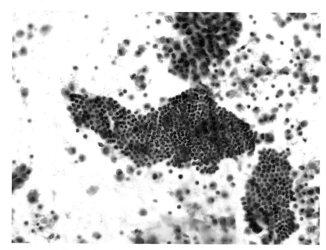

Figure 6.2.10 Endosalpingiosis. Bland-appearing nuclei are seen arranged in a honeycomb structure. While cilia are not seen, the nuclei are round and uniform and have regular nuclear borders. These features favor a benign process, regardless of whether cilia are seen.

	Mesothelial Hyperplasia	Mesothelioma
Age	Usually adults	Older age; usually men
Location	Pericardial, pleural, and peritoneal cavities	Pericardial, pleural, and peritoneal cavities
Signs and symptoms	Often an incidental finding	Dyspnea; chest wall pain; pleural effusion
Etiology	Reactive/reparative process in which hyperplasia of the mesothelial lining	Associated with smoking and asbestos exposure
Cytomorphology	• Small clusters and/or dispersed mesothelial cells; large clusters or fragments not usually seen *(Figures 6.3.1 and 6.3.2)* • Abundant cytoplasm and round nuclei with regular borders *(Figures 6.3.3 and 6.3.4)* • "Lacy skirt" appearance due to two-toned cytoplasm *(Figure 6.3.3)* • Empty spaces ("windows") between adjoining mesothelial cells *(Figure 6.3.5)* • May be multinucleated *(Figure 6.3.3)* • May have nucleoli *(Figure 6.3.2)* • Sometimes associated psammomatous calcification *(Figure 6.3.5)*	• Single cells and/or tissue fragments *(Figures 6.3.6 and 6.3.7)* • Tissue fragments may form "cannonballs" with central ground substance or with bulbous, branching structures *(Figures 6.3.6-6.3.8)* • Typically epithelioid cells in effusions, with abundant amphophilic, vacuolated cytoplasm and round/oval nuclei with prominent nucleoli *(Figure 6.3.9)* • Morphology may overlap with adenocarcinoma in less differentiated mesotheliomas *(Figure 6.3.10)*
Special studies	Negative for BerEP4/MOC-31. Positive for calretinin and often also nuclear WT1. Usually negative for EMA. BAP1 nuclear expression retained	Negative for BerEP4/MOC-31. Positive for calretinin and often also nuclear WT1. Often positive for EMA. BAP1 nuclear expression lost in a subset. p16 homozygous deletion detectable by FISH
Molecular alterations	N/A	Homozygous deletions of p16; NF2 mutations; BAP1 germline mutations
Treatment	None, or tissue biopsy if mesotheliom cannot be excluded	Chemoradiation; surgery; pleurodesis
Clinical implications	N/A	Poor survival; median survival time of less than 12 mo

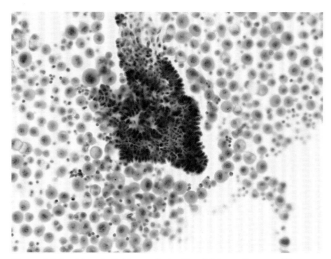

Figure 6.3.1   Mesothelial hyperplasia. The field contains a papillary-shaped fragment of columnar cells with oval to round nuclei. The cells are monotonous and are organized with the fragment. At this magnification, the differential diagnosis includes endosalpingiosis; reactive mesothelial hyperplasia would be negative for MOC-31/BerEP4 and positive for calretinin.

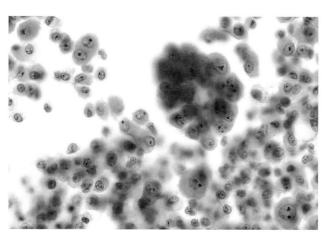

Figure 6.3.2   Mesothelial hyperplasia. A small cluster of enlarged mesothelial cells is seen with numerous mesothelial cells in the background. Some cells have prominent nucleoli. It is difficult to completely exclude mesothelioma using cytomorphology alone; ancillary studies are often helpful.

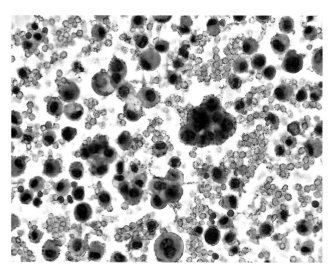

Figure 6.3.3   Mesothelial hyperplasia. Reactive mesothelial cells are present in small clusters as well as singly in the background. The cells are of various sizes, as are their nuclei. Some cells are binucleated, a feature that can be seen in both benign and malignant mesothelial processes.

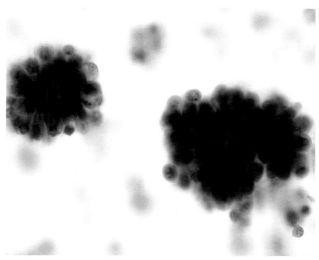

Figure 6.3.4   Mesothelial hyperplasia. These small clusters of mesothelial cells have hobnailed edges. Many of the cells have abundant cytoplasm, and the nuclei are round with regular borders and bland chromatin.

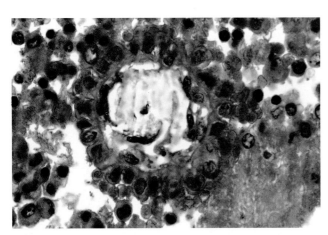

Figure 6.3.5   Mesothelial hyperplasia. This cell block section demonstrates a small fragment of reactive mesothelial cells associated with psammomatous calcification. Psammoma bodies can also be seen in epithelial lesions, such as endosalpingiosis, and this is not specific for mesothelial hyperplasia.

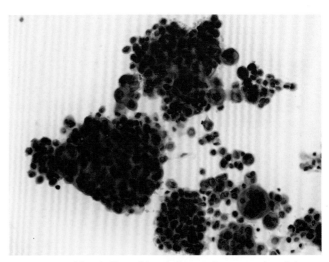

Figure 6.3.6   Mesothelioma. Mesothelioma cells are seen in cellular, three-dimensional fragments as well as dispersed in the background. These large, irregular-shaped fragments containing disorganized nuclei are atypical, and mesothelioma cannot be excluded.

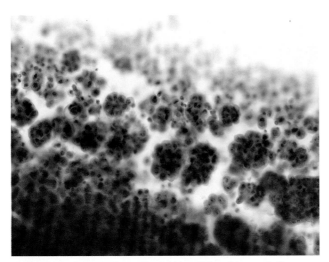

Figure 6.3.7   Mesothelioma. The field is cellular with mesothelioma cells, some in irregularly shaped three-dimensional structures, and others present singly in the background. The cellularity of the specimen and irregularly shaped tissue fragments are suspicious for a mesothelioma.

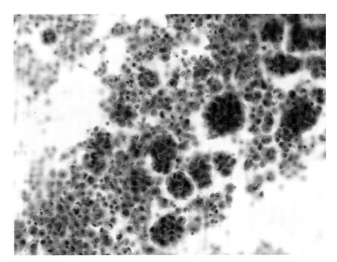

Figure 6.3.8   Mesothelioma. The specimen is very cellular and predominantly with mesothelial cells. It is unusual to see a predominance of mesothelial cells in a cellular specimen, and this finding should raise suspicion for mesothelioma.

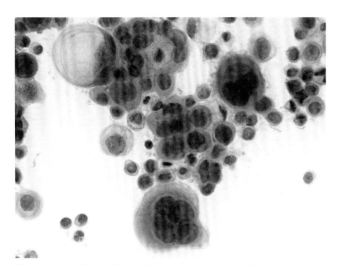

Figure 6.3.9   Mesothelioma. Malignant mesothelial cells often maintain the cytomorphologic features of mesothelial differentiation, such as abundant cytoplasm and "lacy skirt" morphology. The presence of giant cells with mesothelial differentiation is an unusual finding and is suspicious for mesothelioma.

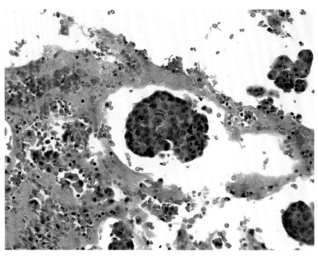

Figure 6.3.10   Mesothelioma. Some mesotheliomas closely resemble adenocarcinoma, such as the tissue fragment seen here containing crowded nuclei with nuclear border irregularities. Once a mesothelial origin is established with immunohistochemistry, additional studies are usually required to confirm the cell as malignant.

	Metastatic Adenocarcinoma	Mesothelioma
Age	Usually older adults	Older age; usually men
Location	Pericardial, pleural, and peritoneal cavities	Pericardial, pleural, and peritoneal cavities
Signs and symptoms	Pleural effusion; ascites; pericardial effusion	Dyspnea; chest wall pain; pleural effusion
Etiology	Metastasis, commonly from lung or breast (pleural and pericardial effusions) or gynecologic, gastrointestinal, or pancreatobiliary tract (ascites)	Associated with smoking and asbestos exposure
Cytomorphology	• Single cells, small fragments, and/or three-dimensional glandular structures *(Figure 6.4.1)* • "Cannonballs" with empty or mucin-containing glandular centers *(Figures 6.4.2 and 6.4.3)* • Single cells with mucinous vacuoles *(Figure 6.4.4)* • Cytomorphology varies with tumor type but classic features of adenocarcinoma: enlarged cells, enlarged nuclei, high N/C ratios, irregular nuclear borders, hyperchromasia, and anisonucleosis *(Figure 6.4.5)*	• Single cells and/or tissue fragments *(Figure 6.4.6)* • Tissue fragments may form "cannonballs" with central ground substance or with bulbous, branching structures *(Figures 6.4.7 and 6.4.8)* • Typically epithelioid cells in effusions, with abundant amphophilic, vacuolated cytoplasm and round/oval nuclei with prominent nucleoli *(Figures 6.4.9 and 6.4.10)* • Morphology may overlap with adenocarcinoma in less differentiated mesotheliomas
Special studies	Usually positive for BerEP4/MOC-31 and negative for calretinin	Negative for BerEP4/MOC-31. Positive for calretinin and often also nuclear WT1. Often positive for EMA. BAP1 nuclear expression lost in a subset. p16 homozygous deletion detectable by FISH
Molecular alterations	Depends on primary tumor site and type	Homozygous deletions of p16; NF2 mutations; BAP1 germline mutations
Treatment	Depends on primary tumor site and type	Chemoradiation; surgery; pleurodesis
Clinical implications	Involvement of serous cavity usually indicates high-stage disease and a poor prognosis	Poor survival; median survival time of less than 12 mo

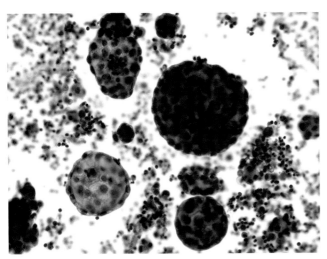

Figure 6.4.1   Metastatic adenocarcinoma. Several large "cannonball" structures are seen, which represent gland-forming adenocarcinoma cells. Ductal breast carcinoma as well as lung adenocarcinoma can form cannonball structures. These structures can also be seen in mesothelioma and thus ancillary studies performed on cell block material can be useful.

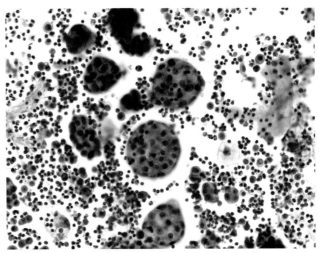

Figure 6.4.2   Metastatic adenocarcinoma. Several "cannonball" structures can be seen in a background of reactive mesothelial cells, histiocytes, and lymphocytes. The cells and their associated nuclei are very large compared with the background benign cells.

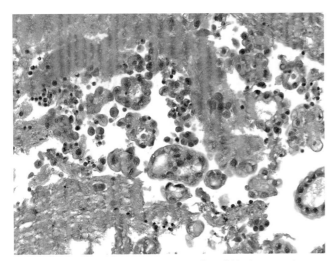

Figure 6.4.3   Metastatic adenocarcinoma. On cell block preparations, the center of "cannonballs" is revealed and may be empty or contain mucin in adenocarcinomas. Mesotheliomas with cannonball structures contain ground substance in the center.

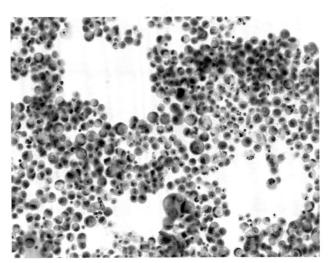

Figure 6.4.4   Metastatic adenocarcinoma. Numerous dispersed large adenocarcinoma cells contain pink-staining mucin vacuoles. The cells have a "signet ring" morphology that is usually associated with metastatic gastric, esophageal, and lobular carcinomas but can sometimes be seen in adenocarcinomas from other sites.

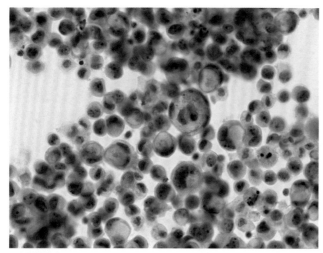

Figure 6.4.5 Metastatic adenocarcinoma. Metastatic adenocarcinoma cells are often high grade and have atypical features seen in adenocarcinomas at other sites: cellular and nuclear enlargement, hyperchromatic nuclei, irregular nuclear contours, and anisonucleosis.

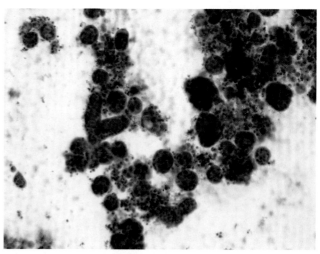

Figure 6.4.6 Mesothelioma. A mixture of cannonball and irregularly shaped, rigid tubular structures are seen. Mesothelioma can present as a predominantly single cell population but may also form cannonballs and structures with rigid, bulbous projections.

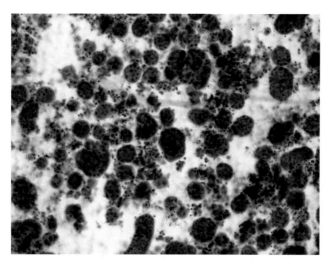

Figure 6.4.7 Mesothelioma. Numerous cannonball structures admixed with bulbous, elongated tissue fragments fill the field. The presence of the former should cause consideration for mesothelioma.

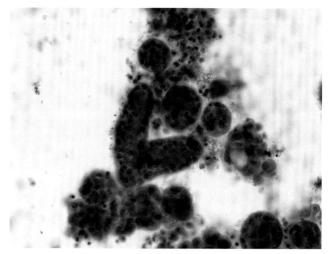

Figure 6.4.8 Mesothelioma. A V-shaped fragment of mesothelioma cells forms bulbous projections and is more suggestive of mesothelioma than an adenocarcinoma. One small tissue fragment appears to contain an empty glandular space, emulating an adenocarcinoma.

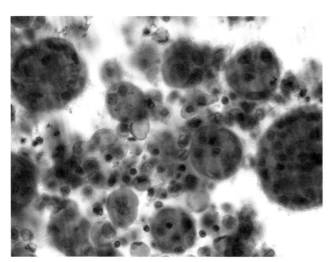

Figure 6.4.9   Mesothelioma. Malignant mesotheliomas may maintain the cytomorphologic features of benign mesothelial cells or appear more atypical. These cells maintain the abundant, amphophilic cytoplasm seen in mesothelial cell but also have some nuclear contour irregularities, anisonucleosis, and nucleoli. Ancillary studies are usually required to make a definitive diagnosis of mesothelioma.

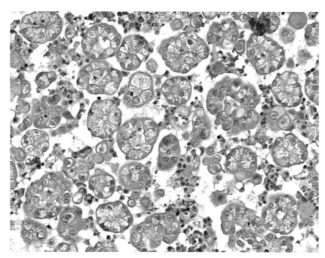

Figure 6.4.10   Mesothelioma. A cell block section of mesothelioma cannonballs highlights their vacuolated cytoplasm, irregular nuclear shapes and sizes, and nucleoli.

	Non-Hodgkin Lymphoma (NHL)	Lymphocytosis
Age	All ages	All ages
Location	Pericardial, pleural, and peritoneal cavities	Pericardial, pleural, and peritoneal cavities
Signs and symptoms	Painless lymphadenopathy, fevers, night sweats, fatigue, weight loss. May initially present as an effusion	Pleural effusion
Etiology	Associated with autoimmune diseases, viruses, radiation, chemotherapy, and immunodeficiencies	Usually unknown. Can be associated with infection (especially tuberculosis) or occult carcinoma
Cytomorphology	• Discohesive population of cells (Figures 6.5.1-6.5.3) • Monotonous or pleomorphic population of cells, depending on lymphoma type (Figures 6.5.1-6.5.3) • Thin cytoplasmic rim (Figure 6.5.2) • Large B-cell lymphoma cells are larger than reactive lymphocytes (Figures 6.5.4 and 6.5.5) • Coarse chromatin or prominent nucleoli (Figure 6.5.4)	• Usually a dispersed population of monotonous, individual small lymphoid cells (Figures 6.5.6 and 6.5.7) • Lymphoid cells have a thin rim of cytoplasm and an angulated nucleus (Figures 6.5.8 and 6.5.9) • Coarse chromatin without prominent nucleoli (Figures 6.5.9 and 6.5.10)
Special studies	Negative for keratin and usually positive for CD45. Most are of B-cell origin and express B-cell markers (eg, CD20). Flow cytometry is the most specific and sensitive method for detecting most small cell lymphomas	Flow cytometry is very helpful in excluding a small cell lymphoma. Cell block material demonstrating a mixture of T- and B-cells on IHC does not entirely exclude lymphoma
Molecular alterations	Various, depending on subtype	N/A
Treatment	Varies	Treatment of etiology, if known
Clinical implication	Missed diagnosis may cause delay in treatment	Depends on etiology

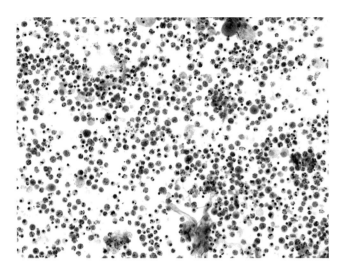

Figure 6.5.1 Large B-cell lymphoma. The field is cellular and contains a mixture of cells. The intact lymphoma cells are large and have high N/C ratios and round nuclei with coarse chromatin. The cells are too large and atypical to represent a small cell lymphoma or reactive lymphoid population.

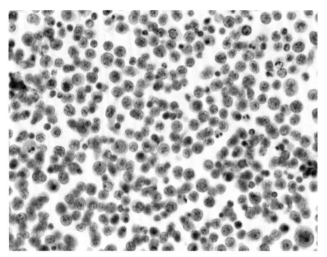

Figure 6.5.2 Large B-cell lymphoma. The field contains cells with nuclei of variable shapes and sizes and irregular contours. The cells maintain a thin rim of blue cytoplasm.

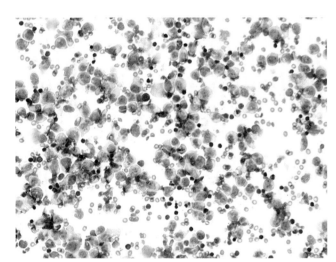

Figure 6.5.3 Large B-cell lymphoma. The field contains pleomorphic single cells and the differential diagnosis includes poorly differentiated adenocarcinoma, melanoma, large cell lymphoma, and, less likely, sarcoma.

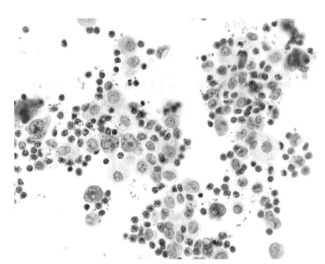

Figure 6.5.4 Large B-cell lymphoma. This large cell lymphoma contains pleomorphic large cells with large nuclei and irregular nuclear contours. Some cells have large nucleoli and are overtly malignant. If positive for lymphoid markers, a lymphoma can be diagnosed without the need for demonstrating clonality.

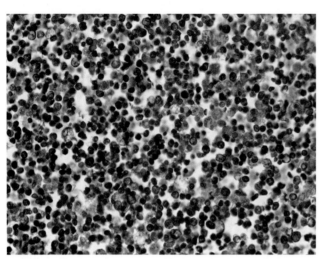

Figure 6.5.5   Large B-cell lymphoma. This cell block material demonstrates large, atypical nuclei without well-defined cytoplasm. The differential diagnosis includes "small" round blue cell tumors such as small cell carcinoma and lymphoma.

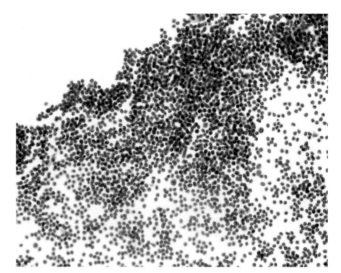

Figure 6.5.6   Lymphocytosis. The field is filled with monotonous-appearing lymphocytes. Reactive lymphocyte populations in serous fluids can look more monotonous than those aspirated from reactive lymph nodes.

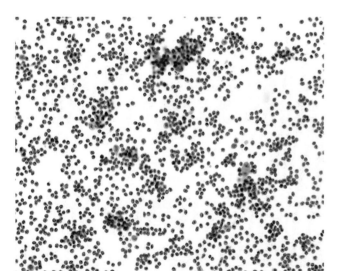

Figure 6.5.7   Lymphocytosis. The field is filled with numerous small lymphocytes, most of which are usually T-cells in reactive serous fluid specimens. A small lymphoma can only be excluded with flow cytometry.

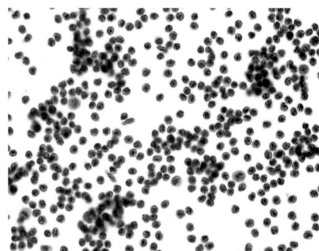

Figure 6.5.8   Lymphocytosis. These small lymphocytes contain a thin rim of blue cytoplasm and angulated nuclei. The chromatin pattern is coarse.

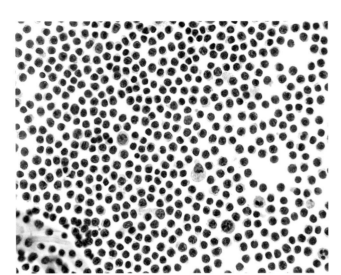

Figure 6.5.9 Lymphocytosis. Lymphocytes are evenly spread over the field, a pattern that sometimes occurs in liquid-based preparations. The lymphocytes are small and have a thin rim of cytoplasm and angulated nuclei.

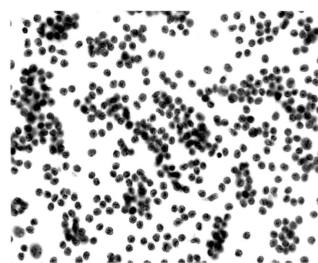

Figure 6.5.10 Lymphocytosis. The field contains numerous small lymphocytes, some of which loosely aggregate and may mimic small cell carcinoma. Lymphoglandular bodies (a feature indicative of a lymphoid population in conventional smear specimens) are not usually seen in liquid based preparations.

7

Cerebrospinal Fluid (CSF)

	Metastatic Carcinoma	Macrophages
Age	Usually older adults	Any age
Location	Cerebrospinal fluid	Cerebrospinal fluid
Signs and symptoms	Meningeal symptoms (headache, seizure, nausea, vomiting) and neurologic deficits	Symptoms of underlying disorder requiring lumbar tap
Etiology	Metastatic carcinoma, commonly from a breast or lung primary	Nonspecific finding
Cytomorphology	• Small three-dimensional clusters and/or individual cells *(Figures 7.1.1 and 7.1.2)* • Large cells with large nuclei and high N/C ratios *(Figures 7.1.3 and 7.1.4)* • Hyperchromasia and irregular nuclear borders *(Figures 7.1.4 and 7.1.5)* • Coarse chromatin *(Figure 7.1.5)*	• Discohesive individual cells *(Figure 7.1.6)* • Usually smaller than carcinoma cells • Cells may artifactually cluster together and create pseudofragments *(Figures 7.1.7 and 7.1.8)* • Abundant, often foamy, cytoplasm *(Figures 7.1.9 and 7.1.10)* • Round or elongated nuclei, often with an indentation or "curve" *(Figures 7.1.9 and 7.1.10)* • Nuclei more uniform than carcinoma cell nuclei
Special studies	Positive for keratins, often negative for CD68	Positive for CD68, negative for keratins
Molecular alterations	Dependent on the primary tumor type	N/A
Treatment	Radiation therapy; intrathecal chemotherapy; systemic therapy with targeted therapies, etc; clinical trials	N/A
Clinical implications	Poor	Dependent on underlying disorder

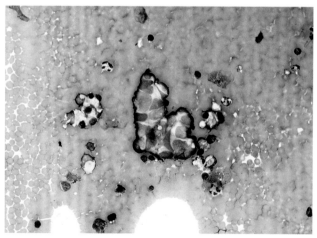

Figure 7.1.1 Metastatic breast carcinoma. The carcinoma cells form a small three-dimensional cluster of cells. The cells are very large and have high N/C ratios, nuclear border irregularities, and irregular nuclear shapes.

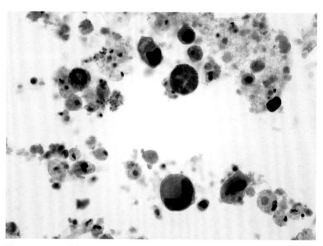

Figure 7.1.2 Metastatic adenocarcinoma. In this case, the cells are overtly malignant and a background of granular debris (likely necrosis) is seen. The cells are pleomorphic, with irregularly shaped, large nuclei and marked hyperchromasia.

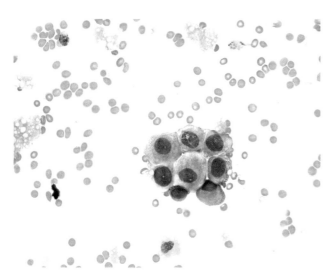

Figure 7.1.3 Metastatic adenocarcinoma. Some of these adenocarcinoma cells have low N/C ratios, but the cells are very large compared with the background red blood cells. The carcinoma cells have slight nuclear border irregularities and vary in size.

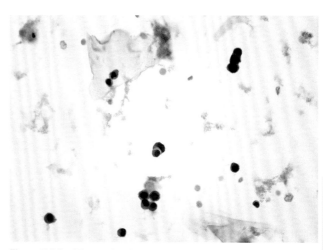

Figure 7.1.4 Metastatic adenocarcinoma. Discohesive cells are present singly and also in loosely cohesive clusters. The nuclei are dark and have marked nuclear border irregularities. The chromatin pattern is coarse.

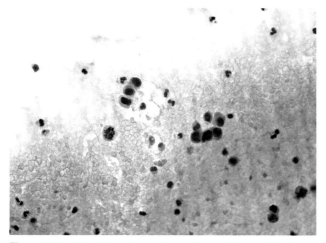

Figure 7.1.5 Metastatic adenocarcinoma. These cells contain dark nuclei with coarse chromatin. The cells have markedly irregular nuclear borders. An atypical mitotic figure can be seen in the center of the field.

Figure 7.1.6 Macrophages. Numerous macrophages are dispersed throughout the field and contain abundant, foamy cytoplasm. This finding is nonspecific.

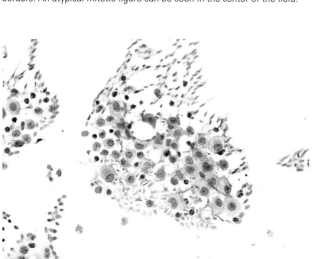

Figure 7.1.7 Macrophages. Macrophages form loose clusters on this preparation. The cells have round-to-elongated nuclei, and some nuclei are curved (indented), a feature that helps identify these cells as macrophages.

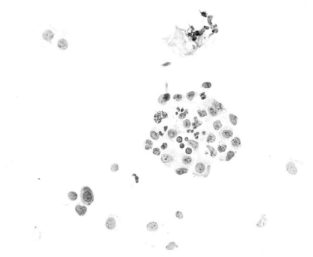

Figure 7.1.8 Macrophages. Several macrophages cluster together in a monolayer to form a false tissue fragment. The cells are intermixed with acute inflammatory cells. The cells have abundant cytoplasm and some have curved nuclei.

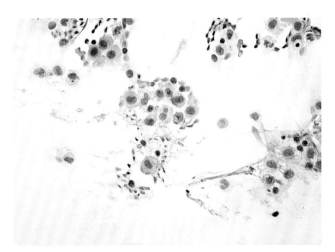

Figure 7.1.9 Macrophages. The field is filled predominantly with loosely cohesive macrophages. Many have a prominent nuclear indentation.

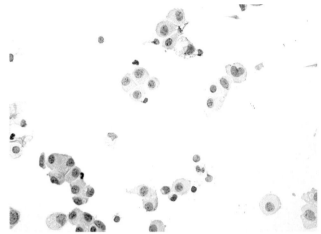

Figure 7.1.10 Macrophages. Macrophages with abundant, foamy cytoplasm. The chromatin pattern is similar among the cells, despite variation in nuclear shapes.

	Lymphoma	Pleocytosis
Age	Any age	Any age
Location	Cerebrospinal fluid	Cerebrospinal fluid
Signs and symptoms	Headache, altered mental status, nausea, vomiting, papilledema, and neurologic deficits	Depends on underlying etiology; may have headaches and neurologic deficits
Etiology	Central nervous involvement by a patient's lymphoma or meningeal dissemination of a primary CNS lymphoma	Many: viral meningitis, Mollaret disease, Lyme disease, autoimmune reponses
Cytomorphology	• Discohesive individual cells *(Figures 7.2.1 and 7.2.2)* • No tissue fragments, but may cluster together into pseudofragments • Morphology varies by lymphoma type, but generally large cells with a thin rim of blue cytoplasm *(Figures 7.2.3 and 7.2.4)*	• Specimen may be highly cellular *(Figures 7.2.5 and 7.2.6)* • A mixture of small lymphocytes, plasma cells, and macrophages *(Figures 7.2.7 and 7.2.8)* • Lymphocytes are polymorphous *(Figure 7.2.7)* • Numerous reactive macrophages, which may appear pleomorphic, especially on Diff-Quik stain *(Figures 7.2.8 and 7.2.9)*
Special studies	Flow cytometry; usually negative for keratin; often insufficient for IHC panel	No clonal population by flow cytometry
Molecular alterations	Dependent on lymphoma type	N/A
Treatment	Systemic chemotherapy, intrathecal chemotherapy, radiation therapy, and/or targeted therapies	Treatment of underlying disease
Clinical implications	Generally poor	Depends on underlying etiology

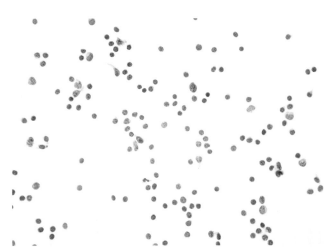

Figure 7.2.1   Plasma cell neoplasm. The cells are discohesive and have variation in cell size. Closer examination will reveal the presence of the coarse, "clockface" chromatin associated with plasma cells. Flow cytometric analysis is the preferred ancillary test to confirm a clonal population.

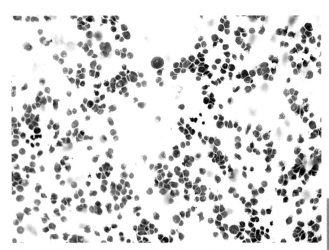

Figure 7.2.2   T-cell lymphoma. The cells are pleomorphic and atypical. The differential includes reactive macrophages, but there is no mixture of cells as is seen in reactive pleocytosis; lymphocytes are missing.

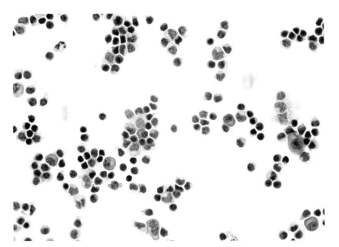

Figure 7.2.3   Plasma cell neoplasm. The specimen contains enlarged cells with perinuclear clearing ("hof"), eccentrically placed nuclei, and clockface chromatin. Some smaller mononuclear cells may represent background lymphocytes or small plasma cells. While an abundance of plasma cells suggests a plasma cell neoplasm, flow cytometry is required to prove clonality.

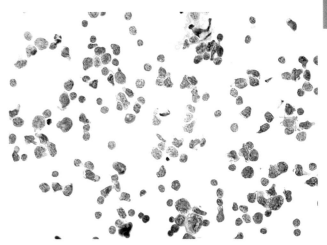

Figure 7.2.4   T-cell lymphoma. The field contains pleomorphic cells with irregularly shaped nuclei. The differential diagnosis includes metastatic adenocarcinoma. The cells are too atypical to represent reactive macrophages or lymphocytes.

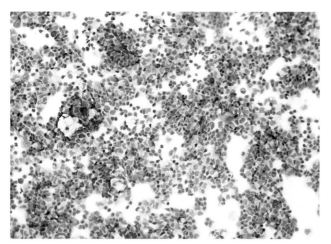

Figure 7.2.5   Pleocytosis. While this very cellular field suggests a malignancy, closer examination will reveal a diverse population of cells. Even at this power, several eosinophils can be identified by their cytoplasmic granules and should suggest the possibility of pleocytosis.

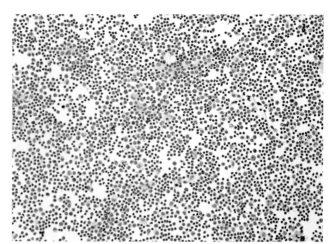

Figure 7.2.6   Pleocytosis. The field is cellular with numerous lymphocytes and larger macrophages. While this mixture of cells suggests a reactive population, flow cytometry analysis can help exclude a subpopulation of clonal cells.

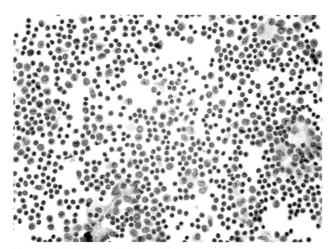

Figure 7.2.7   Pleocytosis. The lymphocytes are pleomorphic, with slight variation in cell and nuclear size. Eosinophils are more difficult to identify on Pap-stained preparations than those stained with Diff-Quik.

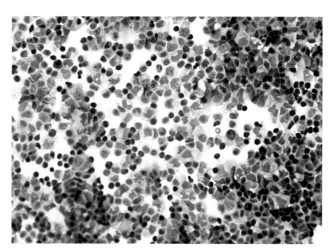

Figure 7.2.8   Pleocytosis. Cells appear larger and more concerning on the Diff-Quik stain. However, small lymphocytes as well as eosinophils can be identified in the background, indicating a mixed population of inflammatory cells.

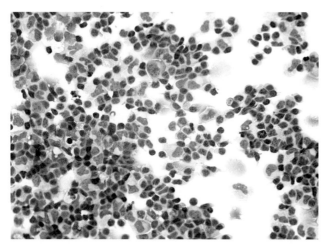

Figure 7.2.9   Pleocytosis. Several macrophages have curved nuclei; these cells have similar quality of chromatin and cytoplasm as the other cells in the field, suggesting that the majority of the large cells are reactive macrophages.

	Hematopoiesis	Leukemia
Age	Any age	Any age
Location	Cerebrospinal fluid	Cerebrospinal fluid
Signs and symptoms	Symptoms of underlying disorder	Headache, altered mental status, nausea, vomiting, papilledema, and neurologic deficits
Etiology	Inadvertently sampled from the spinal column	Central nervous involvement by a patient's leukemia
Cytomorphology	• Myeloid and erythroid precursors, which appear as unusual mononuclear cells on Pap-stained preparations *(Figure 7.3.1)* • A mixture of neutrophils and eosinophils is most readily identifiable *(Figure 7.3.2)* • Megakaryocytes are a specific finding when present *(Figure 7.3.3)* • Other elements from the spinal column (eg, bone) indicating a "missed" tap *(Figure 7.3.4)*	• Cellular specimen containing a single population of atypical large cells *(Figure 7.3.5)* • Cells have scant cytoplasm and irregular nuclear shapes with highly irregular nuclear contours *(Figures 7.3.6-7.3.8)* • Prominent nucleoli may be seen *(Figure 7.3.9)* • Absence of granulocytes and megakaryocytes
Special studies	Flow cytometry (will exclude leukemia) but often can be distinguished on cytomorphology	Flow cytometry
Molecular alterations	None	Depends on type
Treatment	N/A	Systemic chemotherapy, intrathecal chemotherapy, and/or radiation therapy
Clinical implications	N/A	Dependent on underlying disorder

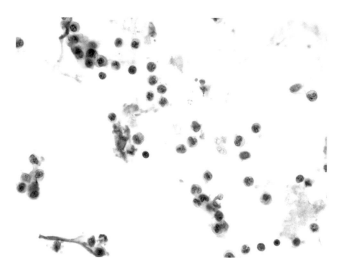

Figure 7.3.1   Hematopoiesis. The field contains a mixture of neutrophils, eosinophils, and mononuclear cells. Several of the mononuclear cells have high N/C ratios with irregular nuclear contours, but the cells are not enlarged; they represent myeloid and lymphoid precursors that are difficult to subclassify on a Pap-stained preparation.

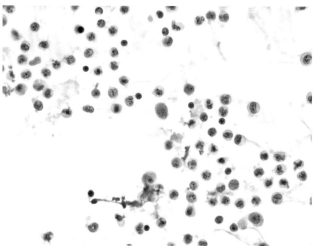

Figure 7.3.2   Hematopoiesis. The field contains a mixture of mononuclear cells, eosinophils, and neutrophils. The identification of both eosinophils and neutrophils in a CSF specimen should raise the possibility of bone marrow elements.

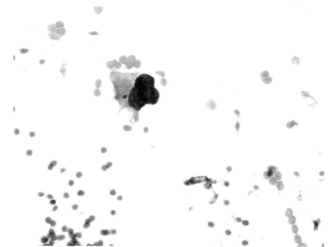

Figure 7.3.3   Hematopoiesis. Megakaryocytes, when present, are a specific finding for hematopoiesis in CSF specimens. Usually the spinal canal has been missed by the needle and the specimen is likely to be nondiagnostic.

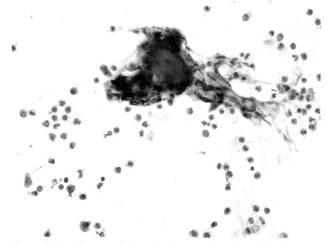

Figure 7.3.4   Hematopoiesis. Other elements from the spinal column, such as fragments of bone, also suggest a fail spinal tap that may have sampled hematopoietic elements.

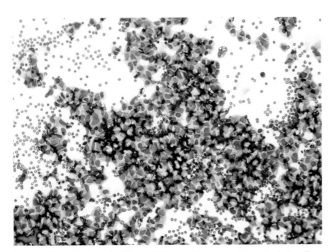

Figure 7.3.5 Leukemia. This cellular specimens contains atypical cells much larger than the background red blood cells. The cells have nuclei with great variation in shape and size. Exact morphology depends in part on the patient's leukemia type.

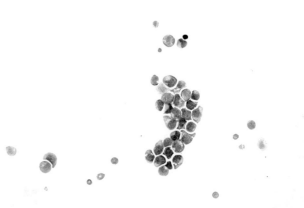

Figure 7.3.6 Leukemia. The field shows numerous leukemia cells which form a loose cluster in this preparation. The cells are large and have nuclei with irregular shapes and irregular contours. While the cells are pleomorphic, they stand out as an atypical population.

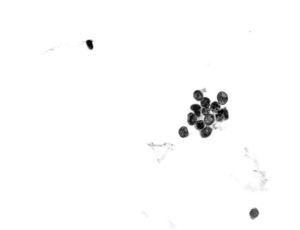

Figure 7.3.7 Leukemia. These cells have highly irregular nuclear borders and coarse chromatin. Flow cytometry is highly specific for identifying leukemia in CSF specimens and can identify markers that have been positive in previous specimens from the patient.

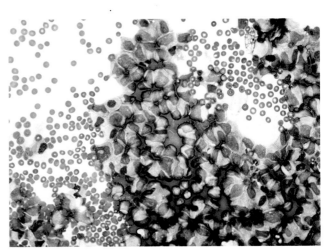

Figure 7.3.8 Leukemia. The cells are large and have large nuclei with irregular shapes and contours.

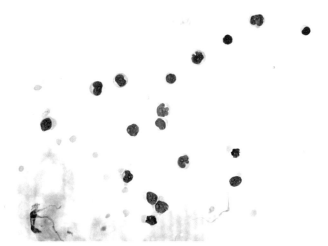

Figure 7.3.9 Leukemia. The cells in this field have prominent nucleoli and highly irregular nuclear contours.

	Metastatic Carcinoma	Lymphoma
Age	Usually older adults	Any age
Location	Cerebrospinal fluid	Cerebrospinal fluid
Signs and symptoms	Meningeal symptoms (headache, seizure, nausea, vomiting) and neurologic deficits	Headache, altered mental status, nausea, vomiting, papilledema, and neurologic deficits
Etiology	Metastatic carcinoma, commonly from a breast or lung primary	Central nervous involvement by a patient's lymphoma or meningeal dissemination of a primary CNS lymphoma
Cytomorphology	• Small three-dimensional clusters and/or individual cells *(Figures 7.4.1* and *7.4.2)* • Morphology depends on primary tumor type • Large cells with large nuclei and high N/C ratios *(Figure 7.4.1)* • Hyperchromasia and irregular nuclear borders *(Figure 7.4.2)* • Coarse chromatin or prominent nucleoli	• Discohesive individual cells *(Figures 7.4.3* and *7.4.4)* • No tissue fragments, but may cluster together into pseudofragments *(Figures 7.4.5* and *7.4.6)* • Morphology varies by lymphoma type, but generally large cells with a thin rim of blue cytoplasm *(Figures 7.4.3-7.4.7)*
Special studies	Negative by flow cytometry; positive for keratin	Flow cytometry; usually negative for keratin; often insufficient for IHC panel
Molecular alterations	Dependent on the primary tumor type	Dependent on lymphoma type
Treatment	Radiation therapy; intrathecal chemotherapy; systemic therapy with targeted therapies, etc; clinical trials	Systemic chemotherapy, intrathecal chemotherapy, radiation therapy, and/or targeted therapies
Clinical implications	Poor	Generally poor

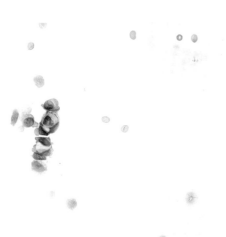

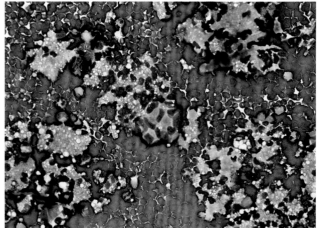

Figure 7.4.1 Metastatic adenocarcinoma. The cells are large compared with the background red blood cells and have irregularly shaped nuclei. The cells have abundant cytoplasm and eccentric nuclei, causing some resemblance to plasma cells, but they lack prominent nucleoli and/or clockface chromatin.

Figure 7.4.2 Metastatic adenocarcinoma. Poorly preserved cells are present singly as well as in small clusters. The cells have irregular nuclei and great variation in N/C ratios. Usually patients with leptomeningeal carcinomatosis have a history of high stage carcinoma, which favors this diagnosis over lymphoma.

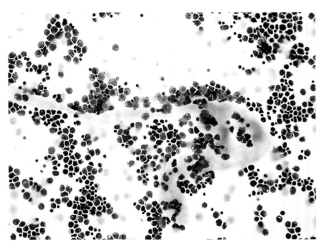

Figure 7.4.3   Plamsa cell neoplasm. A very cellular population of plasma cells is intermixed with smaller lymphocytes. The cells are discohesive, are relatively uniform, and have large amounts of cytoplasm, whereas discohesive adenocarcinoma cells would have less uniformity.

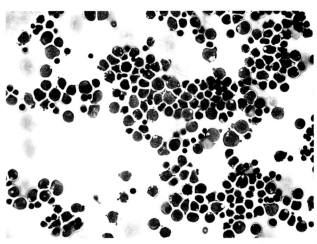

Figure 7.4.4   Plasma cell neoplasm. The cells have eccentrically placed enlarged nuclei and a rim of blue cytoplasm. The clockface chromatin pattern is not seen on this preparation and without a history the differential includes leukemia, lymphoma, carcinoma, and, though unlikely, sarcoma. In this case, the cells are compatible with the patient's history of a plasma cell neoplasm.

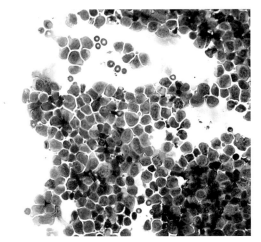

Figure 7.4.5   Plamsa cell neoplasm. Numerous enlarged plasma cells cluster together into a pseudofragment. Flow cytometry would help identify a large population of plasma cells, and also determine whether a clonal population exists.

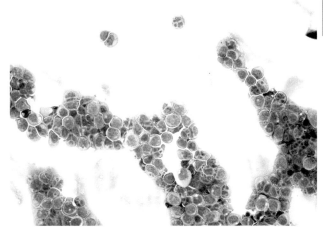

Figure 7.4.6   Plasma cell neoplasm. Poorly preserved enlarged cells are present with irregular nuclear shapes and sizes. The cells are artifactually clustered together to form a pseudofragment. In this case, the patient had a history of a plasma cell neoplasm, otherwise an adenocarcinoma cannot be excluded.

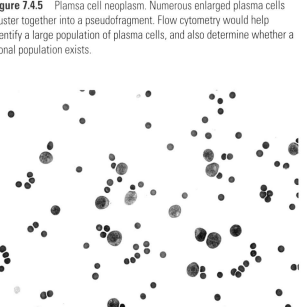

Figure 7.4.7   Plasma cell neoplasm. While some cells maintain classic plasma cell cytomorphology (abundant cytoplasm, eccentric nucleus, perinuclear hof), others have irregularly shaped nuclei and/or minimal cytoplasm.

8

Salivary Gland

	Adenoid Cystic Carcinoma	Pleomorphic Adenoma
Age	Middle-aged adults	Any age; often young adults
Location	Submandibular, sublingual, and minor salivary glands	Usually parotid; rare in sublingual gland
Signs and symptoms	Mass under tongue or in bottom of the mouth or palate; numbness in jaw, palate, mouth, or tongue; dysphagia; facial nerve paralysis	Painless mass that may be long-standing
Etiology	No well-established risk factors	Slow-growing tumor containing epithelial and myoepithelial cells
Cytomorphology	• Basaloid cells in fragments, often with dispersed cells and associated with globular matrix material *(Figure 8.1.1)* • Morphology depends on underlying architecture, such as cribriform or solid growth patterns *(Figures 8.1.2 and 8.1.3)* • Matrix material is best appreciated on Diff-Quik stained preparations and predominantly form spherical globules *(Figures 8.1.4 and 8.1.5)* • The neoplastic cells have round nuclei that may be stripped of cytoplasm, or associated with minimal cytoplasm *(Figure 8.1.4)*	• Small cells with spindled or oval-shaped nuclei associated with fibrillary matrix material *(Figures 8.1.6 and 8.1.7)* • Matrix material appears magenta on Diff-Quik stained preparations *(Figure 8.1.8)* • Monotonous small cells with eccentrically placed nuclei within homogenous-staining cytoplasm (myoepithelial cells) *(Figure 8.1.8)* • The nuclei have bland chromatin and may demonstrate moderate size variation *(Figures 8.1.8 and 8.1.9)* • Cellular pleomorphic adenomas may lack matrix material, causing diagnostic difficulty *(Figure 8.1.10)*
Special studies	May be limited in FNA specimens; positive for MYB nuclear staining; strong and membranous staining for c-kit	Negative for MYB staining; may have weak, membranous c-kit staining
Molecular alterations	t(6;9) translocation leading to *MYB-NFIB* fusion; c-kit mutations	70% have rearrangements involving *PLAG1* or *HMGA2* genes
Treatment	Surgical resection; radiation therapy	Excision
Clinical implications	Slow growing but tends to recur. Solid growth pattern has worst survival, followed by cribriform and then tubular patterns	May recur; may undergo malignant transformation

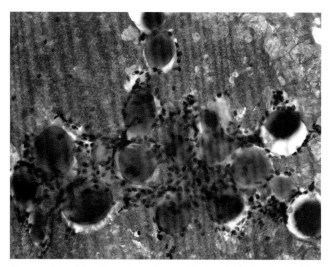

Figure 8.1.1   Adenoid cystic carcinoma. The basaloid cells of adenoid cystic carcinoma are often deceivingly small. They have uniform nuclei and minimal cytoplasm. They are associated with spherical globules of matrix material in this field, a classic morphology of adenoid cystic carcinoma on FNA.

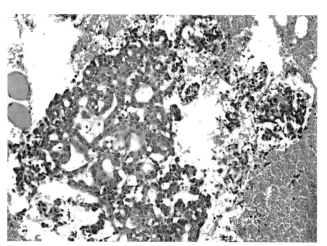

Figure 8.1.2   Adenoid cystic carcinoma. Adenoid cystic carcinoma can have different growth patterns which impact findings on FNA. This cell block section demonstrates a cribriform growth pattern, which often correlates with the presence of globules on fine-needle aspiration, as in the previous image.

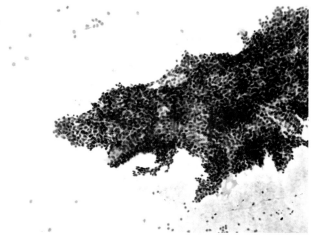

Figure 8.1.3   Adenoid cystic carcinoma. This adenoid cystic carcinoma has a solid growth pattern associated with a small amount of cyanophilic matrix material. The differential diagnosis includes any other basaloid salivary gland neoplasm, such as basal cell adenoma, and cellular (matrix poor) pleomorphic adenoma, which can have a basaloid appearance.

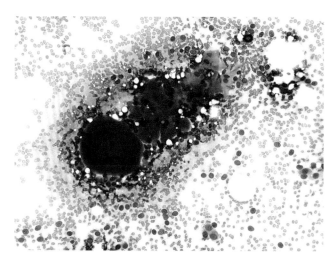

Figure 8.1.4   Adenoid cystic carcinoma. These cells are associated with magenta-colored matrix material. The material is more readily identified on Diff-Quik and related stains. The matrix material of pleomorphic adenoma may look similar in focal areas, a potential pitfall.

8   SALIVARY GLAND

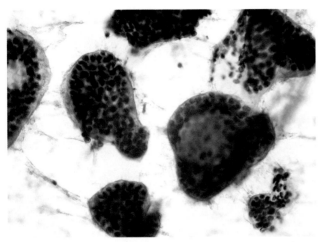

Figure 8.1.5   Adenoid cystic carcinoma. On a Pap-stained preparation, the matrix material is pale-staining and more difficult to identify. The fragments in the field without matrix material simply contain basaloid cells and would raise a broader differential diagnosis if seen on their own.

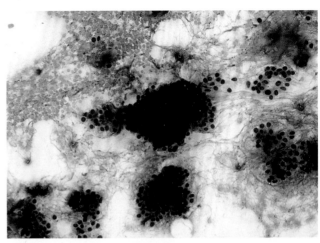

Figure 8.1.6   Pleomorphic adenoma. The cells of pleomorphic adenoma are small but have small variations in nuclear size. The cells alone are not specific to pleomorphic adenoma, while the presence of magenta-colored fibrillary matrix material is essentially diagnostic of pleomorphic adenoma.

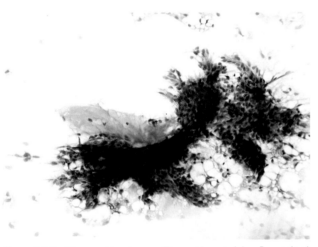

Figure 8.1.7   Pleomorphic adenoma. The matrix material on Pap-stained preparations is less distinctive than on preparations stained with Diff-Quik and related stains. Note the crowded nature of the cells in this field, which confers a basaloid appearance.

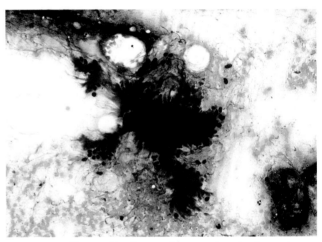

Figure 8.1.8   Pleomorphic adenoma. As opposed to what is seen in adenoid cystic carcinoma in which neoplastic cells surround matrix material, the neoplastic cells of pleomorphic adenoma are embedded in matrix material.

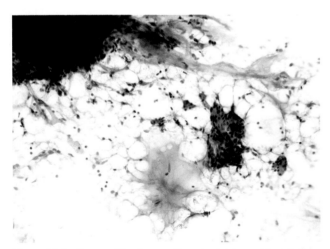

Figure 8.1.9   Pleomorphic adenoma. The pale-staining matrix material of a pleomorphic adenoma is seen in the bottom center of the field, but may be mistaken for nonspecific myxoid material or mucin. However, some stripped nuclei are embedded in the matrix, putting pleomorphic adenoma high on the differential diagnosis.

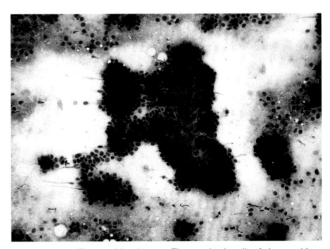

Figure 8.1.10   Pleomorphic adenoma. The neoplastic cells of pleomorphic adenoma often have a plasmacytoid configuration with bland chromatin, homogenous-staining cytoplasm, and oval-to-spindled nuclei. The cells as well as naked nuclei are present as dispersed single cells in the background in addition to being associated in fragments with or without matrix material.

	Mucocele	Mucoepidermoid Carcinoma
Age	Any age	Any age
Location	Often the lower lip. Also inside cheek, floor of mouth, sublingual, neck ("plunging ranula")	Usually parotid. Also found in palate
Signs and symptoms	Mass, sometimes painful but usually asymptomatic	Mass; facial numbness; dysphagia
Etiology	Extravasated mucin with stromal reaction (often secondary to mechanical injury to an excretory duct in children and young adults) or the formation of a retention cyst in older patients	Malignant neoplasm consisting of a mixture of mucous, squamous, intermediate, and clear cells. May be associated with radiation
Cytomorphology	• Paucicellular specimen containing predominantly a myxoid or mucinous background *(Figures 8.2.1-8.2.3)* • Cystic macrophages are present in variable numbers, containing foamy and/or pigmented cytoplasm and hyphen-shaped nuclei *(Figures 8.2.2 and 8.2.3)* • Rare epithelial fragments that may have oncocytic differentiation or squamous metaplasia *(Figures 8.2.3 and 8.2.4)* • The epithelium may contain moderate atypia secondary to reactive changes, including nuclear enlargement and anisonucleosis *(Figures 8.2.3-8.2.5)*	• Neoplasms with variable morphology containing a mixture of epidermoid, intermediate, and goblet cells *(Figures 8.2.6-8.2.9)* • Low-grade neoplasms may contain predominantly mucin and be acellular or paucicellular • Higher-grade neoplasms are often cellular and contain variable epidermoid, intermediate, and goblet cells • Cells may demonstrate oncocytic or clear cell change • Nuclei may be markedly atypical in higher-grade neoplasms *(Figure 8.2.8)*
Special studies	N/A	Positive for p63 and negative for GATA-3 and AR. Special stain for mucin may highlight mucin, if present
Molecular alterations	N/A	Associated with the translocation t(11;19) which results in the *CRTC1-MAML2* fusion oncogene
Treatment	Complete excision; marsupialization; cryosurgery laser ablation, electrocautery; intralesional injection of sclerosing agent or steroids	Complete excision; radiation therapy
Clinical implications	Benign but may recur following treatment	High-grade carcinomas are more likely to recur and have lower survival. Worse prognosis associated with older age, male sex, and submandibular gland location

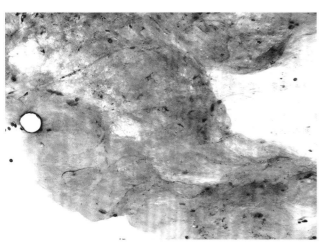

Figure 8.2.1   Mucocele. The field contains abundant mucin-containing rare macrophages and other rare bland mononuclear cells. While this finding would be consistent with a mucocele, a low-grade mucoepidermoid carcinoma cannot be entirely excluded.

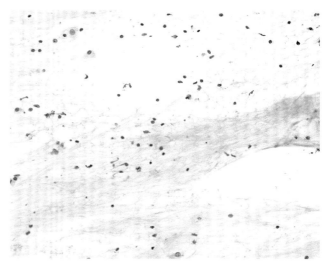

Figure 8.2.2   Mucocele. The field contains abundant mucin-containing macrophages, inflammatory cells, and stripped nuclei. The findings are nonspecific because no definitive lining component is seen.

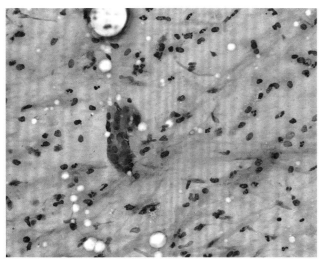

Figure 8.2.3   Mucocele. This aspirate contains mucin, macrophages, and inflammatory cells. A single fragment containing a few oncocytic cells is seen. The cells have ample granular cytoplasm but demonstrate mild anisonucleosis and nuclear contour irregularities, in this case simply reactive changes.

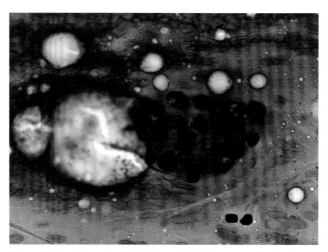

Figure 8.2.4   Mucocele. Markedly atypical cells are seen floating in a background of abundant mucin. Mucocele lesions may occasionally contain atypical epithelial cells, but they are not present in great numbers.

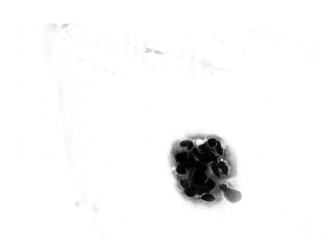

Figure 8.2.5   Mucocele. This aspiration yielded markedly atypical epithelial cells in a background of thin mucin. When presented with a field such as this, it may be difficult to appreciate the mucinous background.

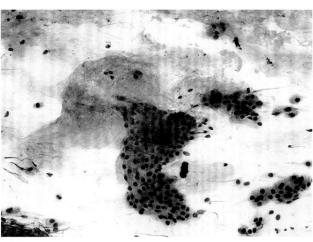

Figure 8.2.6   Low grade mucoepidermoid carcinoma. The field shows several fragments of epidermoid cells in a background of mucin. The fragments also contain rare mucinous cells, as characterized by a purplish blush to their cytoplasm.

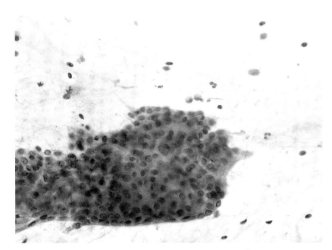

Figure 8.2.7   Low-grade mucoepidermoid carcinoma. Several cells have a faint pink blush in their cytoplasm, indicating they are mucinous cells.

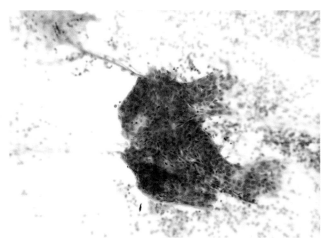

Figure 8.2.8   Mucoepidermoid carcinoma. Intermediate, mucinous, and epidermoid cells are seen within a fragment of low- to intermediate-grade mucoepidermoid carcinoma. The fragment contains areas of red-staining mucin, which would be mucicarmine positive if present on cell block material.

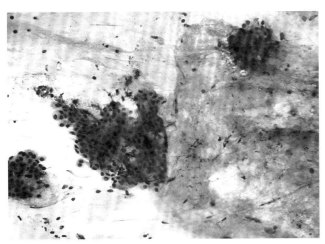

Figure 8.2.9   Low-grade mucoepidermoid carcinoma. The background contains abundant mucin. Epidermoid cells have ample cytoplasm and may be mistaken for an oncocytic cellular proliferation. However, since mucoepidermoid carcinomas may contain cells with oncocytic change, such a misinterpretation should not result in the exclusion of mucoepidermoid carcinoma from the diagnosis.

	Warthin Tumor	Oncocytoma
Age	Usually male adults	Any age; often young adults
Location	Usually parotid gland	Usually parotid; also found in submandibular gland and minor salivary glands
Signs and symptoms	Parotid mass; may be bilateral	Parotid mass
Etiology	Associated with smoking	May be associated with radiation exposure
Cytomorphology	• Oncocytic cells in papillary-shaped fragments *(Figures 8.3.1 and 8.3.2)* • Oncocytic cells have abundant granular cytoplasm, round uniform nuclei, and prominent nucleoli; multinucleation may be seen *(Figures 8.3.3 and 8.3.4)* • Background inflammatory cells with a lymphocyte predominance *(Figures 8.3.1-8.3.5)* • Background granular debris *(Figures 8.3.1 and 8.3.2)* • Background cystic macrophages may be present *(Figure 8.3.5)* • Squamous metaplasia may be present and cause diagnostic difficulties	• Proliferation of oncocytic cells in variably shaped fragments *(Figures 8.3.6-8.3.8)* • Oncocytic cells have abundant granular cytoplasm, round uniform nuclei, and prominent nucleoli *(Figures 8.3.9 and 8.3.10)* • The background does not contain a predominance of lymphocytes or debris *(Figures 8.3.6-8.3.10)*
Special studies	Positive for p63 and negative for p40, S100, mammaglobin, SOX-10, DOG-1, GATA-3, and AR	Positive for p63 and negative for p40, S100, mammaglobin, SOX-10, DOG-1, GATA-3, and AR
Molecular alterations	May not be a neoplastic process	Unknown
Treatment	Surgical resection	Surgical resection
Clinical implications	Recurs rarely; rarely undergoes malignant transformation	Recurs rarely

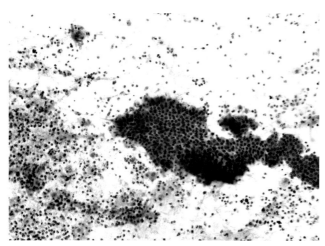

Figure 8.3.1 Warthin tumor. A papillary fragment containing oncocytic cells from the lining of a Warthin tumor. The background contains abundant lymphocytes and granular debris.

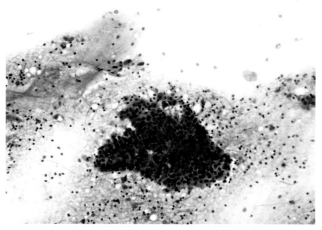

Figure 8.3.2 Warthin tumor. On Pap stain, the cytoplasmic granules may sometimes stain red, which does not indicate keratinization. However, focal keratinization can sometimes occur in Warthin tumor.

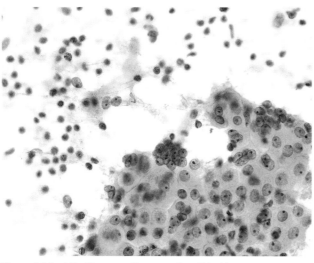

Figure 8.3.3 Warthin tumor. Oncocytes from Warthin tumor appear similar to those seen in oncocytoma and other processes such as oncocytic metaplasia and nodular oncocytic hyperplasia. The cells have abundant, granular cytoplasm with round, regular, and uniform nuclei. Prominent nucleoli are commonly seen.

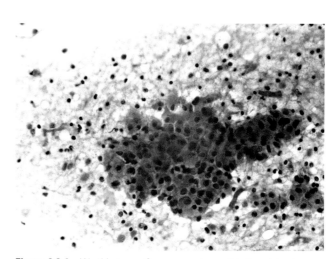

Figure 8.3.4 Warthin tumor. Some oncocytes on this Pap-stained preparation have red granules, which may be mistaken for mucin produced in cells from a mucoepidermoid carcinoma.

8 SALIVARY GLAND

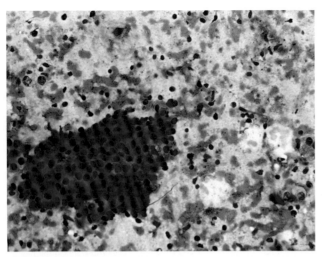

Figure 8.3.5   Warthin tumor. The background of Warthin tumor should contain numerous lymphocytes and granular debris; macrophages may also be seen. It is this background that is most helpful in distinguishing Warthin tumor from other oncocytic lesions.

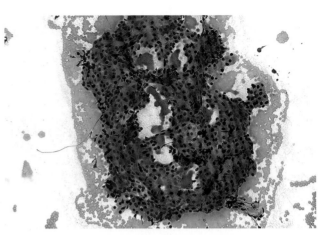

Figure 8.3.6   Oncocytoma. An irregularly shaped fragment with an underlying trabecular architecture is seen. Compared to what is seen in Warthin tumor, the fragment does not have a papillary architecture and the background is clean (lymphocytes and debris are absent).

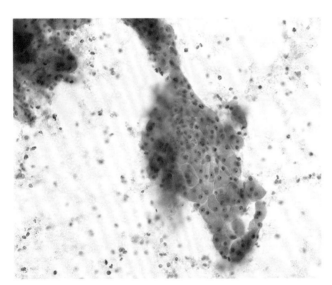

Figure 8.3.7   Oncocytoma. The cells have abundant cytoplasm and small, regular, round, and uniform nuclei with prominent nucleoli. The background contains some nonspecific debris, which may suggest the possibility of a Warthin tumor.

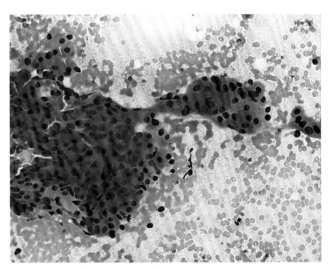

Figure 8.3.8   Oncocytoma. A proliferation of bland-appearing oncocytes in a relatively clean background. Occasional inflammatory cells may be seen on FNA of an oncocytoma, but they should not be seen abundantly.

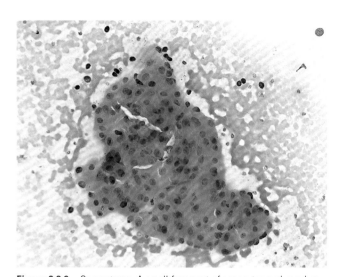

Figure 8.3.9 Oncocytoma. A small fragment of oncocytes and rare lymphocytes in the background. The differential diagnosis includes Warthin tumor, oncocytoma, oncocytic metaplasia, and several other salivary gland neoplasms that can have an oncocytic differentiation.

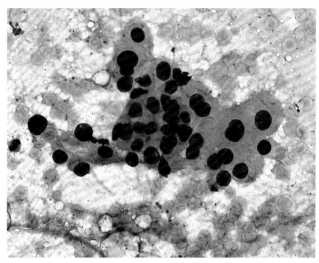

Figure 8.3.10 Oncocytoma. While at high magnification some nuclear size variation may be seen, for the most part the nuclei of oncocytes are round, uniform, and have regular nuclear contours. Nucleoli are usually seen.

8 SALIVARY GLAND

	Benign Acini	Acinic Cell Carcinoma
Age	Any age	Any age
Location	Major and minor salivary glands	Parotid and minor salivary glands
Signs and symptoms	Mass lesion and other symptoms related to the mass lesion	Slow-growing mass lesion that may be painful; facial nerve paralysis; lymphadenopathy if metastases are present
Etiology	Sampled inadvertently during the FNA of a salivary gland mass	May be associated with radiation exposure and/or have a familial predisposition
Cytomorphology	• Paucicellular specimen containing acinar cells in grapelike structures *(Figures 8.4.1 and 8.4.2)* • Acinar cells may be associated with benign ductal elements and adipose tissue *(Figures 8.4.3 and 8.4.4)* • Each grapelike cluster contains approximately 5-10 cells *(Figures 8.4.4 and 8.4.5)* • Acinar cells have small, round, uniform nuclei *(Figures 8.4.4 and 8.4.5)* • Acinar cells have abundant cytoplasm, low N/C ratios, and cytoplasmic vacuoles and/or granules *(Figures 8.4.4 and 8.4.5)*	• Cellular specimen containing numerous neoplastic cells often associated with vessels *(Figure 8.4.6)* • Neoplastic cells are often dispersed individually in the background *(Figure 8.4.6)* • Numerous naked nuclei may be found in the background *(Figures 8.4.6 and 8.4.7)* • Nuclei are often deceivingly round, regular, and uniform *(Figure 8.4.7)* • The neoplastic cells have abundant vacuolated and/or granular cytoplasm *(Figure 8.4.7)*
Special studies	Usually a cytomorphologic diagnosis; stains are not used to differentiate between benign acini and acinic cell carcinoma	Usually a cytomorphologic diagnosis; stains are not used to differentiate between benign acini and acinic cell carcinoma
Molecular alterations	N/A	Under investigation
Treatment	N/A	Excision; radiotherapy
Clinical implications	May indicate the need for re-biopsy if the mass lesion was inadequately sampled	Prognosis depends on stage; recurs if incompletely excised; recurrence and metastatic disease may occur late

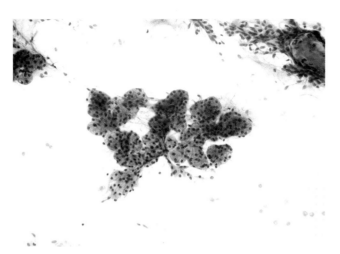

Figure 8.4.1   Benign acini. The cells are similar in appearance and form grapelike clusters.

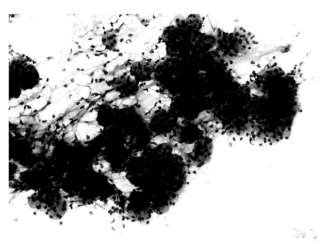

Figure 8.4.2   Benign acini. Numerous grapelike clusters of benign acini are seen, incidentally aspirated during the fine-needle aspiration of a salivary gland mass. The uniform size of each cluster suggests these are simply benign acinar cells.

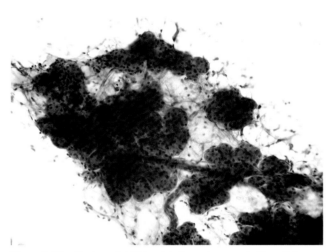

Figure 8.4.3   Benign acini. This acinic tissue is connected to cellular tubular structures, which represent small salivary gland ducts. Both acini and ductular cells are associated with adipocytes.

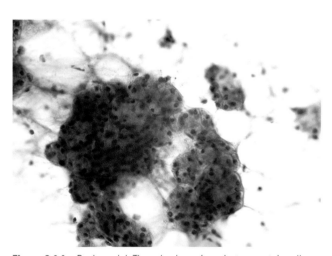

Figure 8.4.4   Benign acini. These benign acinar clusters contain cells with abundant, vacuolated cytoplasm, distinctive cytoplasmic borders, and small, round, regular, and uniform nuclei with small nucleoli. The cells are associated with fat tissue.

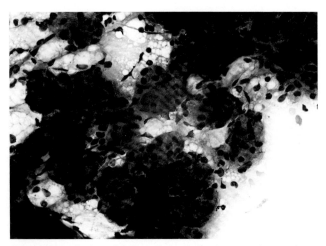

Figure 8.4.5 Benign acini. The cells have abundant, granular cytoplasm and uniform nuclei.

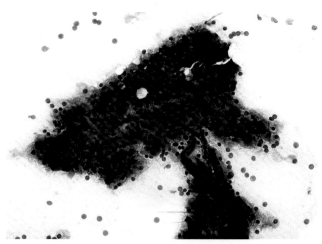

Figure 8.4.6 Acinic cell carcinoma. The cells seen here are associated with irregularly branching vessels. In contrast to benign acini, the cells form solid nests and grapelike structures are not seen. Numerous stripped nuclei can be seen in the background; while these may be mistaken for lymphocytes at low magnification, closer examination reveals they are the same size as the intact tumor cell nuclei and are round, whereas lymphocytes have angulated nuclei.

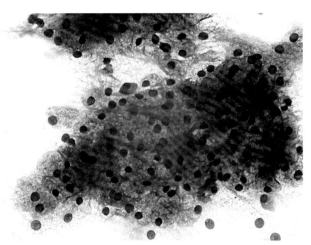

Figure 8.4.7 Acinic cell carcinoma. Acinic cell carcinoma cells often have similar cytomorphology as benign acinar cells, and thus one must rely on other features seen in acinic cell carcinoma, such as hypercellularity, irregular architecture, irregularly branching vessels, and the presence of numerous stripped nuclei in the background.

	Acinic Cell Carcinoma	Oncocytoma
Age	Any age	Any age; often young adults
Location	Parotid and minor salivary glands	Usually parotid; also found in submandibular gland and minor salivary glands
Signs and symptoms	Slow-growing mass lesion that may be painful; facial nerve paralysis; lymphadenopathy if metastases are present	Parotid mass
Etiology	May be associated with radiation exposure and/or have a familial predisposition	May be associated with radiation exposure
Cytomorphology	• Cellular specimen containing numerous neoplastic cells often associated with vessels *(Figures 8.5.1 and 8.5.2)* • Neoplastic cells are often dispersed individually in the background *(Figure 8.5.3)* • Numerous naked nuclei may be found in the background *(Figure 8.5.3)* • Nuclei are often deceivingly round, regular, and uniform *(Figure 8.5.4)* • The neoplastic cells have ample-to-abundant vacuolated and/or granular cytoplasm *(Figure 8.5.4)*	• Proliferation of oncocytic cells in variably shaped fragments *(Figures 8.5.5 and 8.5.6)* • Oncocytic cells have abundant granular cytoplasm, round uniform nuclei, and prominent nucleoli *(Figures 8.5.7 and 8.5.8)* • The background does not contain a predominance of lymphocytes or debris and single neoplastic cells/stripped nuclei are absent *(Figures 8.5.7 and 8.5.8)*
Special studies	Positive for SOX-10 and DOG-1. Negative for p63 and p40	Positive for p63 and negative for p40, SOX-10, and DOG-1
Molecular alterations	Under investigation	Unknown
Treatment	Excision; radiotherapy	Surgical resection
Clinical implications	Prognosis depends on stage; recurs if incompletely excised; recurrence and metastatic disease may occur late	Recurs rarely

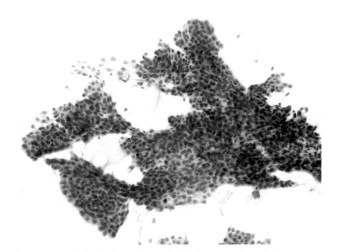

Figure 8.5.1   Acinic cell carcinoma. In this instance, the cells have ample but not abundant cytoplasm and may therefore resemble oncocytic, mucoepidermoid, or basaloid cells seen in other neoplasms. Rare hyphen-shaped nuclei can be seen within the fragment, but otherwise the vessels are obscured by the densely packed tumor cells.

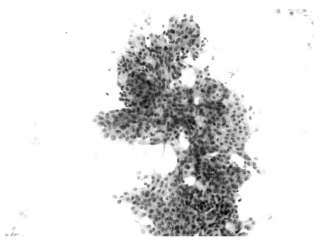

Figure 8.5.2   Acinic cell carcinoma. The cells of acinic cell carcinoma often have prominent nucleoli, a feature seen in oncocytic differentiation. There are several air-dried stripped nuclei in the background which stain faintly; however, they provide one clue that would favor the diagnosis of acinic cell carcinoma.

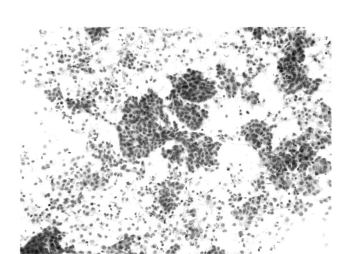

Figure 8.5.3   Acinic cell carcinoma. The field shows several small fragments in a background of numerous carcinoma cells—some dispersed cells are intact, while others are seen as stripped nuclei. At low magnification, these cells may be mistaken for lymphocytes and therefore suggest the incorrect diagnosis of Warthin tumor.

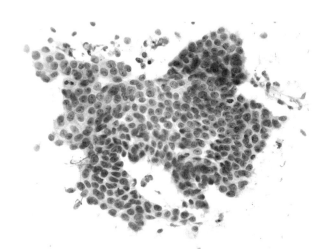

Figure 8.5.4   Acinic cell carcinoma. While many acinic cell carcinomas maintain acinar cell differentiation and have abundant cytoplasm, these carcinoma cells have high N/C ratios. Some cells have strikingly large nucleoli, one feature that should cause consideration for acinic cell carcinoma.

8   SALIVARY GLAND

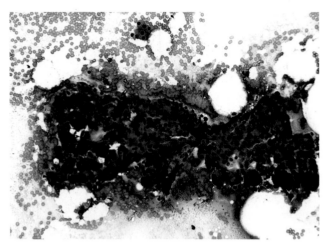

Figure 8.5.5   Oncocytoma. The background is clean, which does not completely eliminate the possibility of a Warthin tumor. However, acinic cell carcinoma usually contains dispersed cells or stripped nuclei in the background. Vessels are also absent, which are often seen associated with tumor cells in acinic cell carcinoma.

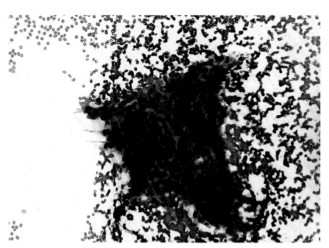

Figure 8.5.6   Oncocytoma. The cells seen here have abundant, granular cytoplasm. The nuclei are more oval-shaped than round and demonstrate some size variation. However, this is within the spectrum of change sometimes seen in oncyctoma and other benign oncocytic lesions.

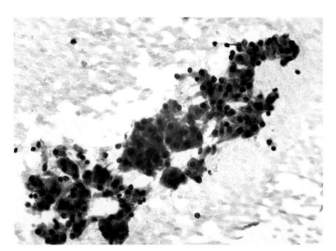

Figure 8.5.7   Oncytoma. The field contains loosely cohesive oncytoma cells with granular cytoplasm, which stains a striking red/pink color on the Pap stain in this preparation. Aspirations containing small numbers of oncocytes may be representative of oncocytic metaplasia.

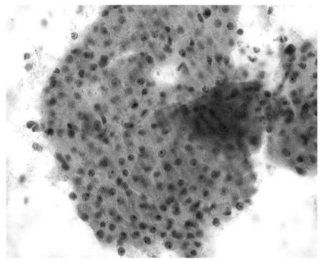

Figure 8.5.8   Oncocytoma. This monolayer sheet contains oncocytes with abundant, granular cytoplasm, distinctive cell borders, small round, uniform nuclei, and prominent nucleoli. While these cells were aspirated from an oncocytoma, a large number of oncocytes can sometimes be aspirated from nodular oncocytic hyperplasia.

9
Kidney

	Oncocytic Neoplasm	Benign Renal Tubular Cells
Age	Usually older adults	Any
Location	Kidney	Kidney
Signs and symptoms	Usually found incidentally on imaging studies	Usually a renal lesion on imaging studies that was the indication for the procedure, as well as any other associated symptoms
Etiology	Depends on neoplasm type; differential includes oncocytoma and renal cell carcinomas such as chromophobe renal cell carcinoma	Benign bystander cells that are incidentally sampled
Cytomorphology	• Cellular specimen *(Figure 9.1.1)* • Discohesive individual cells, which may form small clusters *(Figure 9.1.1)* • Abundant granular cytoplasm and low N/C ratios *(Figures 9.1.2* and *9.1.3)* • Round nuclei with small or indistinct nucleoli and regular nuclear contours *(Figures 9.1.2* and *9.1.3)* • RCC may have enlarged nuclei with irregular borders and nucleolar prominence *(Figure 9.1.4)*	• Paucicellular specimen if lesion of interest is not adequately sampled • Small fragments of cells arranged in a monolayer *(Figures 9.1.5* and *9.1.6)* • Abundant granular cytoplasm with indistinct cytoplasmic borders *(Figures 9.1.7* and *9.1.8)* • Round nuclei with regular nuclear contours *(Figures 9.1.7* and *9.1.8)* • Bland chromatin with absent or small nucleoli; nucleoli should not be prominent *(Figures 9.1.7* and *9.1.8)*
Special studies	Should be distinguished from benign renal tubular cells on cytomorphology; tissue studies usually required to definitively classify neoplasm type	Best identified using cytomorphology, as can express the same markers as renal neoplasms and cells are often too scant for ancillary studies
Molecular alterations	Depends on neoplasm type	N/A
Treatment	Surgical excision via partial nephrectomy or nephrectomy	N/A
Clinical implications	Depends on neoplasm type	N/A

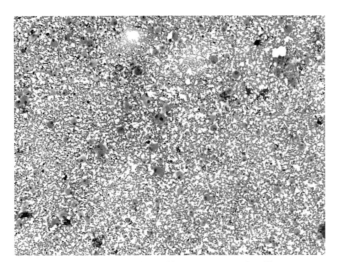

Figure 9.1.1   Oncocytic neoplasm. Numerous oncocytic cells are seen singly dispersed in the background. Renal tubular cells are usually not present singly or present in such great numbers on fine-needle aspiration, indicating that a neoplastic lesion was likely sampled.

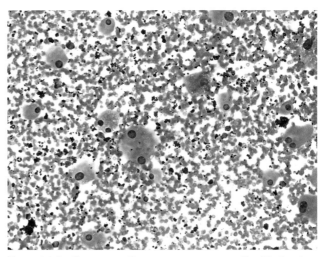

Figure 9.1.2   Oncocytoma. Oncocytoma presents as cells with abundant cytoplasm, low N/C ratios, round nuclei, regular nuclear contours, and small-to-absent nucleoli. However, limited sampling of renal cell carcinomas may appear similarly.

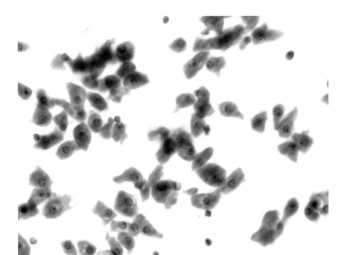

Figure 9.1.3   Oncocytoma. These cells have abundant, granular cytoplasm and uniform, round nuclei with small nucleoli. The cytoplasm has a polygonal shape with distinct borders.

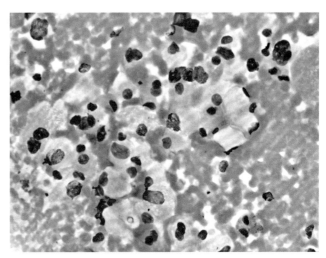

Figure 9.1.4   Chromophobe renal cell carcinoma. Chromophobe renal cell carcinoma as well as other renal cell carcinomas may appear as an oncocytic cell population on fine-needle aspiration. In this case, the nuclei are pleomorphic and enlarged and have irregular nuclear contours, suggesting against an oncocytoma. The features are too atypical for these cells to be renal tubular cells.

9   KIDNEY

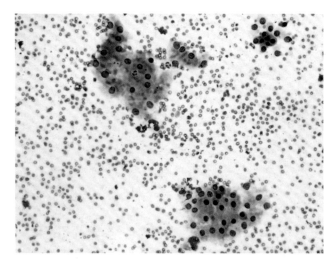

Figure 9.1.5 Benign renal tubular cells. The cells have round nuclei with regular borders and abundant, granular cytoplasm. The cells are generally not present singly and specimens containing only renal tubular cells will be paucicellular, suggesting against the sampling of a neoplasm.

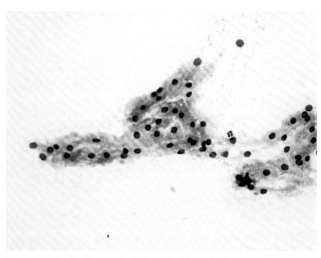

Figure 9.1.6 Benign renal tubular cells. The cells have granular cytoplasm and indistinct cytoplasmic borders. The nuclei are small, round-to-oval, and uniform.

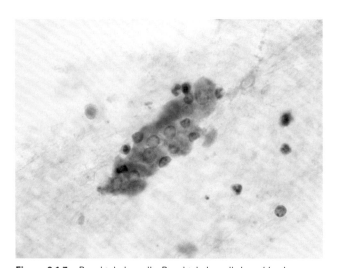

Figure 9.1.7 Renal tubular cells. Renal tubular cells have bland chromatin with small or absent nucleoli (chromocenters). The cytoplasm is abundant and granular.

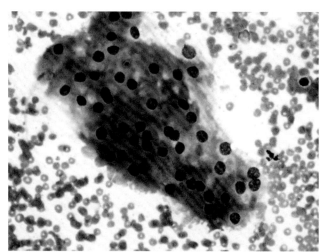

Figure 9.1.8 Renal tubular cells. While the cells resemble the cells in an oncocytoma, oncocytoma cells are usually present individually and in greater numbers.

	Papillary Renal Cell Carcinoma	Glomerulus
Age	Usually older adults	Any
Location	Kidney	Kidney
Signs and symptoms	Mass, flank pain, and hematuria; often found incidentally on imaging studies	Usually a renal lesion on imaging studies that was the indication for the procedure, as well as any other associated symptoms
Etiology	Sporadic but associated with familial papillary renal cell carcinoma syndrome (type 1) and Birt-Hogg-Dube syndrome (type 2)	Benign bystander cells that are incidentally sampled; seen more frequently on touch preparations than fine-needle aspiration specimens
Cytomorphology	• Cellular specimens • Neoplastic cells associated with vessels as well as present singly in the background *(Figure 9.2.1)* • Structures may have a branching, papillary appearance *(Figures 9.2.1 and 9.2.2)* • Pigmented macrophages associated with neoplastic tissue fragments are a specific feature *(Figure 9.2.2)* • Cells may have granular and/or vacuolated cytoplasm, causing overlap with clear cell renal cell carcinoma *(Figures 9.2.3 and 9.2.4)* • Nucleoli range in size from small to prominent	• Usually found in paucicellar specimens in which a lesion went unsampled • Cohesive structures containing folded vessels, which may emulate a papillary architecture *(Figures 9.2.5 and 9.2.6)* • No single cell component in the background • Empty capillary loops at the periphery are a specific feature and may contain red blood cells *(Figures 9.2.5-9.2.8)* • Structures may be associated with renal tubules *(Figures 9.2.6-9.2.8)*
Special studies	Should be distinguished from benign glomerular cells on cytomorphology; tissue studies usually required to definitively classify neoplasm type	Best identified using cytomorphology, as can express the same markers as renal neoplasms and cells are often too scant for ancillary studies
Molecular alterations	*MET* alterations (type 1); chromosomal aberrations (+7, +17, etc) (type 1). Type 2 tumors have a more diverse molecular background	N/A
Treatment	Resection; targeted and systemic therapies	N/A
Clinical implications	Type 1 tumors generally have excellent prognosis; type 2 tumor are more aggressive	N/A

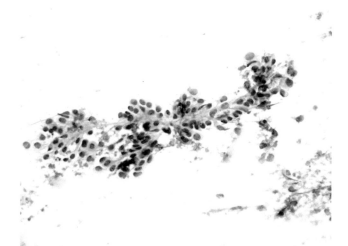

Figure 9.2.1 Low-grade papillary renal cell carcinoma. A papillary stalk is lined by bland neoplastic cells with round-to-oval nuclei, minimal cytoplasm, and indiscernible nucleoli. The more specific features of papillary renal cell carcinoma (such as associated pigment-laden macrophages) are absent.

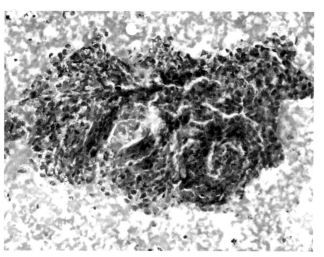

Figure 9.2.2 Papillary renal cell carcinoma. This fragment demonstrates branching papillae containing neoplastic cells with vacuolated cytoplasm. The cells contain green pigment, consistent with a papillary renal cell carcinoma. However, subclassification of renal cell carcinomas on cytomorphology alone is treacherous.

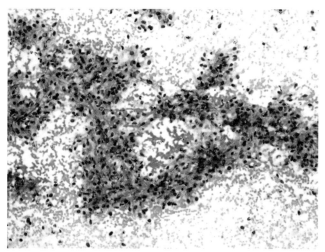

Figure 9.2.3 Clear cell renal cell carcinoma. The vessels surrounding nests of tumor cells have unwound, emulating papillary structures. The neoplastic cells have abundant, vacuolated cytoplasm.

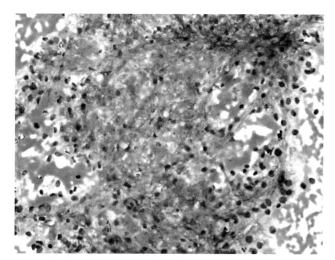

Figure 9.2.4 Clear cell renal cell carcinoma. The neoplastic cells have abundant, vacuolated cytoplasm and can share significant cytomorphologic overlap with other less common entities, such as papillary renal cell carcinoma and clear cell papillary renal cell carcinoma.

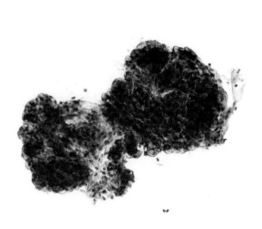

Figure 9.2.5 Glomerulus. This glomerulus contains a mixture of cells (such as mesangial cells and endothelial cells), which appear indistinct from one another at this magnification and may emulate a neoplastic process. Note the empty rings formed at the edges of the glomerulus, a distinctive feature.

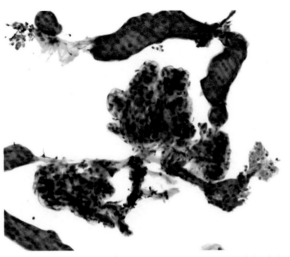

Figure 9.2.6 Glomerulus. A glomerulus is associated with tubular structures in this field and thus should not be mistaken for a neoplasm.

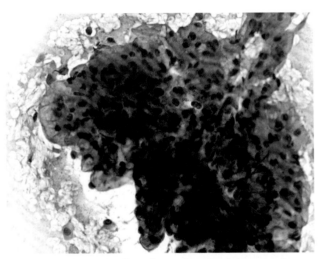

Figure 9.2.7 Glomerulus. The cells seen in a glomerulus are a mixture of types but may appear as a monotonous neoplastic population, causing a diagnostic dilemma.

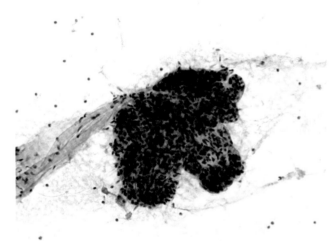

Figure 9.2.8 Glomerulus. This glomerulus forms a three-dimensional structure of crowded nuclei. Typically only a few glomeruli will be seen in any given specimen, a clue that they do not represent a neoplastic process.

	Angiomyolipoma	Papillary Renal Cell Carcinoma
Age	Adults	Usually older adults
Location	Kidney	Kidney
Signs and symptoms	Incidentally discovered; may hemorrhage or invade nearby organs	Mass, flank pain, and hematuria; often found incidentally on imaging studies
Etiology	Benign neoplasm containing a mixture of adipose tissue, smooth muscle, and blood vessels; may be associated with tuberous sclerosis	Sporadic but associated with familial papillary renal cell carcinoma syndrome (type 1) and Birt-Hogg-Dube syndrome (type 2)
Cytomorphology	• Cytomorphology depends on sampling and mixture of components contained by tumor • Tumors with a significant fatty component are usually identified on imaging and do not undergo FNA • Epithelioid and spindled cells in loose clusters and present singly (Figures 9.3.1-9.3.4) • Delicate branching vessels (Figures 9.3.3 and 9.3.4) • Myoid cells with abundant, vacuolated cytoplasm (Figure 9.3.3) • Adipose tissue component may be present • Bland chromatin and inconspicuous nucleoli (Figures 9.3.3 and 9.3.4) • Naked nuclei (Figure 9.3.3) • Occasionally intranuclear inclusions	• Cellular specimens • Neoplastic cells associated with vessels as well as present singly in the background (Figures 9.3.5 and 9.3.6) • Structures may have a branching, papillary appearance (Figure 9.3.5) • Pigmented macrophages associated with neoplastic tissue fragments and/or pigmented neoplastic cells are a specific feature (Figure 9.3.7) • Cells may have granular and/or vacuolated cytoplasm, causing overlap with clear cell renal cell carcinoma (Figures 9.3.8 and 9.3.9) • Nucleoli range in size from small to prominent (Figures 9.3.8 and 9.3.9)
Special studies	Expresses melanocytic and smooth muscle markers (HMB45, MelanA, calponin); negative for pankeratin	Should be distinguished from benign glomerular cells on cytomorphology; tissue studies usually required to definitively classify neoplasm type
Molecular alterations	Under investigation; TSC2 mutations commonly found in sporadic tumors	MET alterations (type 1); chromosomal aberrations (+7, +17, etc) (type 1). Type 2 tumors have a more diverse molecular background
Treatment	Active surveillance; embolization; ablation; resection	Resection; targeted and systemic therapies
Clinical implications	Generally a benign course but may hemorrhage or invade adjacent structures	Type 1 tumors generally have excellent prognosis; type 2 tumor are more aggressive

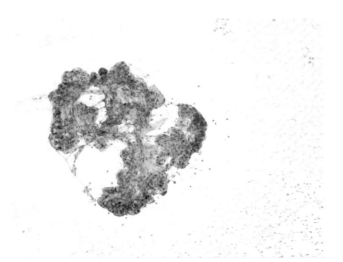

Figure 9.3.1 Angiomyolipoma. This angiomyolipoma is seen as cohesive groups of cells with epithelioid and spindled nuclei. The cellular groups have a papillary appearance and may resemble a renal cell carcinoma.

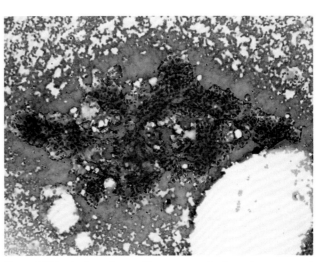

Figure 9.3.2 Angiomyolipoma. These groups of cells are interconnected by small vessels, giving a papillary appearance.

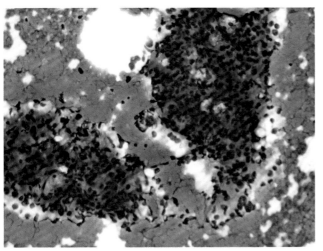

Figure 9.3.3 Angiomyolipoma. At higher magnification, the epithelioid and spindled nuclei can be better appreciated. Nuclei are more densely packed in some areas, whereas in other areas cytoplasm can be better appreciated; cytoplasmic borders are indistinct.

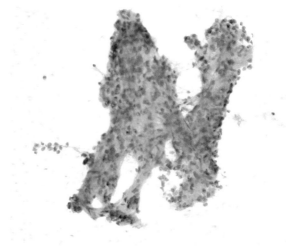

Figure 9.3.4 Angiomyolipoma. Angiomyolipomas sampled by FNA usually have an absent or rare component of adipocytes, otherwise their distinctive radiologic appearance would not require fine-needle aspiration for a diagnosis.

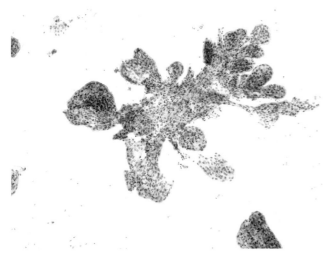

Figure 9.3.5 Papillary renal cell carcinoma. The field shows the classical appearance of branching papillae lined by neoplastic cells. In contrast to angiomyolipoma, the neoplastic cells are more uniform and lack spindled nuclei.

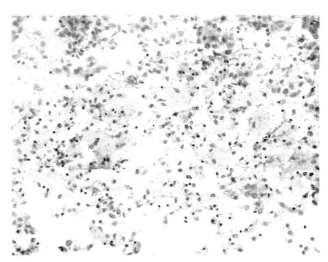

Figure 9.3.6 Papillary renal cell carcinoma. Papillary renal cell carcinoma often contains numerous macrophages, either associated with neoplastic cells or scattered in the background. However, any necrotic renal cell carcinoma may also yield macrophages on fine-needle aspiration.

9 KIDNEY

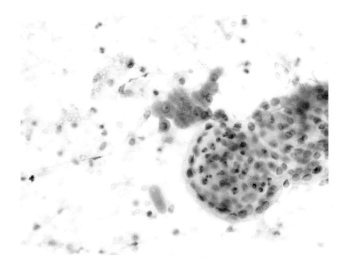

Figure 9.3.7 Papillary renal cell carcinoma. Pigmented macrophages and/or pigmented neoplastic cells are not always seen in papillary renal cell carcinoma fine-needle aspiration, but are a relatively specific feature.

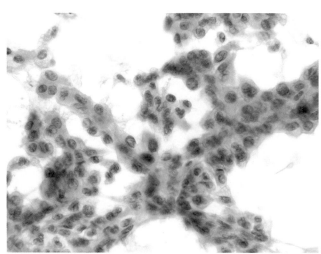

Figure 9.3.8 Papillary renal cell carcinoma. The cells have enlarged epithelioid nuclei with irregular contours and small yet distinct nucleoli. Nucleoli are not seen in angiomyolipoma.

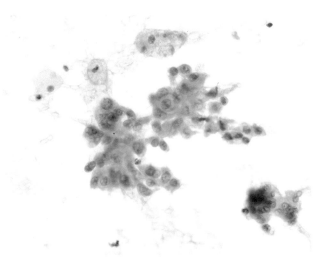

Figure 9.3.9 Papillary renal cell carcinoma. Macrophages are seen adjacent to papillary renal cell carcinoma cells. While the macropahges are not pigment-laden, macrophages are not commonly associated with angiomyolipoma.

	High Grade Urothelial Carcinoma	Clear Cell Renal Cell Carcinoma
Age	Usually older adults (>50 y of age)	Usually older adults
Location	Kidney	Kidney
Signs and symptoms	Asymptomatic or hematuria	Mass, flank pain, and hematuria; usually found incidentally on imaging studies
Etiology	Strong association with tobacco smoking; industrial chemical exposures	Thought to be derived from proximal convoluted tubule cells; associated with smoking, obesity, and hypertension. Associated with von Hippel-Lindau disease
Cytomorphology	• Cellular specimen consisting of single cells as well as tissue fragments • Large cells with hyperchromatic nuclei, coarse chromatin, and irregular nuclear borders (Figure 9.4.1) • Classically associated with cercariform cell morphology: individual cells with eccentrically placed nuclei and tapered cytoplasmic tails (Figures 9.4.1 and 9.4.2) • Nucleolar prominence is not a common feature and more commonly associated with renal cell carcinoma • Squamous differentiation with keratinization may be seen (Figures 9.4.3 and 9.4.4)	• Cellular specimens • Neoplastic cells associated with vessels as well as present singly in the background (Figures 9.4.5 and 9.4.6) • Cells may have granular and/or vacuolated cytoplasm, which may also be seen in some papillary renal cell carcinomas (Figures 9.4.7 and 9.4.8) • Low-grade neoplasms oval-to-round nuclei with mild size variation and moderate contour irregularities (Figures 9.4.7 and 9.4.8) • Nucleoli range in size from small to prominent
Special studies	Positive for GATA-3; may be Pax-8 positive	Typically negative for GATA-3 and positive for Pax-8; diffuse CAIX expression; also positive for CD10 and RCC
Molecular alterations	Aneuploidy; frequently TERT promoter mutations; TP53 mutations	VHL inactivation and/or upregulation of hypoxia inducible factor (HIF)
Treatment	Depending on tumor type and extent of disease (both determined on biopsy), transurethral resection; intravesical BCG; intravesical chemotherapy; cystectomy; and/or chemoradiation	Resection; IL-2 immunotherapy; targeted therapies
Clinical implications	Depends on extent of disease	Depends on stage

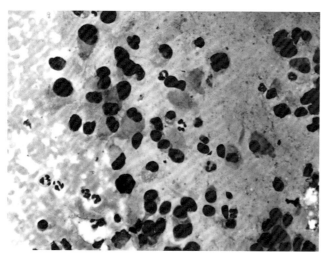

Figure 9.4.1   High-grade urothelial carcinoma. The field contains numerous dispersed cells with eccentrically placed nuclei and tapered cytoplasm ("comet tails"). This cercariform configuration is strongly associated with high-grade urothelial carcinoma when seen on fine-needle aspiration.

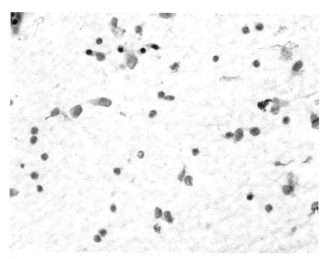

Figure 9.4.2   High-grade urothelial carcinmoma. The cells have enlarged nuclei, irregular nuclear borders, and variation in nuclear sizes. Some cells are cercariform, while others have minimal cytoplasm.

Figure 9.4.3   Keratinizing high-grade urothelial carcinoma. The background contains necrotic and keratinaceous debris. Urothelial carcinoma is the most common cause of squamous differentiation seen on kidney fine-needle aspiration, although rarely metastatic squamous cell carcinomas are found in the kidney.

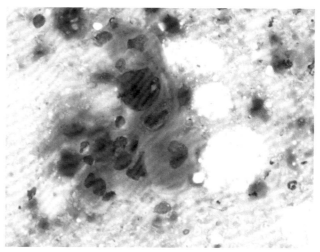

Figure 9.4.4   Keratinizing high-grade urothelial carcinoma. The cells have dense, waxy, blue cytoplasm and highly irregular nuclei. The background contains necrotic debris and a conventional high-grade urothelial component cannot be identified in this field.

9 KIDNEY

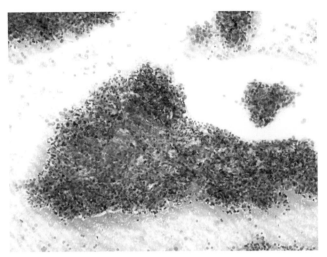

Figure 9.4.5   Clear cell renal cell carcinoma. The field contains nests of cell with vacuolated cytoplasm associated with a network of vasculature. Compared to HGUC, the cells have more uniform nuclei.

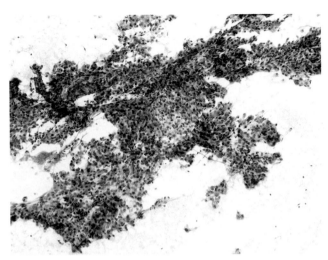

Figure 9.4.6   Clear cell renal cell carcinoma cells. The association with vascular structures may cause a papillary renal cell carcinoma to enter the differential diagnosis.

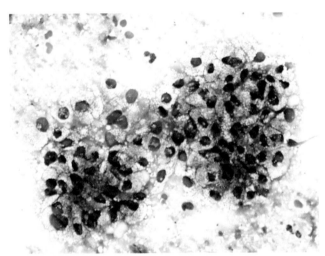

Figure 9.4.7   Clear cell renal cell carcinoma. These cells demonstrate the classic cytomorphologic feature of clear cell renal cell carcinoma—abundant vacuolated cytoplasm, distinct cell borders, round nuclei with slightly irregular contours, and mild anisonucleosis. Nucleoli are more difficult to appreciate on Diff-Quik preparations and vary in size depending on neoplasm grade.

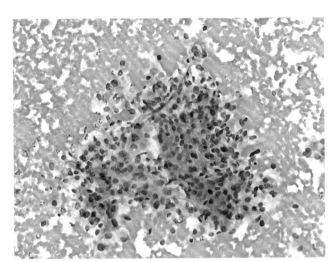

Figure 9.4.8   Clear cell renal cell carcinoma. The cells have abundant, granular cytoplasm and round-to-oval nuclei. The nuclei demonstrate some size variation but are not as pleomorphic as is seen in high-grade urothelial carcinoma.

	Adrenal Tissue	**Clear Cell Renal Cell Carcinoma**
Age	Any	Usually older adults
Location	Kidney	Kidney
Signs and symptoms	Usually asymptomatic; nodular hyperplasia or adrenal neoplasms may be associated with syndromes depending on the hormone elaborated	Mass, flank pain, and hematuria; usually found incidentally on imaging studies
Etiology	Inadvertently sampled during the FNA of a kidney lesion, or intentional sampling of hyperplastic/neoplastic adrenal tissue forming a mass adjacent to the kidney	Thought to be derived from proximal convoluted tubule cells; associated with smoking, obesity, and hypertension. Associated with von Hippel-Lindau disease
Cytomorphology	• Specimen of variable cellularity containing small tissue fragments and/or dispersed cells *(Figure 9.5.1)* • Normal hyperplastic, benign, and malignant processes cannot be reliably distinguished on cytomorphology alone • Typically cells with monotonous, round nuclei with regular contours and variable amounts of granular and/or vacuolated cytoplasm *(Figures 9.5.2 and 9.5.3)* • Anisonucleosis and focal areas of marked nuclear atypia may be seen *(Figure 9.5.4)* • Stripped nuclei in the background *(Figure 9.5.4)* • Distinctive nucleoli may be seen *(Figure 9.5.4)*	• Cellular specimens • Neoplastic cells associated with vessels as well as present singly in the background *(Figure 9.5.5)* • Cells may have granular and/or vacuolated cytoplasm, which may also be seen in some papillary renal cell carcinomas *(Figures 9.5.6-9.5.8)* • Low-grade neoplasms oval-to-round nuclei with mild size variation and moderate contour irregularities *(Figures 9.5.6-9.5.8)* • Nucleoli range in size from small to prominent
Special studies	Positive for MelanA, inhibin, synaptophysin, calretinin, and GATA-3. Negative for PAX-8, CD10, CAIX, and RCC	Positive for PAX-8, CD10, RCC, and CAIX. Negative for MelanA, inhibin, synaptophysin, calretinin, and GATA-3
Molecular alterations	None in benign tissue; tumorigenesis of adrenal neoplasms is under investigation	*VHL* inactivation and/or upregulation of hypoxia inducible factor (HIF)
Treatment	Depends on disease process; resampling of lesion if inadvertently sampled.	Resection; IL-2 immunotherapy; targeted therapies
Clinical implications	Prognosis is usually excellent in most situations, as adrenal malignancies are rare.	Prognosis depends on stage

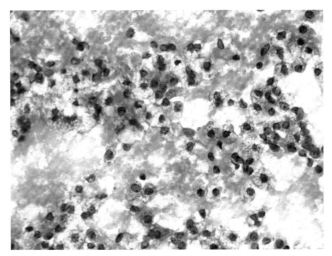

Figure 9.5.1 Adrenal tissue. Loosely cohesive adrenocortical cells with abundant, vacuolated cytoplasm. Their nuclei are round and uniform, with minimal nuclear contour irregularities. Small nucleoli are present.

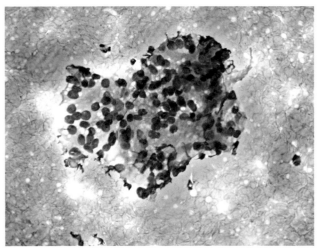

Figure 9.5.2 Adrenal tissue. A small fragment of adrenocortical cells with granular cytoplasm. The cells form an acinar arrangement with the fragment. The nuclei are round and regular.

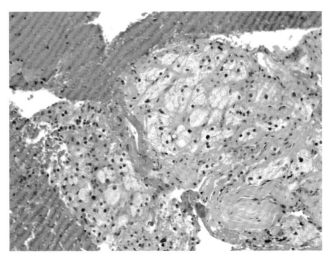

Figure 9.5.3 Adrenal tissue. On a cell block preparation, the adrenal origin of these cells is more easily recognizable.

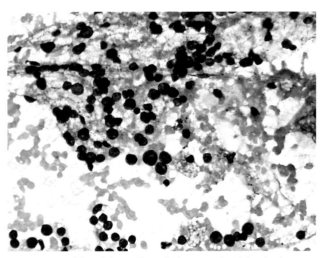

Figure 9.5.4 Adrenal tissue. The cells have round nuclei and anisonucleosis. Stripped nuclei can be seen in the background.

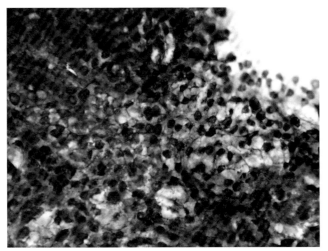

Figure 9.5.5 Clear cell renal cell carcinoma. The associated vessels are difficult to identify in this field, but they are associated with the thickened magenta matrix material seen between some cells.

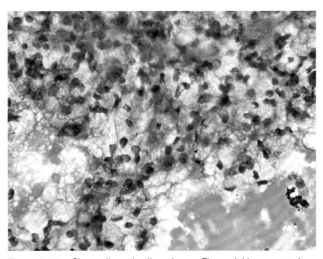

Figure 9.5.6 Clear cell renal cell carcinoma. The nuclei have great size variation and contour irregularities than seen in most adrenocortical cells.

9 KIDNEY

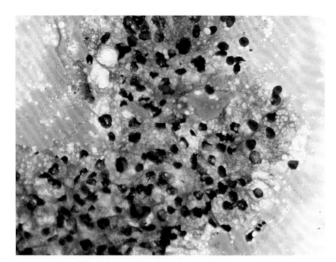

Figure 9.5.7   Clear cell renal cell carcinoma. The cells have marked variation in nuclear sizes and irregularities in nuclear contours. Nucleoli are difficult to assess in this field.

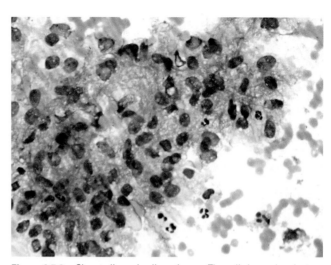

Figure 9.5.8   Clear cell renal cell carcinoma. The cells have abundant, vacuolated cytoplasm. While this feature can be seen in adrenocortical cells, the diffuse nuclear atypia seen here would be unusual for adreno-cortical tissue.

10

Soft Tissue

	Schwannoma	Gastrointestinal Stromal Tumor (GIST)
Age	Any age but most commonly young and middle-aged adults	Older adults
Location	Throughout body; rarely occurs in the stomach	Usually the stomach (60%) or small intestine (35%)
Signs and symptoms	Rare clinical data; often found incidentally	Asymptomatic, abdominal pain, gastrointestinal obstruction
Etiology	Arises from Schwann cells	Arises from the interstitial cell of Cajal often due to an activating *c-kit* mutation
Cytomorphology	• Large cohesive clusters *(Figure 10.1.1)* • Rare to absent single cell population *(Figure 10.1.1)* • Metachromatic fibrillary stroma *(Figure 10.1.2)* • Mostly bland spindle cells with tapered nuclei *(Figures 10.1.3* and *10.1.4)* • Some tumors demonstrate prominent anisonucleosis *(Figure 10.1.5)*	• Tumor cells are in tissue fragments and may be singly dispersed *(Figures 10.1.6-10.1.8)* • Fibrillary stroma may be present • Bland spindle and/or epithelioid cells *(Figure 10.1.9)* • Parallel "side by side" nuclear arrangements • Wavy nuclei with blunt or tapered ends *(Figure 10.1.10)* • Thin wispy bipolar cytoplasm *(Figures 10.1.8* and *10.1.10)*
Special studies	Positive for S-100 protein by IHC and negative for CD34, DOG1, and c-kit	Positive for CD34, c-kit, and DOG1 by IHC; c-kit/PDGFRA mutational panel
Molecular alterations	Inactivation of tumor suppressor gene merlin; may be associated with neurofibromatosis type 2	85% have mutations in c-kit or PDGFRA
Treatment	Surgical excision	Complete surgical resection; targeted therapy in neoplasms with c-kit or PDGFRA mutations
Clinical implications	Rarely recurs	Based on location, size, and mitotic rate

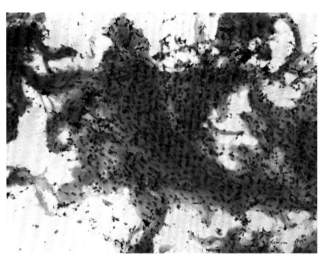

Figure 10.1.1 Schwannoma. Schwannoma cells are usually seen in large tissue fragments with only rare or absent single cells dispersed in the background.

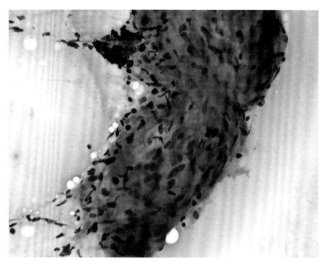

Figure 10.1.2 Schwannoma. Schwannoma can be associated with metachromatic stroma, which is more readily identifiable on smears stained with Diff-Quik.

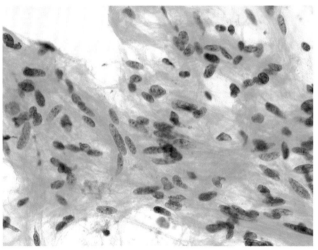

Figure 10.1.3 Schwannoma. Schwannomas usually contains predominantly bland spindle cells with elongated nuclei.

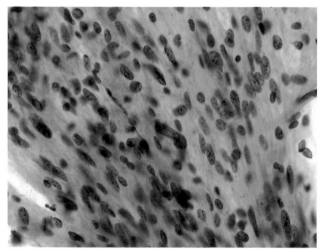

Figure 10.1.4 Schwannoma. The nuclei of schwannoma are often elongated, some with tapered ends. The cytoplasm has a fibrillary appearance and the cellular borders are indistinct, giving a syncytial appearance.

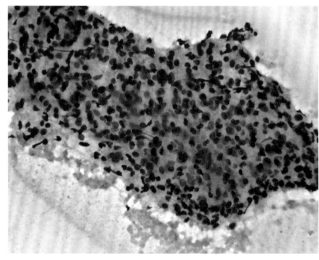

Figure 10.1.5 Schwannoma. Schwannoma may have nuclei that are more epithelioid and with moderate levels of anisonucleosis. Some nuclei in the field are still spindle-shaped with tapered ends.

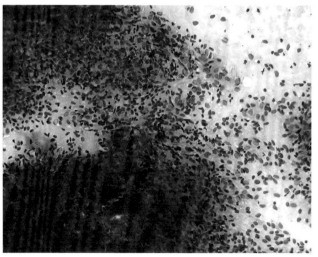

Figure 10.1.6 GIST. GIST typically presents with cells present in tissue fragments as well as single dispersed in the background.

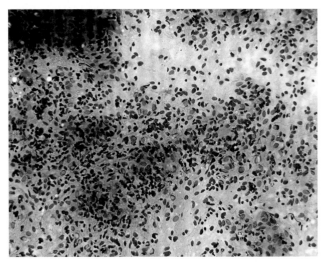

Figure 10.1.7 GIST. While fibrillary metachromatic stroma can occasionally be seen in GIST, most cases demonstrate high cellularity with minimal or absent stroma.

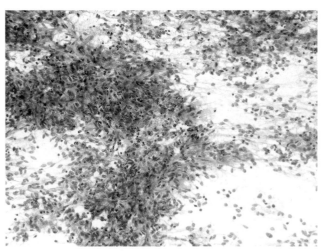

Figure 10.1.8 GIST. The cytoplasm of GIST is wispy and delicate and in this field forms a web between cells, which could be mistaken for stroma.

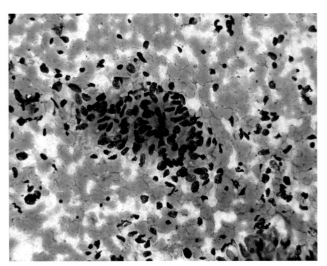

Figure 10.1.9 GIST. GIST may contain predominantly epithelioid or predominantly spindled nuclei. In this case, a mixture of the two can be seen, which is not an uncommon finding.

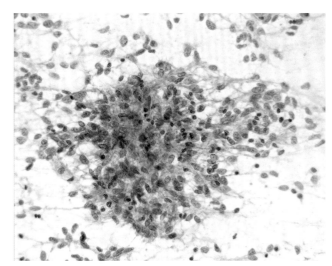

Figure 10.1.10 GIST. GIST often has indistinct and delicate cytoplasm, which forms bipolar processes.

	Leiomyosarcoma	Gastrointestinal Stromal Tumor (GIST)
Age	Middle-aged men	Older adults
Location	Throughout body; in the stomach, represents 1%-3% of malignancies and arises in the body or fundus	Usually the stomach (60%) or small intestine (35%)
Signs and symptoms	Peptic ulcer–like disease; gastric outlet syndrome; gastric perforation	Asymptomatic, abdominal pain, gastrointestinal obstruction
Etiology	In the stomach, arises from the muscularis propria	Arises from the interstitial cell of Cajal often due to an activating *c-kit* mutation
Cytomorphology	• Tissue fragments with variable background of single cells and stripped nuclei *(Figures 10.2.1 and 10.2.2)* • Stroma is often absent *(Figure 10.2.1)* • Spindle cells with blunt-ended or fusiform nuclei, or epithelioid cells with round or indented nuclei *(Figures 10.2.3 and 10.2.4)* • Anisonucleosis and marked nuclear border irregularities *(Figure 10.2.4)* • Some tumors demonstrate prominent pleomorphism with multinucleated cells *(Figure 10.2.5)*	• Tumor cells are in tissue fragments and may be singly dispersed *(Figures 10.2.6 and 10.2.7)* • Fibrillary stroma may be present • Bland spindle and/or epithelioid cells *(Figures 10.2.8 and 10.2.9)* • Parallel "side by side" nuclear arrangements *(Figure 10.2.10)* • Wavy nuclei with blunt or tapered ends *(Figures 10.2.9 and 10.2.10)* • Thin wispy bipolar cytoplasm
Special studies	Positive for SMA and focally positive for desmin by IHC. Negative for CD34, DOG1, and c-kit	Positive for CD34, c-kit, and DOG1 by IHC; c-kit/PDGFRA mutational panel
Molecular alterations	Typically complex karyotypic alterations	85% have mutations in c-kit or PDGFRA
Treatment	Resection with or without radiation/chemotherapy	Complete surgical resection; targeted therapy in neoplasms with c-kit or PDGFRA mutations
Clinical implications	50% 5-y survival rate; size of >5 cm confers a poor prognosis	Based on location, size, and mitotic rate

Figure 10.2.1   Leiomyosarcoma. A fascicular fragment of tumor cells with indistinct cytoplasmic borders and fusiform nuclei.

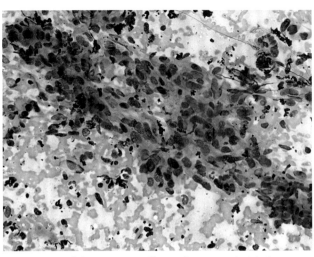

Figure 10.2.2   Leiomyosarcoma. These cells are seen both in fragments as well as individually dispersed in the background.

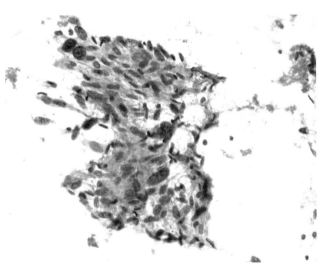

Figure 10.2.3   Leiomyosarcoma. This fragment contains cells with predominantly spindle-shaped nuclei. Some have blunt ends while others appear more fusiform.

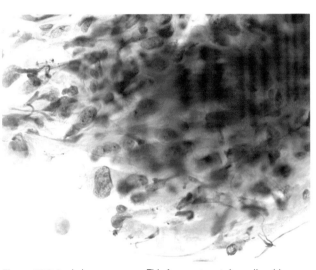

Figure 10.2.4   Leiomyosarcoma. This fragment contains cells with nuclei that are more round in appearance, although they mostly maintain an oval elongated shape. Some nuclei have indentations.

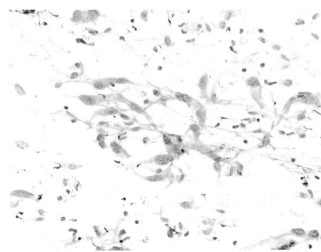

Figure 10.2.5   Leiomyosarcoma. The field shows dispersed pleomorphic cells demonstrating multinucleated, anisonucleosis, and marked nuclear border irregularities.

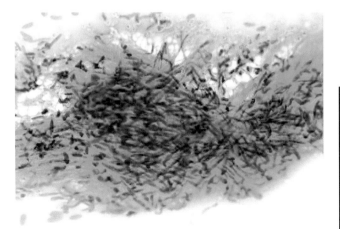

Figure 10.2.6   GIST. A large tissue fragment of spindle cells with dispersed individual cells in the background.

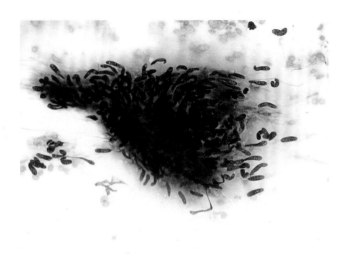

Figure 10.2.7   GIST. A tissue fragment of spindle cells with dispersed individual cells in the background.

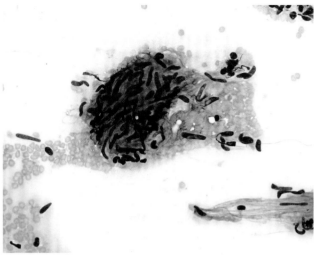

Figure 10.2.8   GIST. The tumor cells are bland, predominantly containing spindle-shaped nuclei with blunt ends.

Figure 10.2.9   GIST. The tumor cells are bland and the nuclei appear arranged in a parallel to one another in some areas.

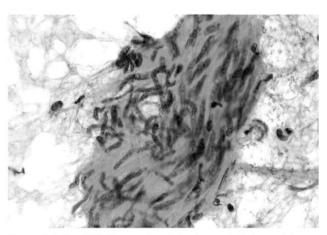

Figure 10.2.10   GIST. The cytoplasmic borders are indistinct and the cytoplasm is delicate in appearance. Note how the nuclei stream together and appear to run parallel to one another in some areas.

	Fibromatosis (Desmoid Type)	Schwannoma
Age	Young adults	Most commonly young and middle-aged adults
Location	Head and neck; abdomen; pelvis; retroperitoneal; near proximal muscles	Extremities, head and neck, mediastinum, and retroperitoneum
Signs and symptoms	Depends on location; in head and neck, can compromise critical structures	Generally asymptomatic
Etiology	Can be associated with trauma, FAP syndrome, and familial desmoid syndrome	Arises from Schwann cells
Cytomorphology	• Tumor cells embedded in matrix material forming fascicles and/or present singly in the background *(Figures 10.3.1-10.3.3)* • Associated with metachromatic matrix material *(Figure 10.3.4)* • Bland spindle cells with long, fusiform nuclei *(Figure 10.3.5)*	• Large cohesive clusters *(Figure 10.3.6)* • Rare to absent single cell population • Metachromatic fibrillary stroma • Mostly bland spindle cells with tapered nuclei *(Figures 10.3.7-10.3.8)* • Some tumors demonstrate prominent anisonucleosis
Special studies	May demonstrate variable positivity for SMA and c-kit; negative for CD34, S-100 protein, DOG-1, and keratin	Positive for S-100 protein by IHC and negative for CD34, DOG1, and c-kit
Molecular alterations	Alterations in APC-Beta catenin pathway	Inactivation of tumor suppressor gene merlin; may be associated with neurofibromatosis type 2
Treatment	Excision with wide margins; observation if asymptomatic	Surgical excision
Clinical implications	May recur; locally aggressive	Rarely recurs

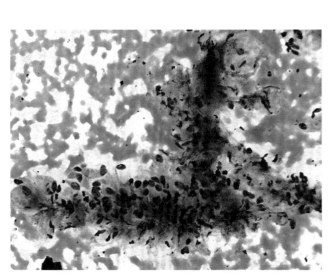

Figure 10.3.1 Fibromatosis. The cells are associated with metachromatic matrix material and form a fascicular tissue fragment.

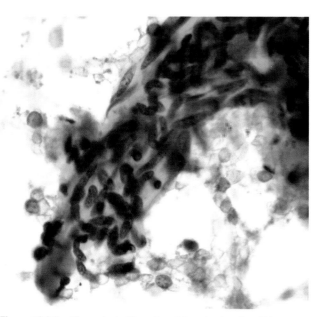

Figure 10.3.2 Fibromatosis. The cells exist predominantly within a tissue fragment and contain long, fusiform nuclei.

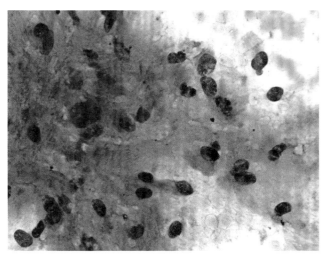

Figure 10.3.3 Fibromatosis. Some cells are embedded in metachromatic matrix while one (upper right) is disassociated in the background.

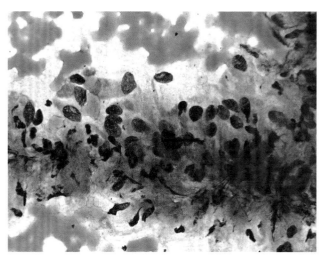

Figure 10.3.4 Fibromatosis. The cells have fusiform nuclei, which is eccentrically placed within delicate, elongated cytoplasm.

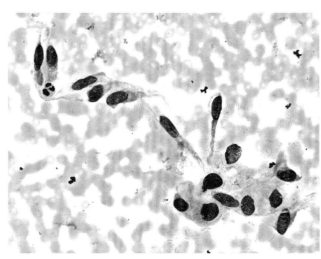

Figure 10.3.5 Fibromatosis. Some of the cell cytoplasm forms bipolar processes. The nuclei are predominantly fusiform, with some nuclei appearing round or oval.

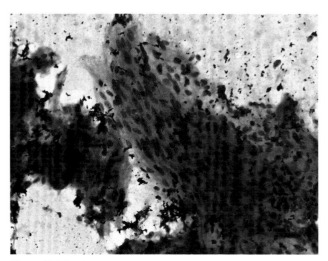

Figure 10.3.6 Schwannoma. A large cohesive tissue fragment containing schwannoma cells. Only rare cells are present singly in the background.

10 SOFT TISSUE

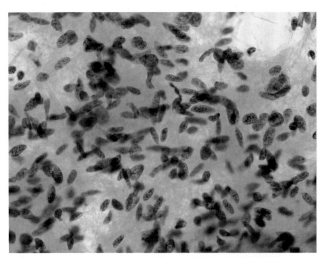

Figure 10.3.7   Schwannoma. The cells are bland, containing spindle-shaped nuclei, many with tapered ends.

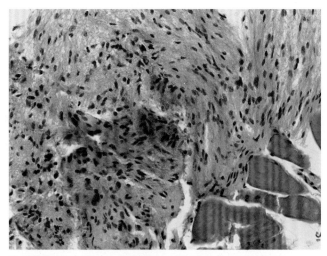

Figure 10.3.8   Schwannoma. This cell block section demonstrates schwannoma cells, which have indistinct cytoplasmic borders and spindle-shaped nuclei.

	Nodular Fasciitis	Malignant Peripheral Nerve Sheath Tumor
Age	Young adults	Adults; plexiform variant in children
Location	Forearm, chest, back, head and neck	Neck, forearm, lower torso
Signs and symptoms	Rapidly growing mass	Enlarging palpable mass
Etiology	Reactive proliferation of fibroblasts and myofibroblasts thought to be secondary to trauma	50% arise de novo and 50% in association with NF1
Cytomorphology	• Often hypercellular with fragments of loosely associated and/or dispersed cells (*Figures 10.4.1* and *10.4.2*) • Associated myxoid matrix material (*Figure 10.4.1*) • Spindled and/or epithelioid cells with cytoplasmic tails (*Figures 10.4.3* and *10.4.4*) • Eccentrically placed nuclei (*Figure 10.4.3*) • Marked nuclear atypia may be present (*Figure 10.4.3*)	• Large cohesive clusters (*Figures 10.4.5* and *10.4.6*) • Rare to absent single cell population • Metachromatic fibrillary stroma (*Figures 10.4.5* and *10.4.7*) • Mostly bland spindle cells with tapered nuclei (*Figures 10.4.8* and *10.4.9*) • Some tumors demonstrate prominent anisonucleosis
Special studies	Positive for SMA and calponin; negative for keratin, desmin, S-100 protein, and c-kit	Positive for CD99; only 60% express S-100 protein; negative for keratin, SMA, desmin, and c-kit
Molecular alterations	Possibly associated with a t(17; 22) translocation	Molecular heterogeneity
Treatment	Observation or resection	Complete excision with wide margins and radiation; chemotherapy for systemic disease
Clinical implications	Benign; typically does not recur	Recurs locally and often metastasizes

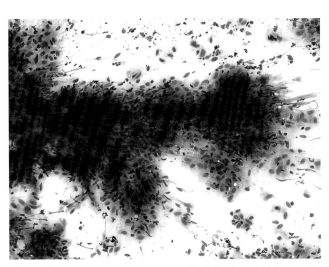

Figure 10.4.1 Nodular fasciitis. Nodular fasciitis often yields hypercellular smears, emulating a neoplastic process.

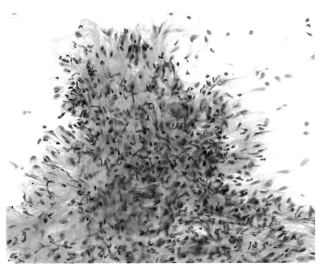

Figure 10.4.2 Nodular fasciitis. The field shows cells in a loosely cohesive tissue fragment as well as dispersed individual cells in the background.

Figure 10.4.3 Nodular fasciitis. The individually dispersed cells of NF have unipolar cytoplasmic tails and eccentrically placed nuclei. Nuclear pleomorphism may be marked in some cases.

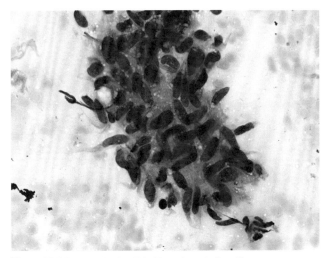

Figure 10.4.4 Nodular fasciitis. Here, the spindle cells appear more bland and monotonous. Cytoplasmic tails are prominent.

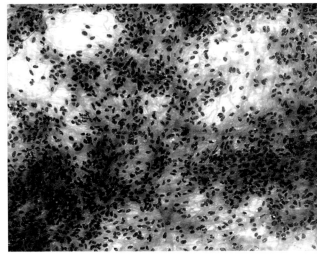

Figure 10.4.5 MPNST. MPNST cells and associated matrix material form a large fragment with rare dispersed single cells.

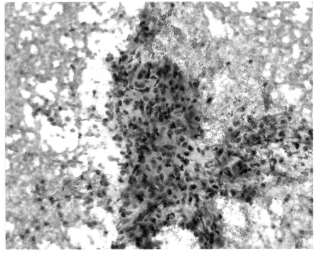

Figure 10.4.6 MPNST. A large cellular, cohesive fragment of cells with few discohesive cells in the background.

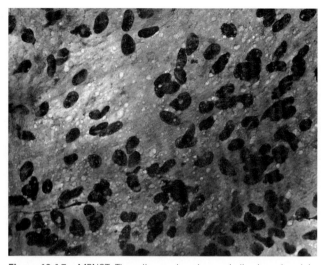

Figure 10.4.7   MPNST. The cells seen here have spindle-shaped nuclei and anisonucleosis. The cells are associated with fibrillary matrix material and their cytoplasm is difficult to define.

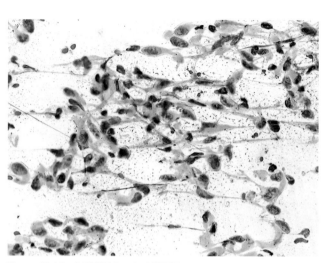

Figure 10.4.8   MPNST. Rarely, MPNST may present with discohesive single cells. The chromatin pattern is coarse and the nuclear borders are irregular.

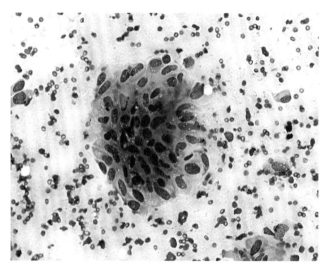

Figure 10.4.9   MPNST. This small fragment contains cells with elongated nuclei and associated magenta matrix material.

	Myxoid Liposarcoma	Myxoma
Age	Young and middle-aged adults	Middle-aged and older adults
Location	Extremity, especially posterior thigh	Thigh, shoulder, and upper arm
Signs and symptoms	Slow-growing tumor on an extremity	Enlarging palpable mass
Etiology	Mesenchymal neoplasm that occurs secondary to FUS-DDIT3 or EWSR1-DDIT3 rearrangements	Unknown
Cytomorphology	• Often presents as small fragments with or without dispersed single cells *(Figures 10.5.1 and 10.5.2)* • Oval-to-round tumor cells embedded in a myxoid background *(Figures 10.5.3 and 10.5.4)* • Arborizing (bifuracating) capillary vascular network *(Figure 10.5.5)* • Microvacuolated or univacuolated lipoblasts with scalloped nuclei may be present in 50% of cases *(Figures 10.5.1, 10.5.3 and 10.5.4)*	• Few spindled or histiocytoid cells in a myxoid background *(Figures 10.5.6-10.5.8)* • Rare vessels that do not branch *(Figure 10.5.9)* • Long cytoplasmic processes *(Figure 10.5.8)* • Oval-to-spindled bland nuclei *(Figure 10.5.10)*
Special studies	Positive for S-100 protein. Tests for associated translocations	Spindle cells positive for CD34; myxoid matrix positive by mucicarmine and Alcian blue special stains
Molecular alterations	t(12; 16) [FUS-DDIT3] in most; rarely t(12; 22) EWSR1-DDIT3	60% have GNAS1 mutations
Treatment	Complete excision	Excision
Clinical implications	Metastases are common and can occur following treatment; a round cell component is associated with poor prognosis	Rarely recurs

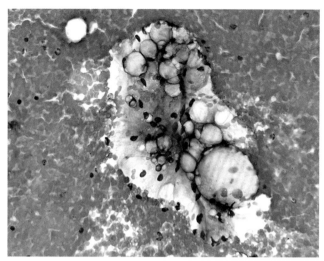

Figure 10.5.1   MLS. The field shows bland oval-shaped tumor cells embedded in matrix material.

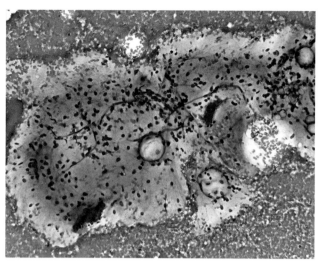

Figure 10.5.2   MLS. These bland oval-shaped tumor cells are embedded in matrix material. Note the branching vasculature in the center of the fragment.

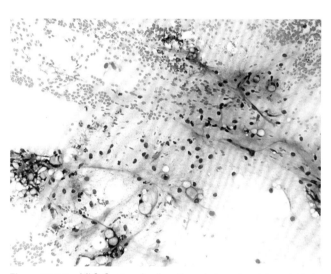

Figure 10.5.3   MLS. Scattered cells with oval-shaped nuclei emebdded in a myxoid matrix. Some cells are vacuolated.

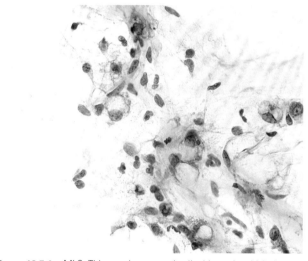

Figure 10.5.4   MLS. This neoplasm contains lipoblasts, in which the cytoplasm vacuoles indent the nuclei.

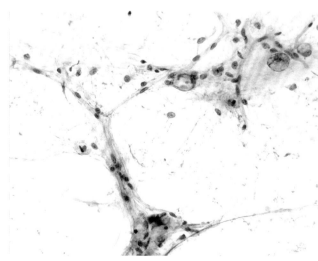

Figure 10.5.5   Branching MLS. This branching (arborizing) vasculature pattern is distinctive of MLS and is often refered to as a "chicken wire" appearance.

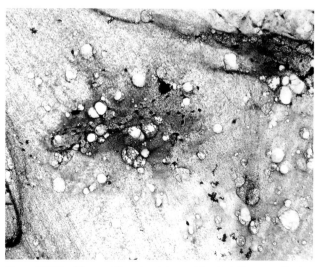

Figure 10.5.6   Myxoma. Granular pink mucoid material is present in the background, characteristic of myxoma.

10 SOFT TISSUE

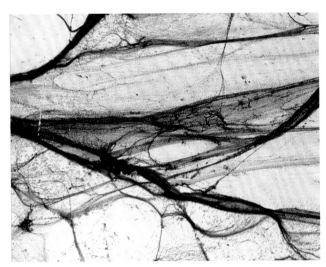

Figure 10.5.7 Myxoma. This FNA of a myxoma yielded a paucicellular field with strands of mucoid material.

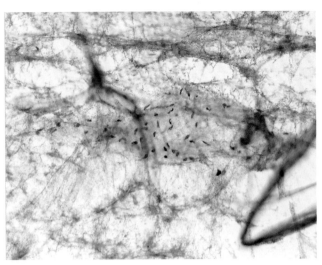

Figure 10.5.8 Myxoma. The rare tumor cells of myxoma have delicate cytoplasm that may have long cytoplasmic processes, as seen projecting from the edges of this tissue fragment.

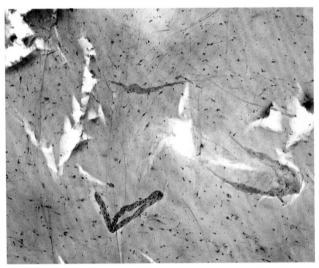

Figure 10.5.9 Myxoma. While myxoma may contain vasculature, it should be rare and not branch.

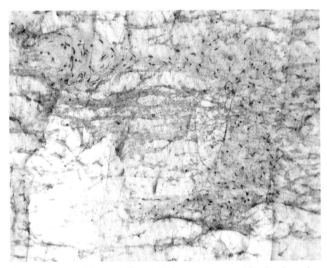

Figure 10.5.10 Myxoma. The nuclei in a myxoma are bland and may be spindle-shaped or oval-shaped.

	Malignant Peripheral Nerve Sheath Tumor	Spindle Cell Melanoma
Age	Adults; plexiform variant in children	Incidence increases with age but can affect young adults
Location	Neck, forearm, lower torso	Anywhere
Signs and symptoms	Enlarging palpable mass	Lymphadenopathy; depends on location of metastases
Etiology	50% arise de novo and 50% in association with NF1	UV light exposure
Cytomorphology	• Large cohesive clusters *(Figure 10.6.1)* • Rare to absent single cell population *(Figure 10.6.1)* • Metachromatic fibrillary stroma *(Figure 10.6.2)* • Mostly bland spindle cells with tapered nuclei *(Figures 10.6.3* and *10.6.4)* • Some tumors demonstrate prominent anisonucleosis	• Often single dispersed cells but may form large fragments *(Figures 10.6.5* and *10.6.7)* • Spindled nucleus with delicate cytoplasm *(Figure 10.6.8)* • No background stroma • May have abundant cytoplasm *(Figure 10.6.9)* • Some tumors demonstrate prominent anisonucleosis *(Figure 10.6.9)*
Special studies	Positive for CD99; only 60% express S-100 protein; negative for keratin, SMA, desmin, and c-kit	Positive for S-100 protein (sensitive but not specific); spindle cell variant often negative for other melanoma markers such as HMB45, Melan-A, Sox-10, MITF. Negative for keratin
Molecular alterations	Molecular heterogeneity	Most commonly BRAF and NRAS hotspot mutations
Treatment	Complete excision with wide margins and radiation; chemotherapy for systemic disease	For metastatic disease, chemotherapy, immunotherapy, and targeted therapy (BRAF and MEK inhibitors)
Clinical implications	Recurs locally and often metastasizes	Poor for metastatic disease, especially if spread outside of lymph nodes

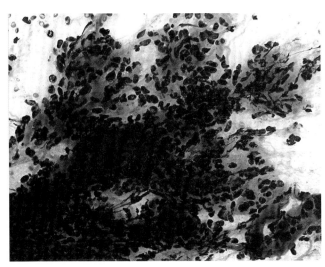

Figure 10.6.1   MPNST. This cohesive fragment of cells demonstrates pleomorphic nuclei and indistinct nuclear borders. Thin magenta-colored matrix material is associated with the fragment.

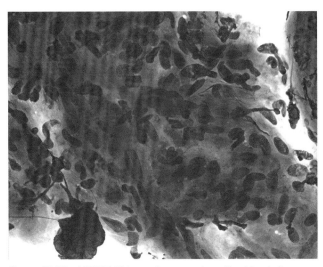

Figure 10.6.2   MPNST. This neoplasm contains cells with spindle-shaped nuclei and regular nuclear borders. Thin wisps of magenta-colored matrix are interspersed among the cells.

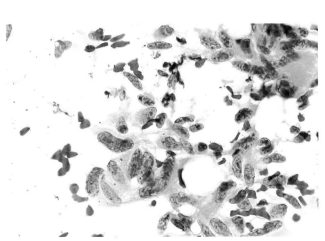

Figure 10.6.3   MPNST. The field shows markedly atypical nuclei that have irregular borders and great size variation. The chromatin is coarse.

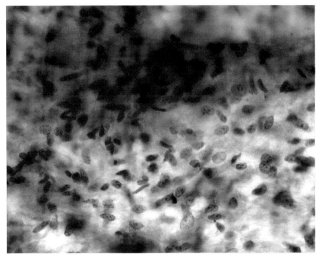

Figure 10.6.4   MPNST. These cells show variation in nuclear size and shape. The cytoplasmic borders are indistinct.

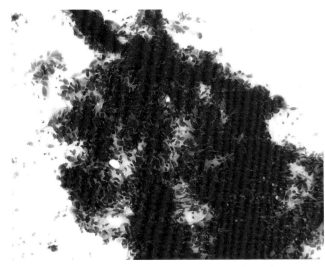

Figure 10.6.5   Melanoma. A large fragment of cohesive melanoma cells. Many of the cells contain oval- to spindle-shaped nuclei.

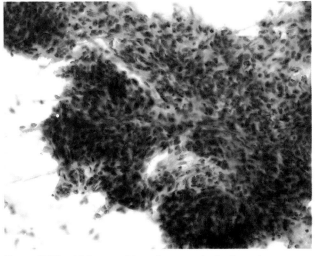

Figure 10.6.6   Melanoma. A large fragment of cohesive melanoma cells. The spindle cell variant of melanoma should always be on the differential when a spindle cell lesion is encountered.

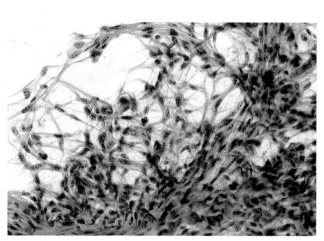

Figure 10.6.7   Melanoma. These cells have thin wispy cytoplasm and coarse chromatin.

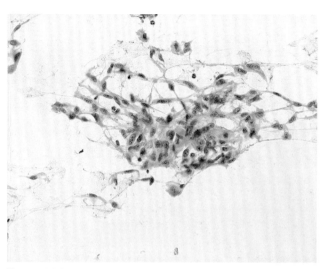

Figure 10.6.8   Melanoma. These cells have thin wispy cytoplasm and coarse chromatin. A few singly dispersed cells are present in the background.

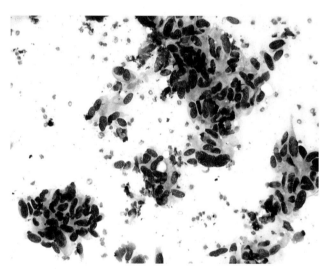

Figure 10.6.9   Melanoma. Some of the melanoma cells seen here demonstrate the classical features of melanoma not seen in the previous photographs: binucleation, prominent nucleoli, and abundant granular cytoplasm.

	Synovial Sarcoma	Adenocarcinoma
Age	All ages; median age is 35 y	Incidence increases with age but can affect young adults
Location	All locations; two-thirds occur in the extremities	Anywhere, but primarily in organs (thorax, abdomen, pelvis)
Signs and symptoms	Enlarging palpable mass; depends on location	Depends on location of primary tumor and/or metastases
Etiology	Caused by translocation t(X; 18); unknown cell of origin	Diverse
Cytomorphology	• Moderate to marked cellularity • Cohesive clusters of cells *(Figures 10.7.1 and 10.7.2)* • Cells may be epithelioid, spindled, or both, depending on both sampling and tumor subtype *(Figures 10.7.3 and 10.7.4)* • Spindle cells with ovoid nuclei and scant, tapered cytoplasm *(Figure 10.7.3)* • Epithelioid cells with eccentrically placed nuclei *(Figure 10.7.4)* • Discohesive cells and prominent nucleoli are uncommon features *(Figure 10.7.5)*	• Moderate to marked cellularity *(Figure 10.7.6)* • Cells in three-dimensional tissue fragments and/or singly dispersed *(Figure 10.7.6)* • Gland formation *(Figure 10.7.6)* • Large cells with large, hyperchromatic, and eccentrically placed nuclei *(Figures 10.7.7 and 10.7.8)* • Irregular nuclear borders *(Figure 10.7.9)* • Anisonucleosis and nuclear pleomorphism *(Figures 10.7.9 and 10.7.10)* • May contain mucin vacuoles *(Figure 10.7.9)* • Coarse chromatin and/or prominent nucleoli *(Figures 10.7.9 and 10.7.10)*
Special studies	Positive for TLE1, keratin, bcl-2, CD99. Negative for desmin, CD34, myogenin. RT-PCR for specific translocations	Positive for keratin; specific markers available for differentiation and/or primary site. Special chemical stains for mucin (mucicarmine)
Molecular alterations	Translocation involving SS18 with SSX1, SSX2, or SSX4	Diverse
Treatment	Complete excision, sometimes with radiation therapy or chemotherapy	Generally, resection. For metastatic disease, chemotherapy and/or radiation therapy. Targeted therapy and immunotherapy in certain instances
Clinical implications	Variable depending on tumor size, patient age, and presence of metastatic disease	Under most circumstances, poor for disease that cannot be surgically removed

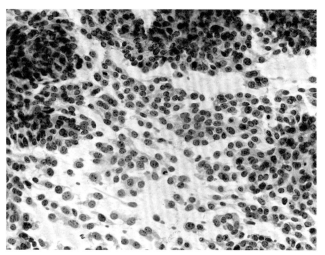

Figure 10.7.1 Synovial sarcoma. Synovial sarcoma may be biphasic (spindled and epithelioid) or monophasic. Here the tumor cells have a mixture of spindled and epithelioid nuclei and appear predominantly in tissue fragments, with some loosely dispersed cells.

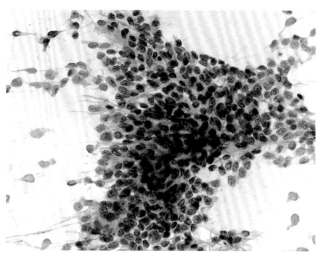

Figure 10.7.2 Synovial sarcoma. This tissue fragment contains cells with both epithelioid and spindled morphologies. The cytoplasm is scant and tapered.

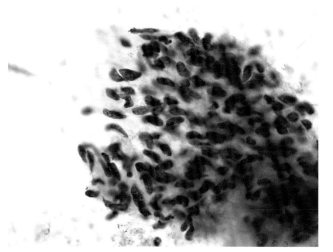

Figure 10.7.3 Synovial sarcoma. Spindle cells often dominate biphasic tumors and thus the presence of one morphology on FNA does not necessarily indicate a monophasic neoplasm.

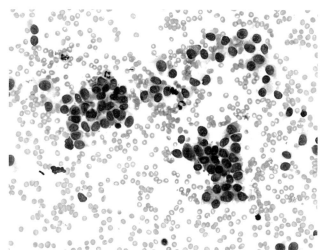

Figure 10.7.4 Synovial sarcoma. This cells in this field are predominantly epithelioid and have eccentrically placed nuclei. The nuclear borders are quite regular, as opposed to most adenocarcinomas.

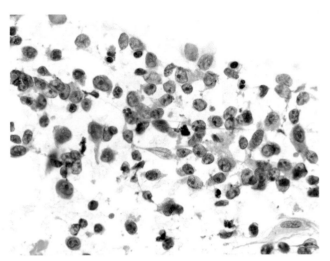

Figure 10.7.5 Synovial sarcoma. This field contains dispersed cells with prominent nucleoli. These features are more commonly seen in adenocarcinoma than synovial sarcoma.

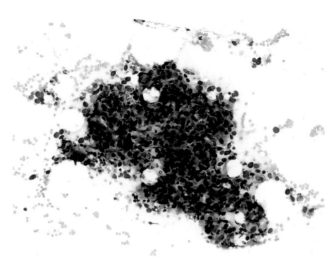

Figure 10.7.6 Adenocarcinoma. This adenocarcinoma forms a three-dimensional fragment with occasional single cells in the background. Several circular empty spaces are seen, indicating the formation of glandular structures.

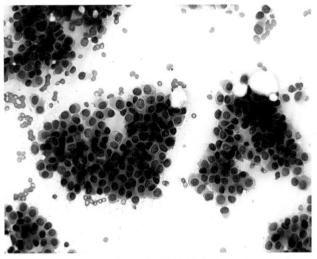

Figure 10.7.7 Adenocarcinoma. In this field, the tissue fragments form flat monolayers rather than three-dimensional fragments.

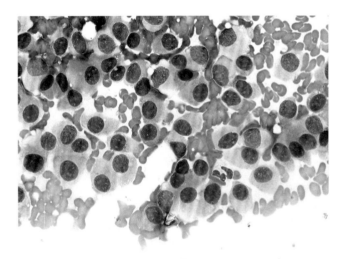

Figure 10.7.8 Adenocarcinoma. Loosely cohesive cells with eccentrically placed nuclei and foamy cytoplasm. Some cells have nuclear membrane irregularities.

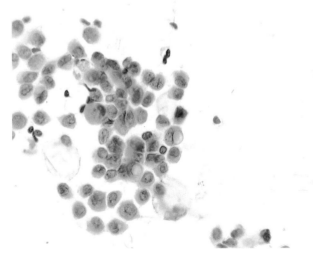

Figure 10.7.9 Adenocarcinoma. These cells demonstrate anisonucleosis, nuclear pleomorphism, irregular nuclear borders, and coarse chromatin. Several cells contain mucin vacuoles.

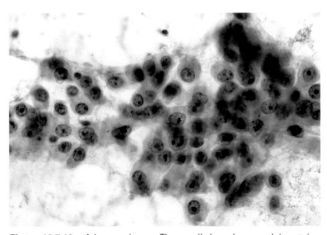

Figure 10.7.10 Adenocarcinoma. These cells have large nuclei containing prominent nucleoli and/or coarse chromatin.

	Conventional Chondrosarcoma	Chordoma
Age	Young and middle-aged adults	Most commonly middle-aged adults
Location	Ribs, pelvis, vertebrae, humerus, femur; rarely skull	Midline, often vertebrae, clivus, or sacrococcyx
Signs and symptoms	Dull pain, worst at night	Depends on location; neurologic deficits and spinal cord compression symptoms
Etiology	Unknown	May arise from fetal remnants of notochord
Cytomorphology	• Clusters and sheets of atypical chondro-cytes associated with background chon-dromyxoid matrix *(Figures 10.8.1-10.8.4)* • Neoplastic chondrocytes may be nested within chondroid matrix *(Figure 10.8.3)* • Eccentric nuclei and abundant, vacuolated cytoplasm *(Figure 10.8.5)* • High-grade tumors may have high N/C ratios and nuclear pleomorphism	• Fragments of fibrillary matrix associated with epithelioid tumor cells *(Figures 10.8.6 and 10.8.7)* • Tumor cells may be present singly in the background *(Figure 10.8.8)* • Tumor cells may stretch the matrix to form projections *(Figures 10.8.9 and 10.8.10)* • Physaliferous cells are usually present and contain intracytoplasmic vacuoles, which displace the nucleus *(Figure 10.8.6)*
Special studies	Positive for S-100 protein; negative for brachyury and cytokeratin; diagnosis should be made in conjunction with imaging studies	Positive for S-100 protein, cytokeratin, EMA, and brachyury
Molecular alterations	Gain of 8q and 20q	Tandem duplication of brachyury gene in famil-ial cases; brachyury gene amplification in some sporadic cases
Treatment	Wide excision	Resection with radiation therapy
Clinical implications	May recur or metastasize years later	Recurs locally; rarely metastasizes. Prognosis mproves with complete removal; skull-based tumors have poorer prognosis

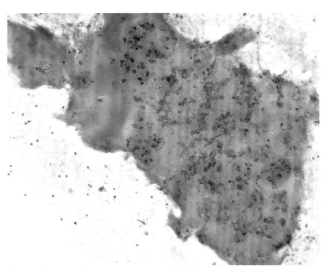

Figure 10.8.1   Chondrosarcoma. A large fragment of cartilage containing malignant chondrocytes. While this suggests a chondroid neoplasm, correlation with imaging studies is required to make a definitive diagnosis of chondrosarcoma.

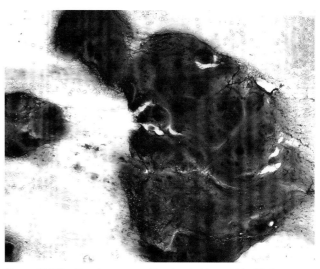

Figure 10.8.2   Chondrosarcoma. The chondroid myxoid in this fragment of chondrosarcoma appears more myxoid with wispy edges. It is difficult to assess the cytomorphology of the embedded cells at this low magnification.

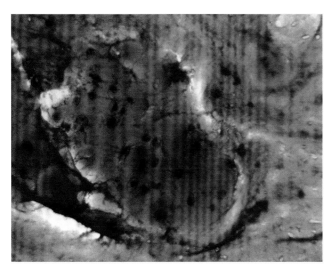

Figure 10.8.3   Chondrosarcoma. The malignant chondrocytes are interspersed throughout chondromyxoid matrix and are deceptively bland-appearing.

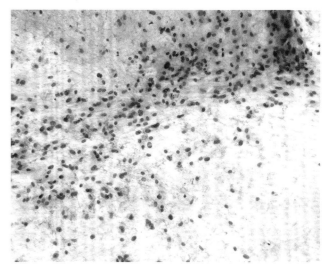

Figure 10.8.4   Chondrosarcoma. The neoplastic cells are dispersed throughout the field and appear bland, as they demonstrate minimal pleomorphism and regular nuclear contours. The background myxoid matrix is thin and is difficult to identify definitively as chondroid.

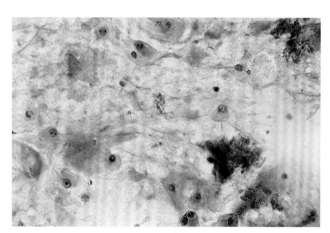

Figure 10.8.5 Chondrosarcoma. Low-grade chondrosarcoma cells contain abundant cytoplasm with an eccentrically placed nucleus. They are closely associated with chondromyxoid matrix material.

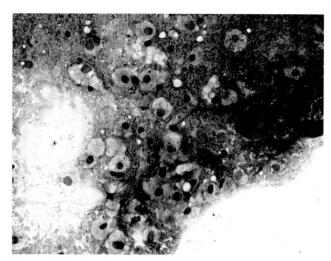

Figure 10.8.6 Chordoma. Chordoma cells are dispersed throughout the field and loosely associated with fibrillary magenta material. Several physaliferous cells can be seen; these cells contain large intracytoplasmic vacuoles, which displace the nucleus.

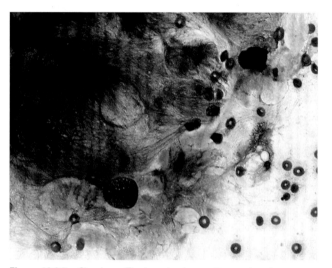

Figure 10.8.7 Chordoma. The two chordoma cells seen here have large nuclei and abundant cytoplasm which forms projections. They are intimately associated with the background matrix material.

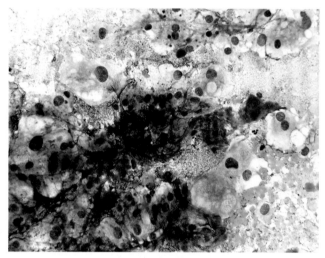

Figure 10.8.8 Chordoma. Chordoma often contains cells of varying size. This field demonstrates several large cells with voluminous cytoplasm as well as smaller cells with higher N/C ratios.

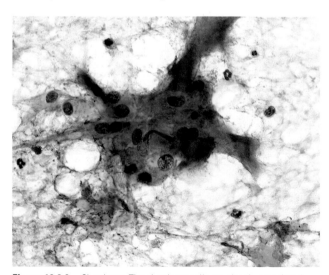

Figure 10.8.9 Chordoma. The chordoma cells are closely associated with matrix material; both the matrix material and cell cytoplasm form outward projections.

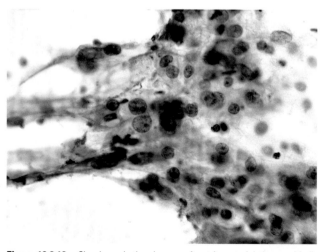

Figure 10.8.10 Chordoma. In the absence of matrix material, these epithelioid cells emulate non-mesenchymal neoplasms that may contain abundant cytoplasm, such as renal cell carcinoma, melanoma, and prostate carcinoma.

11

Liver

	Benign Hepatocytes	Well-Differentiated Hepatocellular Carcinoma
Age	Any age	Older adults (with cirrhosis) or young adults (without cirrhosis)
Location	Liver	Liver
Signs and symptoms	Any symptoms related to the etiology of the mass on imaging studies being sampled	Abdominal pain; jaundice; ascites; hepatomegaly; elevated AFP (nonspecific finding)
Etiology	Inadvertent sampling of benign background hepatocytes	Associated with hepatitis B, hepatitis C, cirrhosis, and aflatoxins
Cytomorphology	• Hypocellular or moderately cellular sample • Cells present singly or in small cohesive groups *(Figures 11.1.1 and 11.1.2)* • Polygonal cells with abundant, granular cytoplasm that may also contain pigment *(Figure 11.1.3)* • Round, uniform nuclei with regular contours and small nucleoli *(Figures 11.1.2 and 11.1.4)* • Intermixed rare fragments of benign ductal cells suggest the sampling of benign liver tissue *(Figure 11.1.5)*	• Hypercellular specimen with cells present in loosely cohesive fragments and/or singly dispersed in the background *(Figures 11.1.6 and 11.1.7)* • Fragments of hepatocytes with thickened plates (>2 cells thick) *(Figure 11.1.8)* • Polygonal cells with abundant, granular cytoplasm *(Figure 11.1.6)* • Nuclei may become oval with nuclear contour irregularities *(Figure 11.1.8)* • Transgressing vessels with nests of tumor cells *(Figures 11.1.9 and 11.1.10)*
Special studies	Negative for CK7 and positive for hepatocytic markers (HepPar1, arginase). Usually negative for glypican-3	Negative for CK7 and positive for hepatocytic markers (HepPar1, glypican-3, arginase)
Molecular alterations	N/A	Chromosomal aberrations
Treatment	N/A	Resection; transplantation; ablation/embolization
Clinical implication	The patient may need a repeat biopsy if the mass lesion was not sampled	Prognosis depends on stage; the fibrolamellar variant has better survival

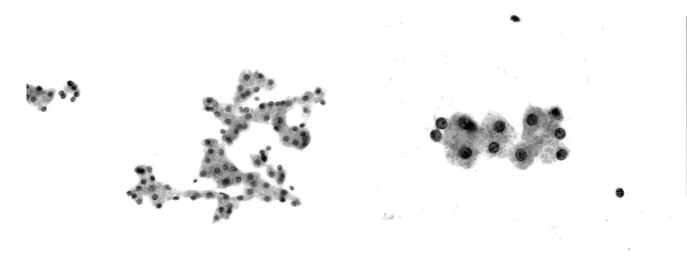

Figure 11.1.1   Benign hepatocytes. The cells have uniform, round nuclei and abundant and granular cytoplasm. Small nucleoli can also be seen.

Figure 11.1.2   Benign hepatocytes. A small group of benign hepatocytes is seen with abundant, polygonal cytoplasm. The cells have distinct and uniform nucleoli; nuclear contours are regular. Nonneoplastic hepatocytes should not be seen in layers greater than two hepatocytes thick.

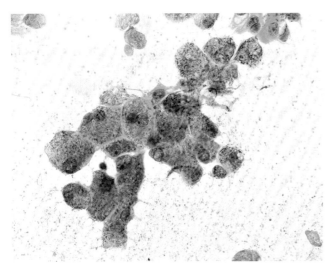

Figure 11.1.3   Benign hepatocytes. These hepatocytes contain green-yellow cytoplasmic pigment consistent with bile and abundant, granular cytoplasm. Cell borders are well-defined, and some cells are binucleated.

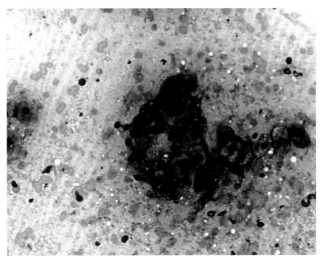

Figure 11.1.4   Benign hepatocytes. There is a small amount of variation in nuclear size, but most nuclei are round with regular borders.

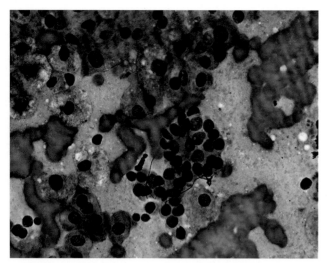

Figure 11.1.5 Benign hepatocytes. A small fragment of benign ductal cells is seen surrounded by benign hepatocytes. The nuclei are uniform and have regular contours, and the cells are not present in great numbers. A mixture of two components (ductal cells and hepatocytes) suggests the sampling of benign liver.

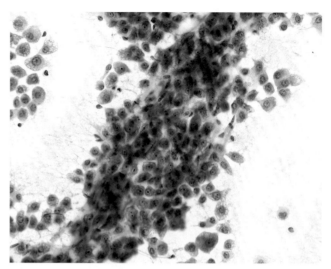

Figure 11.1.6 Hepatocellular carcinoma. Well-differentiated hepatocellular carcinoma cells can be difficult to distinguish from benign hepatocytes, but specimens are generally more cellular. In addition, this fragment of hepatocytes is thickened, suggesting a neoplastic process. Small spindle-shaped nuclei can also be seen within the fragment, indicating the presence of a transgressing vessel, a finding associated with hepatocellular carcinoma.

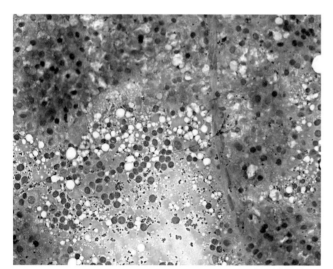

Figure 11.1.7 Hepatocellular carcinoma. A fragment of carcinoma is present in a background of single neoplastic cells and stripped nuclei. A vessel passes vertically at the right side of the field, further suggesting a neoplastic process.

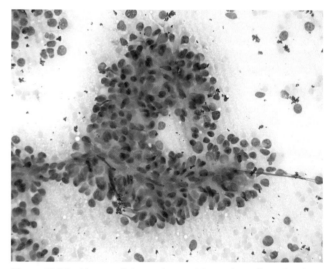

Figure 11.1.8 Hepatocellular carcinoma. A large, three-dimensional fragment of hepatocytes. The nuclei are more pleomorphic than benign, reactive hepatocytes and have irregular shapes.

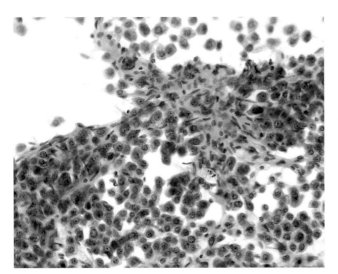

Figure 11.1.9   Hepatocellular carcinoma. Several vessels transgress the field and are associated with nests of proliferative hepatocytes. Despite maintaining abundant, granular cytoplasm, these hepatocytes have formed thickened layers, indicating a neoplastic process.

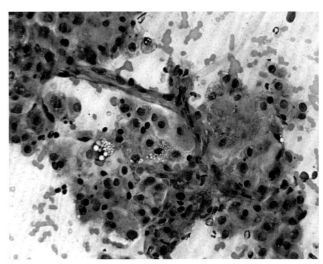

Figure 11.1.10   Hepatocellular carcinoma. Malignant hepatocytes form thickened nests associated with a vessel. The cells demonstrate anisonucleosis and irregular nuclear contours. Some nucleoli are quite prominent.

	Cholangiocarcinoma	Hepatocellular Carcinoma
Age	Older adults	Older adults (with cirrhosis) or young adults (without cirrhosis)
Location	Liver	Liver
Signs and symptoms	May be asymptomatic and identified on imaging studies; abdominal pain; cachexia; elevated serum liver enzymes	Abdominal pain; jaundice; ascites; hepatomegaly; elevated AFP (nonspecific finding)
Etiology	Secondary to chronic inflammation of intrahepatic bile ducts; most cases have no known etiology but can be associated with primary sclerosing cholangitis, Thorotrast contrast agent, hepatitis C, cirrhosis, and liver fluke infection in endemic areas of East Asia	Associated with hepatitis B, hepatitis C, cirrhosis, and aflatoxins
Cytomorphology	• Predominantly cohesive cells in tissue fragments, but individual cells may be dispersed in poorly differentiated neoplasms *(Figures 11.2.1 and 11.2.2)* • Nuclei are disorganized within tissue fragment ("drunken honeycomb") *(Figure 11.2.3)* • Nuclear size variation (usually greater than 4:1) and nuclear border irregularities *(Figure 11.2.4)* • Hyperchromasia, coarse chromatin, and high N/C ratios *(Figures 11.2.3 and 11.2.4)* • Nucleoli may be seen	• Hypercellular specimen with cells present in loosely cohesive fragments and/or singly dispersed in the background *(Figures 11.2.5 and 11.2.6)* • Fragments of hepatocytes with thickened plates (>2 cells thick) *(Figure 11.2.7)* • Polygonal cells with abundant, granular cytoplasm *(Figure 11.2.8)* • Nuclei may become oval with nuclear contour irregularities *(Figure 11.2.9)* • Transgressing vessels with nests of tumor cells *(Figures 11.2.7 and 11.2.8)*
Special studies	Positive for CK7 and negative for markers of hepatic differentiation; loss of DPC4 expression in a subset of tumors	Negative for CK7 and positive for hepatocytic markers (HepPar1, glypican-3, arginase)
Molecular alterations	Diverse. Mutations in KRAS, IDH1, IDH2, BRAF, EGFR. Chromosomal aberrations	Chromosomal aberrations
Treatment	Surgical resection; targeted therapies	Resection; transplantation; ablation/embolization
Clinical implication	Poor prognosis	Prognosis depends on stage; the fibrolamellar variant has better survival

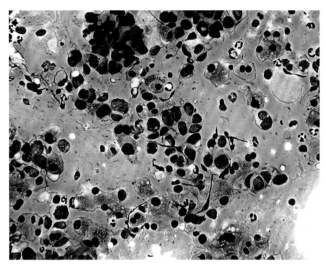

Figure 11.2.1   Cholangiocarcinoma. This carcinoma is poorly differen-tiated and seen as loosely cohesive cells in tissue fragments. The cells are large, have high N/C ratios, and markedly irregular borders. The background contains benign hepatocytes, which have abundant, granular cytoplasm, small, round nuclei, and prominent nucleoli.

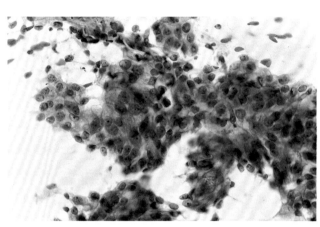

Figure 11.2.2   Cholangiocarcinoma. The cells have large and variably sized nuclei with coarse chromatin or nucleoli. The cell cytoplasm has a foamy quality, indicating the glandular nature of this carcinoma, a feature not seen in hepatocellular carcinoma.

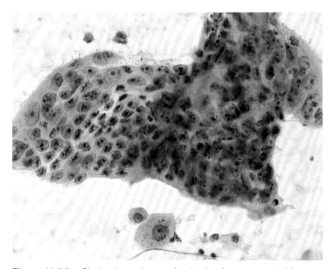

Figure 11.2.3   Cholangiocarcinoma. A cohesive fragment containing enlarged nuclei with coarse chromatin. The nuclei are arranged in a disorderly fashion within the fragment.

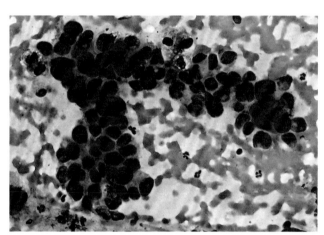

Figure 11.2.4   Cholangiocarcinoma. A papillary fragment contains cells with high N/C ratios, large nuclei, and irregular nuclear borders. Features of hepatocellular differentiation are lacking, and the three-dimensional nature of the fragment favors an adenocarcinoma.

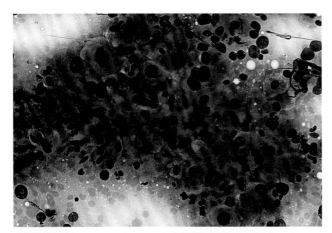

Figure 11.2.5 Hepatocellular carcinoma. The field contains loosely cohesive cells with pleomorphic nuclei. Despite the marked nuclear atypia, many cells maintain large amounts of granular cytoplasm, which should cause consideration for a hepatocellular origin.

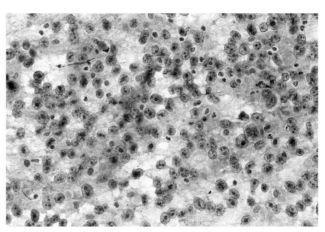

Figure 11.2.6 Hepatocellular carcinoma. The cells have coarse chromatin or prominent nucleoli and indistinct cytoplasm. A poorly differentiated adenocarcinoma is in the differential diagnosis and should be evaluated with ancillary immunohistochemical studies in the proper clinicoradiologic context.

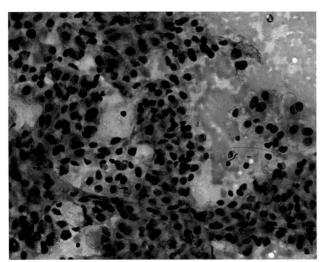

Figure 11.2.7 Hepatocellular carcinoma. This hepatocellular carcinoma mimics an adenocarcinoma given its cohesive nature and the appearance of the cell cytoplasm, which could be mistaken for having a mucinous rather than granular quality. However, close examination reveals magenta-colored material associated with spindled nuclei, indicating the presence of transgressing vessels.

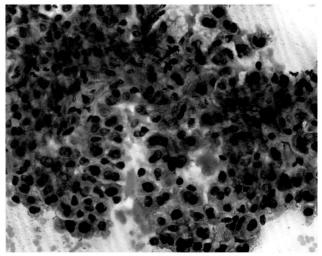

Figure 11.2.8 Hepatocellular carcinoma. The transgressing vessels in this field are more obvious and should raise consideration for a hepatocellular carcinoma. In addition, the cells have ample, granular cytoplasm and some cells are binucleated, additional features suggestive of hepatocellular carcinoma.

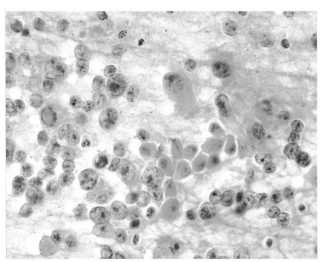

Figure 11.2.9   Hepatocellular carcinoma. These pleomorphic cells have cytomorphologic overlap with a poorly differentiated adenocarcinoma. A prominent intranuclear inclusion is seen in the left center field. Intranuclear inclusions can be seen in hepatocellular carcinoma; while they are not a specific feature, when seen in the liver, they raise the possibility of a hepatocellular carcinoma.

	Cholangiocarcinoma	Benign Hepatocytes and Ductal Cells
Age	Older adults	Any age
Location	Liver	Liver
Signs and symptoms	May be asymptomatic and identified on imaging studies; abdominal pain; cachexia; elevated serum liver enzymes	Any symptoms related to the etiology of the mass on imaging studies being sampled
Etiology	Secondary to chronic inflammation of intrahepatic bile ducts; most cases have no known etiology but can be associated with primary sclerosing cholangitis, Thorotrast contrast agent, hepatitis C, cirrhosis, and liver fluke infection in endemic areas of East Asia	Inadvertent sampling of benign background hepatocytes and ductal cells
Cytomorphology	• Predominantly cohesive cells in tissue fragments *(Figures 11.3.1* and *11.3.2)* • Nuclei are disorganized within tissue fragment ("drunken honeycomb") *(Figures 11.3.3-11.3.5)* • Nuclear size variation and nuclear border irregularities *(Figure 11.3.4)* • Hyperchromasia, coarse chromatin, and high N/C ratios *(Figures 11.3.3* and *11.3.4)* • Prominent nucleoli may be seen *(Figure 11.3.5)*	• Hypocellular or moderately cellular sample • Hepatocytes present singly or in small cohesive groups *(Figures 11.3.6* and *11.3.7)* • Hepatocytes are polygonal with abundant, granular cytoplasm that may also contain pigment *(Figures 11.3.6* and *11.3.7)* • Hepatocytes with round, uniform nuclei with regular contours and small nucleoli *(Figures 11.3.6* and *11.3.7)* • Intermixed rare small fragments of benign ductal cells in an organized, honeycomb configuration *(Figures 11.3.6-11.3.8)* • Benign ductal cells have uniform nuclei with regular nuclear contours *(Figures 11.3.6-11.3.8)*
Special studies	Positive for CK7 and negative for markers of hepatic differentiation; loss of DPC4 expression in a subset of tumors	Benign hepatocytes are negative for CK7 and positive for hepatocytic markers (HepPar1, arginase). Usually negative for glypican-3. Benign ductal cells are positive for CK7 and negative for markers of hepatic differentiation
Molecular alterations	Diverse. Mutations in KRAS, IDH1, IDH2, BRAF, EGFR. Chromosomal aberrations	N/A
Treatment	Surgical resection; targeted therapies	N/A
Clinical implication	Poor prognosis	The patient may need a repeat biopsy if the mass lesion was not sampled

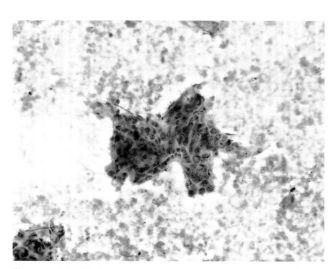

Figure 11.3.1   Cholangiocarcinoma. A three-dimensional fragment containing cells with enlarged nuclei, high N/C ratios, coarse chromatin, and irregular nuclear contours is seen, consistent with an adenocarcinoma. The background is necrotic.

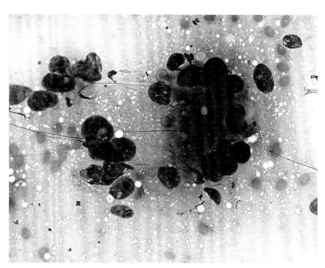

Figure 11.3.2   Cholangiocarcinoma. The field demonstrates a poorly differentiated adenocarcinoma cells with large, irregularly shaped nuclei and minimal-to-absent cytoplasm. Some cells have prominent nucleoli, while others have coarse, clumpy chromatin.

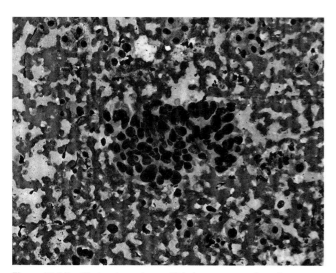

Figure 11.3.3   Cholangiocarcinoma. This fragment contains adenocarcinoma cells in which the nuclei are arranged in a disorderly ("drunken honeycomb") fashion. However, other features are also sufficient for a diagnosis of adenocarcinoma, including the pleomorphic nature of the nuclei. Several benign hepatocytes are present at the top of the field and provide a morphologic comparison.

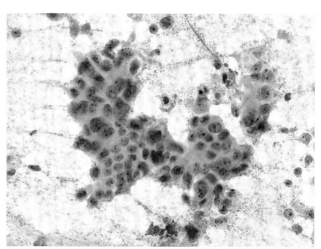

Figure 11.3.4   Cholangiocarcinoma. The neoplastic cells are disorderly arranged within a tissue fragment and have high N/C ratios. Some cells have notches in their nuclear membranes, an atypical feature. Anisonucleosis is present, but a 4:1 variation in size between neighboring nuclei is not seen. Regardless, the atypia is sufficient for a diagnosis of adenocarcinoma.

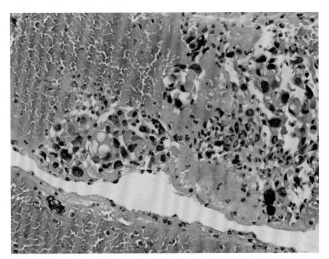

Figure 11.3.5 Cholangiocarcinoma. This cell block preparation contains overtly malignant cells, some with prominent nucleoli. There is great variation in nuclear size.

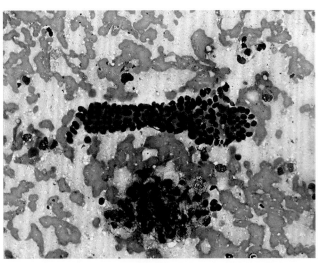

Figure 11.3.6 Benign liver elements. The field contains both benign ductal cells and hepatocytes. The ductal cells are well-organized within a tubular structure and have uniform nuclei. The hepatocytes contain cytoplasmic vacuoles and round, regular nuclei. In contrast to a neoplastic process, benign elements are usually not present in great numbers.

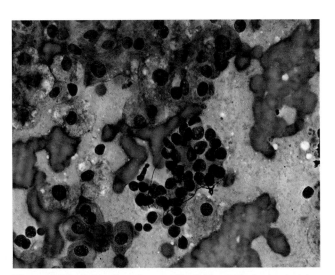

Figure 11.3.7 Benign liver elements. The field contains benign ductal cells surrounded by benign hepatocytes. The ductal cells are present in a small fragment and contain uniform nuclei. The hepatocytes have abundant, granular cytoplasm and round nuclei with minimal size variation.

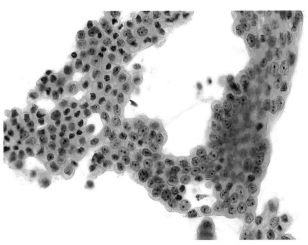

Figure 11.3.8 Benign ductal cells. While mild anisonucleosis and nuclear contour irregularities are both present, the nuclei are organized in a honeycomb fashion within the fragment. If the specimen contained numerous fragments such as this, a well-differentiated adenocarcinoma would be in the differential diagnosis.

12
Breast

	Apocrine Metaplasia	**Ductal Adenocarcinoma**
Age	Adults	Middle-aged and older women
Location	Breast	Breast
Signs and symptoms	Part of fibrocystic change; may form a mass	Breast mass; skin dimpling, swelling, redness, and/or pain; nipple discharge and/or retraction; axillary lymphadenopathy
Etiology	Unknown	Numerous contributing environmental and lifestyle factors; inherited mutations in BRCA1/BRCA2, TP53, PTEN, or mismatch repair genes, among others
Cytomorphology	• Monolayer sheets of epithelial cells (*Figures 12.1.1* and *12.1.2*) • Nuclei are regularly spaced within fragments (*Figure 12.1.3*) • Cells have abundant, granular cytoplasm (*Figure 12.1.4*) • Nuclei are round-to-oval (*Figure 12.1.5*) • Anisonucleosis is common, but nuclei maintain regular contours (*Figures 12.1.3-12.1.5*) • Bland chromatin with small chromocenters or nucleoli (*Figures 12.1.4* and *12.1.5*)	• Cells in fragments and/or singly dispersed (*Figures 12.1.6* and *12.1.7*) • Disorderly nuclei within fragments (*Figures 12.1.7* and *12.1.8*) • Formation of three-dimensional structures (*Figure 12.1.9*) • Increased N/C ratios (*Figures 12.1.8* and *12.1.9*) • Greater nuclear size variation and irregularity in nuclear shapes and/or contours (*Figure 12.1.10*) • Overlapping nuclei (*Figures 12.1.8* and *12.1.9*) • Coarse chromatin (*Figure 12.1.10*)
Special studies	N/A	N/A
Molecular alterations	N/A	Complex due to heterogeneity of disease
Treatment	N/A	Surgical removal, axillary lymph node dissection, chemoradiation, hormonal therapy, and/or targeted therapies
Clinical implications	N/A	Varies

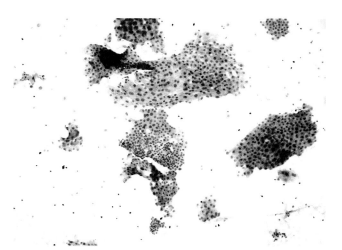

Figure 12.1.1   Apocrine metaplasia. Several fragments contain cells with abundant, granular cytoplasm. The nuclei are organized within the fragments and are generally round with regular contours. Anisonucleosis is a common feature of apocrine metaplasia.

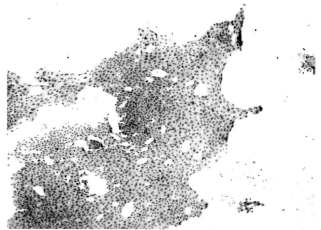

Figure 12.1.2   Apocrine metaplasia. A large monolayer fragment has "punched out" spaces containing cells with abundant, granular cytoplasm. The nuclei are organized within the fragment.

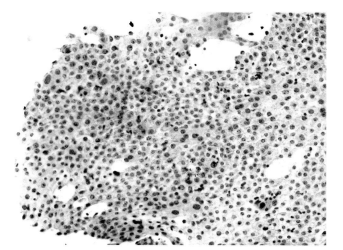

Figure 12.1.3   Apocrine metaplasia. Despite some nuclear size variation, the nuclei remain round with regular nuclear borders. The cells have small nucleoli or chromocenters.

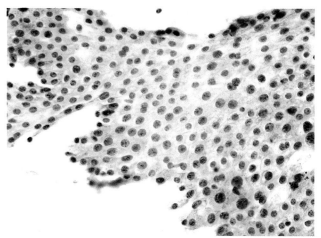

Figure 12.1.4   Apocrine metaplasia. At high magnification, distinct cell borders can be seen between cells. Some cells are binucleated. The cells are evenly arranged within the fragment and have round nuclei with regular borders.

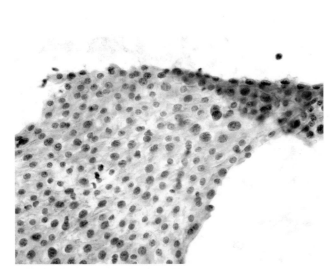

Figure 12.1.5   Apocrine metaplasia. The nuclei are round-to-oval and have regular contours and bland chromatin. The N/C ratios are low due to increased amounts of granular cytoplasm.

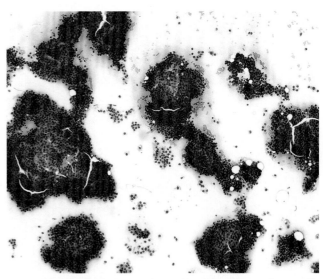

Figure 12.1.6   Ductal adenocarcinoma. Numerous adenocarcinoma cells are arranged in papillary fragments as well as singly dispersed in the background.

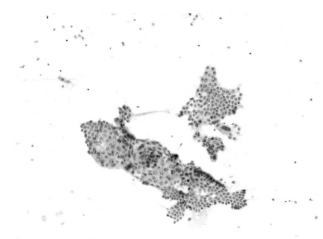

Figure 12.1.7   Adenocarcinoma. Two papillary fragments contain adenocarcinoma cells within high N/C ratios. Some cells demonstrate significant nuclear size variation, and the cells are disorganized within the fragments. An atypical mitotic figure can be seen.

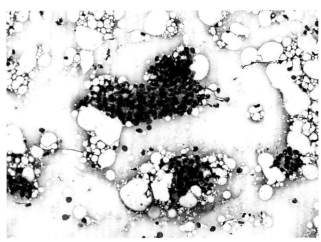

Figure 12.1.8   Adenocarcinoma. These fragments contain cells with high N/C ratios, overlapping nuclei, and nuclei with irregular shapes.

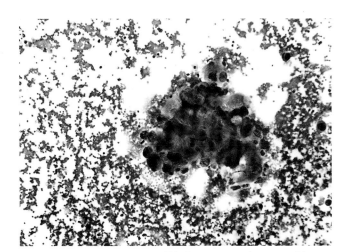

Figure 12.1.9   Adenocarcinoma. This fragment contains many of the features diagnostic of carcinoma: three-dimensionality, high N/C ratios, irregular nuclear borders, anisonucleosis, prominent nucleoli, and overlapping nuclei.

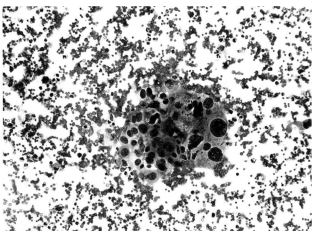

Figure 12.1.10   Adenocarcinoma. These cells are overtly malignant and demonstrate great variation in nuclear sizes. Some cells have markedly irregular nuclear borders, and a coarse chromatin pattern can be seen in some of the cells. Some nuclei are many times larger than the inflammatory cells seen in the background.

	Fibroadenoma	Ductal Adenocarcinoma
Age	Young women	Middle-aged and older women
Location	Breast, often upper outer quadrant	Breast
Signs and symptoms	Part of fibrocystic change; may form a mass	Breast mass, dimpling, swelling, redness, and/or pain; nipple discharge and/or retraction; axillary lymphadenopathy
Etiology	Benign neoplasm containing both epithelial and stromal components	Numerous contributing environmental and lifestyle factors; inherited mutations in BRCA1/BRCA2, TP53, PTEN, or mismatch repair genes, among others
Cytomorphology	• Cellular papillary ("staghorn") fragments of elongated epithelial (ductal) cells *(Figures 12.2.1 and 12.2.2)* • Ductal cells are well organized within the fragments *(Figure 12.2.3)* • Singly dispersed spindle (myoepithelial) cells in the background *(Figure 12.2.1)* • Uniform ductal cells with oval nuclei with regular borders and powdery chromatin *(Figure 12.2.4)* • Associated stroma material *(Figure 12.2.5)*	• Cells in fragments and/or singly dispersed *(Figures 12.2.6 and 12.2.7)* • Disorderly nuclei within fragments *(Figure 12.2.8)* • Formation of three-dimensional structures *(Figure 12.2.9)* • Increased N/C ratios *(Figures 12.2.8 and 12.2.9)* • Greater nuclear size variation and irregularity in nuclear shapes and/or contours *(Figure 12.2.8)* • Overlapping nuclei *(Figures 12.2.8 and 12.2.9)*
Special studies	N/A	N/A
Molecular alterations	N/A	Complex due to heterogeneity of disease
Treatment	Usually surgical excision	Surgical removal, axillary lymph node dissection, chemoradiation, hormonal therapy, and/or targeted therapies
Clinical implications	Excellent; sometimes recurs	Varies

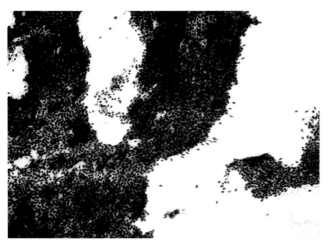

Figure 12.2.1 Fibroadenoma. The field contains a large branching ("staghorn") fragment of ductal cells with scattered spindled myoepithelial cells in the background. The ductal cells have similarly sized, oval-shaped nuclei with regular borders.

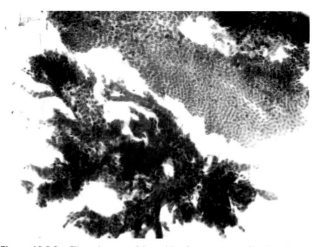

Figure 12.2.2 Fibroadenoma. A branching fragment contains ductal cells with elongated nuclei. The cells have high N/C ratios, but regular nuclear borders and stream within the fragment in an organized fashion.

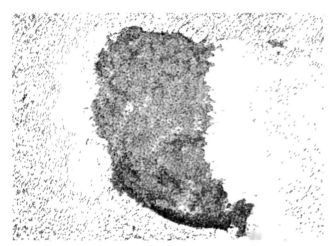

Figure 12.2.3 Fibroadenoma. Ductal cells are well-organized within this monolayer fragment. The nuclei are round-to-oval, uniform, and have regular contours. Rare spindled myoepithelial cells can be seen at the edge of the fragment as well as in the background.

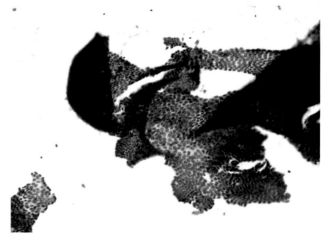

Figure 12.2.4 Fibroadenoma. The field shows a papillary ("staghorn") fragment of ductal cells. The cells resemble papillary thyroid carcinoma due to their elongated nuclei with powdery chromatin.

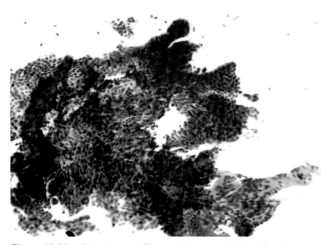

Figure 12.2.5 Fibroadenoma. The nuclei are crowded, oval, and over-lapping, but are uniform in size and shape. The fragment is attached to a cyanophilic stromal fragment (bottom right).

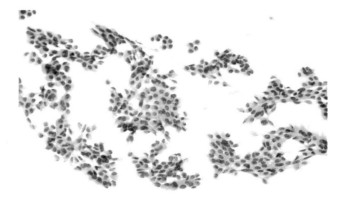

Figure 12.2.6 Ductal adenocarcinoma. Some nuclei are irregularly shaped and larger than adjacent nuclei. Some cells have increased N/C ratios. Myoepithelial cells are absent. Mild atypia such as this is seen in well-differentiated adenocarcinomas and may be difficult to distinguish from benign processes.

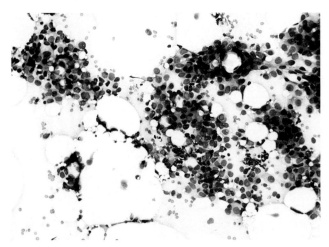

Figure 12.2.7   Ductal adenocarcinoma. These tissue fragments contain discohesive adenocarcinoma cells. The cells are large and have high N/C ratios. Some cells have irregular shapes and anisonucleosis is present. Myoepithelial cells are absent.

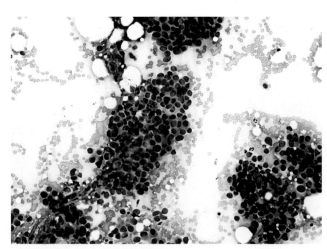

Figure 12.2.8   Ductal adenocarcinoma. The field shows cellular fragments containing enlarged adenocarcinoma cells with overlapping nuclei. The nuclei have irregular shapes and vary in size. Several cells are individually dispersed adjacent to the fragments.

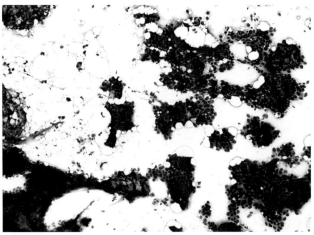

Figure 12.2.9   Ductal adenocarcinoma. The cells form three-dimensional areas and have little cytoplasm; even at this low magnification, variations in nuclear size and shape can be seen.

	Papilloma	Ductal Adenocarcinoma
Age	Adult women	Middle-aged and older women
Location	Breast	Breast
Signs and symptoms	Mammographic calcifications (peripheral) or nipple discharge (central)	Breast mass, dimpling, swelling, redness, and/or pain; nipple discharge and/or retraction; axillary lymphadenopathy
Etiology	Intraductal proliferation of epithelial and myoepithelial cells	Numerous contributing environmental and lifestyle factors; inherited mutations in BRCA1/BRCA2, TP53, PTEN, or mismatch repair genes, among others
Cytomorphology	• Cellular papillary fragments of elongated epithelial (ductal) cells *(Figures 12.3.1 and 12.3.2)* • Bipolar nuclei present at fragment borders and in the background *(Figures 12.3.3 and 12.3.4)* • Ductal cells have elongated, uniform nuclei and bland chromatin *(Figure 12.3.5)* • Background foamy macrophages *(Figure 12.3.5)*	• Cells in fragments and/or singly dispersed *(Figures 12.3.6 and 12.3.7)* • Disorderly nuclei within fragments *(Figure 12.3.8)* • Formation of three-dimensional structures *(Figure 12.3.9)* • Increased N/C ratios *(Figures 12.3.8 and 12.3.9)* • Greater nuclear size variation and irregularity in nuclear shapes and/or contours *(Figure 12.3.10)* • Overlapping nuclei *(Figure 12.3.9)*
Special studies	N/A	N/A
Molecular alterations	N/A	Complex due to heterogeneity of disease
Treatment	Usually surgical excision	Surgical removal, axillary lymph node dissection, chemoradiation, hormonal therapy, and/or targeted therapies
Clinical implications	Excellent; the presence of multiple papillomas is associated with risk of subsequent malignancy	Varies

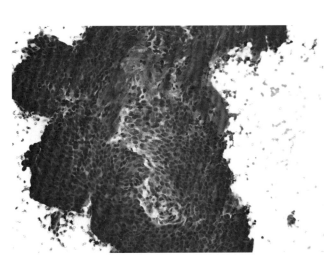

Figure 12.3.1   Papilloma. The field contains a large fragment containing elongated epithelial cells with uniform nuclei. The cells have high N/C ratios but regular nuclear borders and they are well organized within the fragment.

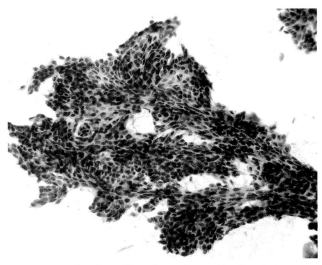

Figure 12.3.2   Papilloma. The cells are elongated but have little variation in nuclear size and shape. Small spindle cells can be seen at the edges of the tissue fragment (bottom right corner).

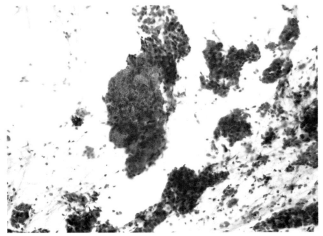

Figure 12.3.3   Papilloma. Small papillary fragments are seen intermixed with dispersed myoepithelial cells. The ductal cells are crowded with high N/C ratios but are similar in size and shape. Nuclear borders are regular.

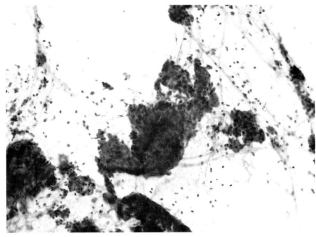

Figure 12.3.4   Papilloma. Several papillary fragments are intermixed with dispersed myoepithelial cells. The presence of numerous myoepithelial cells is generally reassuring.

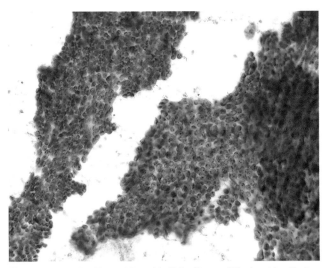

Figure 12.3.5   Papilloma. Myoepithelial cells are difficult to identify, but the cells contain uniform nuclei and bland chromatin.

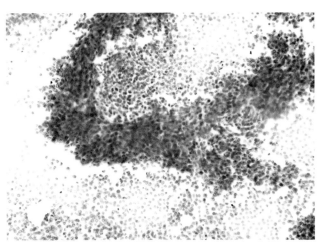

Figure 12.3.6   Ductal adenocarcinoma. The field is cellular with adenocarcinoma cells present singly as well as in large tissue fragments. The tissue fragment is three-dimensional and has a disorganized cellular architecture.

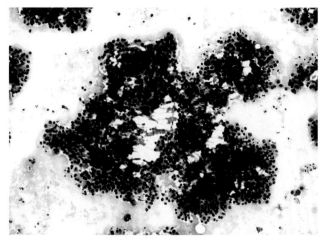

Figure 12.3.7   Ductal adenocarcinoma. These three-dimensional papillary structures contain discohesive adenocarcinoma cells. The cells have nuclei with varied shapes and sizes.

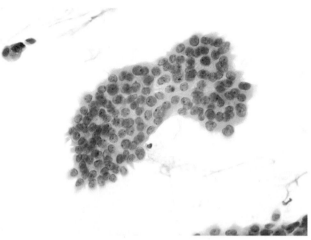

Figure 12.3.8   Ductal adenocarcinoma. This small fragment contains disorganized nuclei. The nuclei vary in size and shape, and some have irregular nuclear contours as well as nuclear grooves.

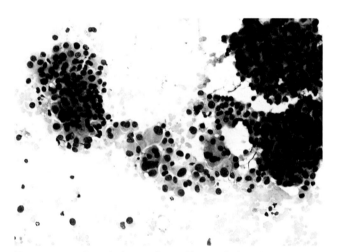

Figure 12.3.9   Ductal adenocarcinoma. These cells form three-dimensional fragments as well as present singly in the background. The cells are enlarged and have eccentric nuclei that are quite varied in size and shape.

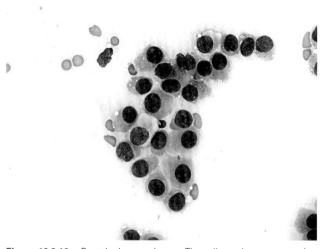

Figure 12.3.10   Ductal adenocarcinoma. The cells are large compared to background red blood cells. Despite their low N/C ratios, the cells are concerning due to their nuclei with irregular borders and coarse chromatin.

	Papilloma	Fibroadenoma
Age	Adult women	Young women
Location	Breast	Breast, often upper outer quadrant
Signs and symptoms	Mammographic calcifications (peripheral) or nipple discharge (central)	Part of fibrocystic change; may form a mass
Etiology	Intraductal proliferation of epithelial and myo-epithelial cells	Benign neoplasm containing both epithelial and stromal components
Cytomorphology	• Cellular papillary fragments of elongated epithelial (ductal) cells *(Figures 12.4.1 and 12.4.2)* • Bipolar nuclei present at fragment borders and in the background *(Figure 12.4.3)* • Ductal cells have elongated, uniform nuclei and bland chromatin *(Figure 12.4.4)* • Background foamy macrophages *(Figure 12.3.4)*	• Cellular papillary ("staghorn") fragments of elongated epithelial (ductal) cells *(Figures 12.4.5 and 12.4.6)* • Ductal cells are well organized within the fragments *(Figure 12.4.7)* • Singly dispersed spindle (myoepithelial) cells in the background *(Figure 12.4.8)* • Uniform ductal cells with oval nuclei with regular borders and powdery chromatin *(Figures 12.4.8 and 12.4.9)* • Associated stroma material *(Figure 12.4.9)*
Special studies	N/A	N/A
Molecular alterations	N/A	N/A
Treatment	Usually surgical excision	Usually surgical excision
Clinical implications	Excellent; the presence of multiple papillomas is associated with risk of subsequent malignancy	Excellent; sometimes recurs

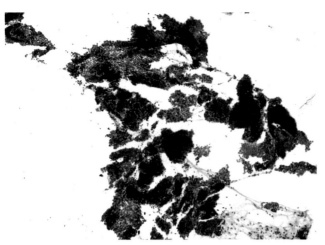

Figure 12.4.1   Papilloma. The fragments contain densely packed nuclei, but the nuclei are uniform and well-organized within the fragments. Rare myoepithelial cells are present in the background.

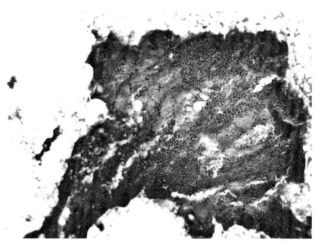

Figure 12.4.2   Papilloma. Even at this magnification, the nuclei appear uniform and do not overlap within the fragment.

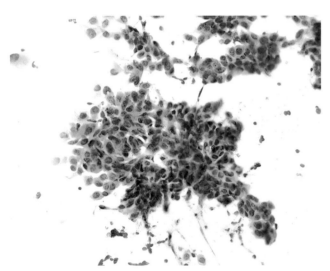

Figure 12.4.3   Papilloma. Rare spindle-shaped myoepithelial cells can be seen in association with the fragment.

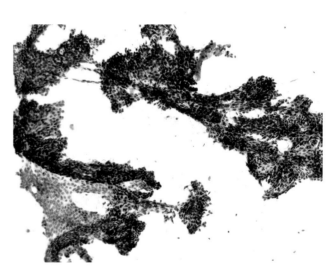

Figure 12.4.4   Papilloma. The nuclei are oval shaped and uniform. Rare myoepithelial cells can be seen in the background as spindle-shaped and bipolar cells.

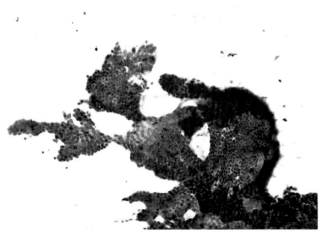

Figure 12.4.5   Fibroadenoma. The cytomorphology is very similar to that seen in papilloma.

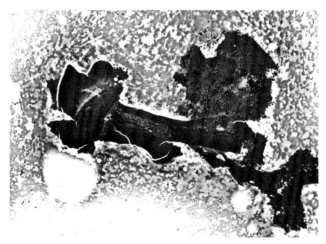

Figure 12.4.6   Fibroadenoma. The cells are arranged in a "staghorn" architecture. configuration. The cells have oval-shaped, uniform nuclei, which are arranged in an organized fashion.

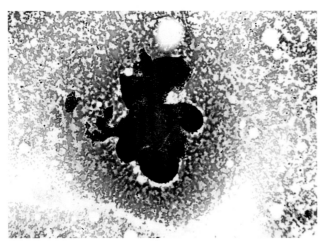

Figure 12.4.7   Fibroadenoma. In this field, the cells form bulbous projections. These structures, which resemble those seen in papillary thyroid carcinoma, are commonly seen in fibroadenoma.

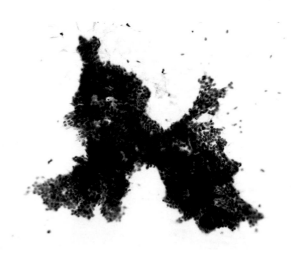

Figure 12.4.8   Fibroadenoma. The cells seen here have high N/C ratios and elongated nuclei containing powdery chromatin. The cells are uniform and do not vary in size or shape.

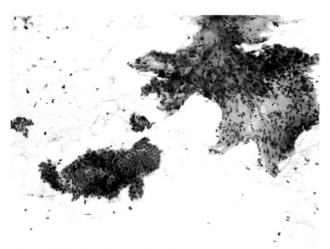

Figure 12.4.9   Fibroadenoma. Bland ductal cells are seen adjacent to a stromal fragment, which contains cellular and acellular zones. Spindle-shaped myoepithelial cells can be seen in association with the stromal fragment as well as dispersed in the background, where some have bipolar processes.

	Mucocele-like Lesion	Colloid Carcinoma
Age	Middle-aged women	Older women
Location	Breast	Breast
Signs and symptoms	Mass or radiologic lesion	Breast mass or radiologic lesion; uncommonly metastasizes
Etiology	Rare entity; unknown cause	Numerous contributing environmental and lifestyle factors; inherited mutations in BRCA1/BRCA2, TP53, PTEN, or mismatch repair genes, among others
Cytomorphology	• Mucin containing rare or absent cells *(Figures 12.5.1-12.5.5)* • Macrophages *(Figure 12.5.3)* • Rare, bland epithelial cells may be present in sheets or degenerated in the background *(Figures 12.5.3-12.5.5)*	• Cellular specimen with predominantly dis-cohesive individual cells and cells in small nests *(Figures 12.5.6-12.5.8)* • Nuclear atypia may be bland *(Figure 12.5.8)* or severe *(Figure 12.5.9)* • Mucinous background *(Figures 12.5.6-12.5.10)*
Special studies	N/A	N/A
Molecular alterations	N/A	Under investigation; generally have fewer alterations than conventional ductal carcinoma
Treatment	Complete excision, or surveillance if no atypia seen on core biopsy, no irregular margins on imaging studies, and no mass formation	Surgical removal, chemoradiation, hormonal therapy, and/or targeted therapies. Sentinel lymph node biopsy may be performed but usually does not require removal of lymph nodes
Clinical implications	Excellent; can be associated with adjacent ADH/DCIS	Better than for conventional ductal carcinoma if pure colloid carcinoma; >90% survival at 10 y

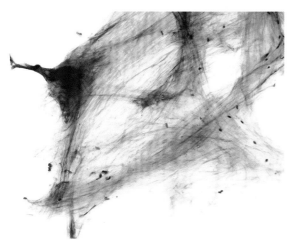

Figure 12.5.1   Mucocele. Thick mucin containing relatively few cells. The cells are predominantly macrophages. As opposed to colloid carcinoma, pure mucocele-like lesions are generally paucicellular.

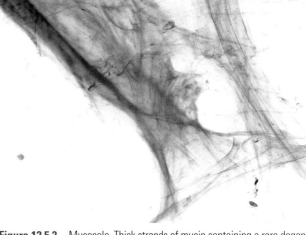

Figure 12.5.2   Mucocele. Thick strands of mucin containing a rare degenerated cell with an oval nuclei. The epithelial cells seen in mucocele-like lesions are usually not intact and may only be present as stripped nuclei.

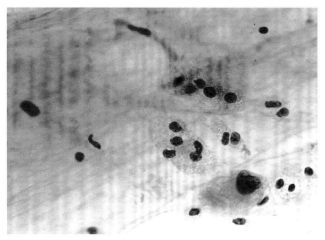

Figure 12.5.3   Mucocele. Numerous macrophages in a background of thick proteinaceous material (mucin). The cells have abundant, foamy cytoplasm and oval, indented nuclei.

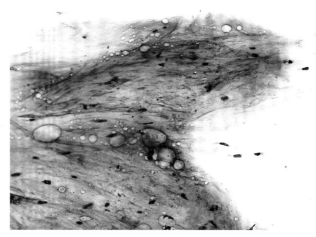

Figure 12.5.4   Mucocele. As opposed to serum, mucin is thick enough to have bubbles. Rare macrophages and bland epithelioid cells can be seen.

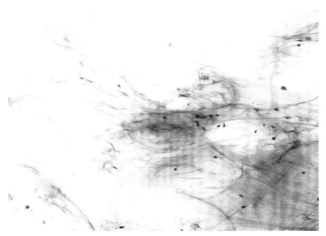

Figure 12.5.5   Mucocele. Thick mucin containing bubbles and rare bland cells. A specimen containing an increased number of cells raises concern for an atypical lesion or colloid carcinoma.

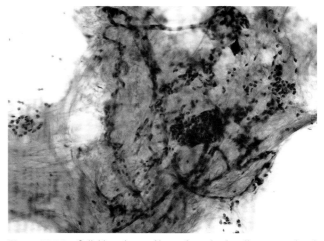

Figure 12.5.6   Colloid carcinoma. Nests of neoplastic cells are associated with abundant mucin. The cells are forming three-dimensional clusters and are discohesive at the edges. Intact tumor cells can also be seen singly in the background. In this case, the nuclei are uniform and deceivingly bland. The appearance of "tangled up" capillary vessels is a classic finding.

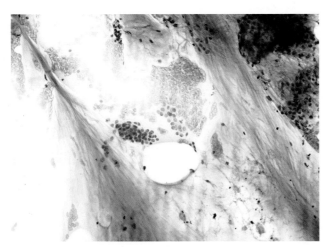

Figure 12.5.7 Colloid carcinoma. The cells form nests and intact single cells within a mucinous matrix. The nuclei are round, uniform in size, and have regular borders. However, the cellularity is too much for this to be a simple mucocele-like lesion.

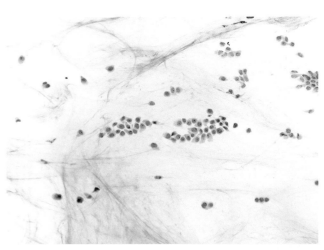

Figure 12.5.8 Colloid carcinoma. Monotonous epithelioid cells float in a mucinous matrix. The cells are discohesive and loosely cluster together. They demonstrate some mild nuclear atypia, such as mild anisonucleosis and contour irregularities.

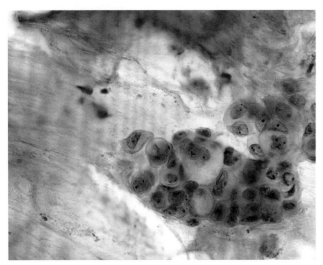

Figure 12.5.9 Colloid carcinoma. The colloid carcinoma cells seen here are less bland than the previous examples and have enlarged nuclei with coarse chromatin, size variation, and border irregularities. Some cells contain mucinous vacuoles. The morphology suggests a malignancy, and the abundant colloid in the background would be consistent with a colloid carcinoma.

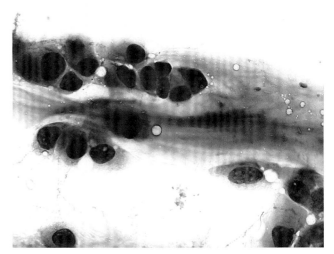

Figure 12.5.10 Colloid carcinoma. Large tumor cells are associated with thick, purple-staining mucin. The cells are loosely associated and have overtly malignant features: coarse chromatin, irregular nuclear borders, and variation in size and shape.

INDEX

Note: Page numbers followed by "f" indicate figures.